theclinics.com

ANESTHESIOLOGY CLINICS

Monitoring

GUEST EDITORS
Jeffrey S. Vender, MD
Joseph W. Szokol, MD, and
Glenn S. Murphy, MD

CONSULTING EDITOR
Lee A. Fleisher, MD

December 2006 • Volume 24 • Number 4

SAUNDERS

An Imprint of Elsevier, Inc.
PHILADELPHIA   LONDON   TORONTO   MONTREAL   SYDNEY   TOKYO

W.B. SAUNDERS COMPANY
A Division of Elsevier Inc.

1600 John F. Kennedy Boulevard, Suite 1800 • Philadelphia, Pennsylvania 19103-2899

http://www.theclinics.com

ANESTHESIOLOGY CLINICS Volume 24, Number 4
December 2006 ISSN 0889-8537
Editor: Rachel Glover ISBN 1-4160-3789-6

Copyright © 2006 by Elsevier Inc. All rights reserved. No part of this publication may be reproduced or transmitted in any form or by any means, electronic or mechanical, including photocopy, recording, or any information retrieval system, without written permission from the Publisher.

Single photocopies of single articles may be made for personal use as allowed by national copyright laws. Permission of the publisher and payment of a fee is required for all other photocopying, including multiple or systematic copying, copying for advertising or promotional purposes, resale, and all forms of document delivery. Special rates are available for educational institutions that wish to make photocopies for non-profit educational classroom use. Permissions may be sought directly from Elsevier's Rights Department in Philadelphia, PA, USA; phone: (215) 239-3804, fax: (215) 239-3805, e-mail: healthpermissions@elsevier.com. Requests may also be completed on-line via the Elsevier home page (http://www.elsevier.com/locate/permissions). In the USA, users may clear permissions and make payments through the Copyright Clearance Center, Inc., 222 Rosewood Drive, Danvers, MA 01923, USA; phone: (978) 750-8400, fax: (978) 750-4744, and in the UK through the Copyright Licensing Agency Rapid Clearance Service (CLARCS), 90 Tottenham Court Road, London W1P 0LP, UK; phone: (+44) 171 436 5931; fax: (+44) 171 436 3986. Other countries may have a local reprographic rights agency for payments.

The ideas and opinions expressed in *Anesthesiology Clinics* do not necessarily reflect those of the Publisher. The Publisher does not assume any responsibility for any injury and/or damage to persons or property arising out of or related to any use of the material contained in this periodical. The reader is advised to check the appropriate medical literature and the product information currently provided by the manufacturer of each drug to be administered to verify the dosage, the method and duration of administration, or contraindications. It is the responsibility of the treating physician or other health care professional, relying on independent experience and knowledge of the patient, to determine drug dosages and the best treatment for the patient. Mention of any product in this issue should not be construed as endorsement by the contributors, editors, or the Publisher of the product or manufacturers' claims.

Anesthesiology Clinics (ISSN 0889-8537) is published quarterly by Elsevier Inc., 360 Park Avenue South, New York, NY 10010-1710. Months of issue are March, June, September, and December. Business and Editorial Offices: 1600 John F. Kennedy Blvd., Suite 1800, Philadelphia, PA 19103-2899. Customer Service Office: 6277 Sea Harbor Drive, Orlando, FL 32887-4800. Periodicals postage paid at New York, NY and additional mailing offices. Subscription prices are $101.00 per year (US student/resident), $202.00 per year (US individuals), $246.00 per year (Canadian individuals), $302.00 per year (US institutions), $366.00 per year (Canadian institutions), $134.00 per year (Canadian and foreign student/resident), $263.00 per year (foreign individuals), and $366.00 per year (foreign institutions). To receive student and resident rate, orders must be accompanied by name of affiliated institution, date of term, and the *signature* of program/residency coordinator on institutions letterhead. Orders will be billed at individual rate until proof of status is received. Foreign air speed delivery is included in all *Clinics'* subscription prices. All prices are subject to change without notice. POSTMASTER: Send address changes to *Anesthesiology Clinics*, Elsevier Periodicals Customer Service, 6277 Sea Harbor Drive, Orlando, FL 32887-4800. **Customer Service: 1-800-654-2452** (US). From outside of the US, call **1-407-345-4000**. E-mail: hhspcs@wbsaunders.com.

Anesthesiology Clinics, is also published in Spanish by McGraw-Hill Inter-americana Editores S. A., P.O. Box 5-237, 06500 Mexico D. F., Mexico.

Anesthesiology Clinics, is covered in *Index Medicus, Current Contents/Clinical Medicine, Excerpta Medica, ISI/BIOMED*, and *Chemical Abstracts*.

Printed in the United States of America.

MONITORING

CONSULTING EDITOR

LEE A. FLEISHER, MD, Robert D. Dripps Professor and Chair, Department of Anesthesiology and Critical Care, The University of Pennsylvania School of Medicine, Philadelphia, Pennsylvania

GUEST EDITORS

JEFFREY S. VENDER, MD, Professor and Associate Chairman, Department of Anesthesiology, Feinberg School of Medicine, Northwestern University, Chicago; Chairman, Department of Anesthesiology, Director, Critical Care Services, Evanston Northwestern Healthcare, Evanston, Illinois

JOSEPH W. SZOKOL, MD, Vice Chairman, Department of Anesthesiology, Evanston Northwestern Healthcare, Evanston; Associate Professor, Northwestern University, Feinberg School of Medicine, Chicago, Illinois

GLENN S. MURPHY, MD, Associate Professor, Department of Anesthesiology, Feinberg School of Medicine, Northwestern University, Chicago; Director of Cardiovascular Anesthesia and Clinical Research, Evanston Northwestern Healthcare, Evanston, Illinois

CONTRIBUTORS

J.P. ABENSTEIN, MSEE, MD, Associate Professor of Anesthesiology, Mayo Clinic College of Medicine, Rochester, Minnesota

ATILIO BARBEITO, MD, Assistant Professor, Department of Anesthesiology, Duke University Medical Center, Durham, North Carolina

T. ANDREW BOWDLE, MD, PhD, Professor of Anesthesiology and Pharmaceutics, (Adjunct) Chief of the Division of Cardiothoracic Anesthesiology, Department of Anesthesiology, University of Washington, Seattle, Washington

MICHAEL K. CAHALAN, MD, Professor and Chair, Department of Anesthesiology, University of Utah School of Medicine, Salt Lake City, Utah

GERALDINE DIAZ, DO, Fellow in Critical Care, Assistant Professor of Anesthesiology, Department of Anesthesiology, College of Physicians & Surgeons of Columbia University, New York, New York

LEE A. FLEISHER, MD, Robert D. Dripps Professor and Chair, Department of Anesthesiology and Critical Care, The University of Pennsylvania School of Medicine, Philadelphia, Pennsylvania

STEVEN R. INSLER, DO, Staff Anesthesiologist, Department of Cardiothoracic Anesthesia, The Cleveland Clinic, Cleveland, Ohio

LESLIE C. JAMESON, MD, Associate Professor of Anesthesiology, University of Colorado at Denver and Health Sciences Center, Denver, Colorado

A.D. JOHN, MD, Assistant Professor, Department of Anesthesia and Critical Care, Johns Hopkins University School of Medicine, Baltimore, Maryland

JONATHAN B. MARK, MD, Professor and Vice Chairman, Department of Anesthesiology, Duke University Medical Center, North Carolina; Chief, Anesthesiology Service, Veterans Affairs Medical Center, Durham, North Carolina

JESSE MARYMONT, MD, Departments of Anesthesiology and Medicine (Cardiology), Evanston Northwestern Healthcare; Assistant Professor, Northwestern University, Feinberg School of Medicine, Evanston, Illinois

VIVEK MOITRA, MD, Fellow in Critical Care, Assistant Professor of Anesthesiology, Department of Anesthesiology, College of Physicians & Surgeons of Columbia University, New York, New York

GLENN S. MURPHY, MD, Director, Cardiovascular Anesthesia, Evanston Northwestern Healthcare, Evanston; and Associate Professor, Northwestern University, Feinberg School of Medicine

DAVID H. ODELL, MD, Adjunct Assistant Professor, Department of Internal Medicine, Division of Cardiology; Co-Director of Perioperative Echocardiography Service, University of Utah School of Medicine, Salt Lake City, Utah

JAMES RAMSAY MD, FRCP(C), Professor of Anesthesiology, Program Director, Anesthesiology Critical Care Medicine, Emory University School of Medicine; Anesthesiology Service Chief, Emory University Hospital, Atlanta, Georgia

ANTOINE G. ROCHON, MD, FRCPC, Assistant Professor, Department of Anesthesiology, Montreal Heart Institute, Montreal, Canada

DANIEL I. SESSLER, MD, Chair, Department of Outcomes Research, The Cleveland Clinic, Cleveland, Ohio; L&S Weakley Professor of Anesthesiology and Director of Outcomes Research Institute, University of Louisville, Louisville, Kentucky

LINDA SHORE-LESSERSON, MD, Associate Professor, Department of Anesthesiology; Chief, Cardiothoracic Anesthesiology, Montefiore Medical Center, Bronx, New York

ROBERT N. SLADEN, MB,ChB, MRCP(UK), FRCP(C), FCCM, Professor and Vice Chair, Chief, Division of Critical Care, Department of Anesthesiology, College of Physicians & Surgeons of Columbia University, New York, New York

TOD B. SLOAN, MD, MBA, PhD, Professor of Anesthesiology, University of Colorado at Denver and Health Sciences Center, Denver, Colorado

MONITORING

CONTENTS

Foreword xi
Lee A. Fleisher

Preface xiii
Jeffrey S. Vender, Joseph W. Szokol, and Glenn S. Murphy

Technology Assessment for the Anesthesiologist 677
J.P. Abenstein

> This article discusses new and interesting technologies. When considering whether to incorporate a new medical technology into one's practice both the health care-related and economic consequences of that decision should be evaluated. In this article, the basic principles of health care technology assessment are discussed. It is unlikely that a practicing anesthesiologist or even a large academic department will have all the tools or data to conduct a formal technology assessment before purchase. Still, these principles can be applied to most new technologies and can assist anesthesiologists in making sound decisions grounded on the available science.

Electrocardiography: The ECG 697
A.D. John and Lee A. Fleisher

> This article examines the role of electrocardiography in patient monitoring during an operative procedure. In addition to providing a wealth of physiological information, including information on the electrical activity of the heart, the ECG assists in monitoring and detecting a variety of changes, such as cardiac arrhythmias, electrolyte changes, and ischemia. Information presented on an ECG should be analyzed systematically with an understanding of the constituent elements of an ECG, the rate, the rhythm, the

morphology, the axis, the presence of conduction abnormalities, electrolyte changes, and ischemic changes. To assess accurately the information presented, hemodynamic information and cardiac-risk analysis should be integrated to have a complete picture.

Arterial and Central Venous Pressure Monitoring 717
Atilio Barbeito and Jonathan B. Mark

Pressure monitoring systems influence the contour of the displayed waveforms and, on occasion, can introduce significant artifact in the pressure traces. Careful observation of the arterial pressure waveform can provide information about ventricular function, the arterial system, and ventricular preload. In particular, systolic pressure variation during the respiratory cycle in mechanically ventilated patients is a clinically useful indicator of volume status. Central venous pressure (CVP) monitoring is also used to assess intravascular volume, but this measurement is significantly influenced by ventricular compliance and intrathoracic pressure. A trend in CVP values or its change with therapeutic maneuvers is usually more reliable than a single measurement. Like arterial pressure waveforms, CVP waveform morphology can provide important information about clinical pathophysiology.

Intraoperative Monitoring with Transesophageal Echocardiography: Indications, Risks, and Training 737
Jesse Marymont and Glenn S. Murphy

This article discusses three areas of intraoperative transesophageal echocardiography (TEE): indications, risks, and training. The discussion incorporates four current guidelines for use of TEE in the perioperative period. These are (1) the "Practice Guidelines for Perioperative Transesophageal Echocardiography" from the American Society of Anesthesiologists (ASA) and the Society of Cardiovascular Anesthesiologists (SCA) Task Force on TEE; (2) guidelines from the American College of Cardiology (ACC), the American Heart Association (AHA), and the American Society of Echocardiography (ASE) about transthoracic and transesophageal echocardiography; (3) guidelines from the ASE and SCA about the training requirements for anesthesiologists performing perioperative echocardiography; and (4) guidelines from the ASE and SCA on how to perform an intraoperative multiplane transesophageal examination.

Assessment of Left Ventricular Global and Segmental Systolic Function with Transesophageal Echocardiography 755
David H. Odell and Michael K. Cahalan

In this article, the authors review a systematic approach to using transesophageal echocardiography for the evaluation of global and segmental left ventricular systolic function. The authors describe the necessary cross sections for the evaluation as well as practical and common techniques to estimate global left ventricular ejection and to detect segmental wall-motion abnormalities, which are sensitive and specific signs of myocardial ischemia. In addition, the authors delineate the advantages and limitations of the techniques. The evaluation of left ventricular global and segmental systolic function is a primary application for perioperative transesophageal echocardiography. Although the practical techniques customarily used for these applications have limitations, they afford direct measures of function not otherwise available in the operating room or intensive care setting.

Noninvasive Technologies for Tissue Perfusion 763
James Ramsay

In the clinical setting, the perfusion of vital organs usually is assessed by measuring the cardiac output (CO), and usually by thermodilution using a pulmonary artery catheter (PAC). This article describes four techniques of measuring CO without the need for a PAC: indirect partial rebreathing Fick, blood flow velocity measurement by Doppler, arterial pressure waveform analysis, and thoracic bioimpedance. Most clinical assessments have compared less invasive or noninvasive techniques with thermodilution to achieve clinical relevance and acceptability. In the absence of another readily available standard this is probably appropriate; however there is some variability inherent with thermodilution itself.

Monitoring of the Brain and Spinal Cord 777
Leslie C. Jameson and Tod B. Sloan

Over the last 30 years, intraoperative neurophysiologic monitoring (IOM) of the brain and spinal cord has become an established technique to provide functional neurologic assessment during axial skeletal, head and neck, spinal cord, and some intracranial procedures. IOM techniques have been developed to assess neuronal electrophysiology, blood flow, oxygenation, and even specific tissue-specific values. Changing surgical techniques and the necessity to prevent new injuries or prevent exacerbation of existing neurologic injury have driven refinement and innovation. This article focuses on the commonly used intraoperative monitoring modalities: somatosensory evoked potential, motor evoked potential, electromyography, and brain stem auditory evoked responses.

Depth of Anesthesia Monitoring 793
T. Andrew Bowdle

Depth-of-anesthesia monitoring with electroencephalography (EEG) or EEG in combination with middle-latency auditory evoked response is becoming widely used in anesthesia practice. The BIS monitor is the most thoroughly studied and most widely used depth-of-anesthesia monitor, but there is a growing amount of information about other monitors. Evidence shows that EEG monitoring improves outcome by reducing the incidence of intraoperative awareness (specifically for the BIS monitor) while reducing the average amount of anesthesia administered, resulting in faster wake-up and recovery, and perhaps reduced nausea and vomiting. As with any monitoring device, there are significant limitations in the use of the monitors, and the anesthesiologist must be able to interpret the data accordingly.

Perioperative Thermoregulation and Temperature Monitoring 823
Steven R. Insler and Daniel I. Sessler

Surgery and general anesthesia impair the normal balance between heat production and loss. Anesthetic agents, opioids, and sedatives inhibit behavior and autonomic responses. Thus when patients are exposed to cool ambient operating room environments, mild-to-moderate hypothermia is the usual result. Although hypothermia may provide protection against ischemia, there is clinical evidence showing that even mild perioperative hypothermia causes multiple physiologic derangements and leads to adverse outcomes. Conversely, hyperthermia also can occur within the perioperative environment, indicating that heat production exceeds heat loss. Because temperature disturbances are common, multi-factorial, and serious, it is important that clinicians understand the impact of general anesthesia and surgery on the human thermoregulatory system. Similarly, monitoring temperature accurately is required to make correct diagnoses and provide timely intervention. This article covers normal physiologic temperature regulation, perioperative thermal stress, and techniques of intraoperative temperature monitoring.

Coagulation Monitoring 839
Antoine G. Rochon and Linda Shore-Lesserson

This article discusses the many different tests currently available to the anesthesiologist to monitor hemostasis in the perioperative period. An updated concept of hemostasis is reviewed briefly. Preoperative and point-of-care monitors and the literature currently available supporting their use are presented.

Monitoring Hepatic and Renal Function 857
Vivek Moitra, Geraldine Diaz and Robert N. Sladen

Liver disease represents a serious risk factor for patients requiring anesthesia and surgery. Even subclinical liver disease increases perioperative morbidity and mortality. Perioperative renal dysfunction and failure have similar implications. Thus, detection of early hepatic and renal dysfunction and monitoring of their progress is essential. This article discusses methods for monitoring hepatic and renal function in patients who have high risk for liver or renal injury in the perioperative period.

Index   **881**

FORTHCOMING ISSUES

March 2007
Trauma
Micha Y. Shamir, MD, and
Yoram G. Weiss, MD, FCCM, *Guest Editors*

June 2007
Patient Safety and Simulation
W. Andrew Kofke, MD, MBA, FCCM, and
Vinay Nadkarni, MD, *Guest Editors*

September 2007
Neurosurgical Anesthesia
Jeffrey R. Kirsch, MD, *Guest Editor*

RECENT ISSUES

September 2006
Common Medical Problems and Anesthesia
Stanley H. Rosenbaum, MD, *Guest Editor*

June 2006
Influence of Perioperative Care on Outcome
Steffen E. Meiler, MD, *Guest Editor*

March 2006
Palliative Care
Jonathan R. Gavrin, MD, *Guest Editor*

THE CLINICS ARE NOW AVAILABLE ONLINE!

For more information about Clinics:
http://www.theclinics.com

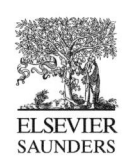

Foreword

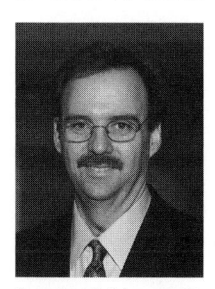

Lee A. Fleisher, MD
Consulting Editor

Appropriate monitoring of the surgical patient is one of very few "standards" for the anesthesiologist. Since Cushing [1] first established the utility of measuring and recording blood pressure, there has been a constant effort to develop new and better modalities to assess all aspects of physiologic functions under anesthesia. New technology has advanced and allowed better insight into normal and abnormal physiology. For this issue of the *Anesthesiology Clinics of North America*, the editors asked a group of authors, including myself, to address the interpretation and use of a wide variety of monitoring technologies.

As guest editor for this issue, we are pleased to have Jeffrey S. Vender, FCCM, FCCP, MD. Dr. Vender is the Chairman of the Department of Anesthesiology, Evanston Northwestern Health Care, as well as Director of the Medical-Surgical Intensive Care Unit and Professor and Associate Chairman of the Department of Anesthesiology at Northwestern University's Feinberg School of Medicine. Among other issues, he has published extensively on pulmonary artery catheter (PAC) use.

To assist him with this issue, Dr. Vender chose as his co-editors Joseph W. Szokol, MD and Glenn S. Murphy, MD. Both associate professors at Evanston Northwestern Health Care, Drs. Szokol and Murphy have worked with Dr. Vender on numerous publications related to cardiopulmonary bypass and PAC. Their collaboration has brought us an excellent edition of *Anesthesiology Clinics*.

Lee A. Fleisher, MD
Department of Anesthesiology and Critical Care
The University of Pennsylvania School of Medicine
3400 Spruce Street
Philadelphia, PA 19104, USA

E-mail address: Lee.fleisher@uphs.upenn.edu

Reference

[1] Cushing H. On routine determination of arterial tension in operating room and clinic. Boston Med Surg J 1903;148:250–6.

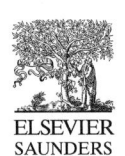

Preface

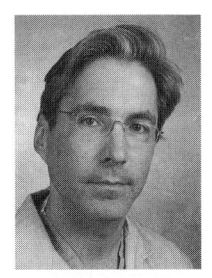

Jeffrey S. Vender, MD Joseph W. Szokol, MD Glenn S. Murphy, MD
Guest Editors

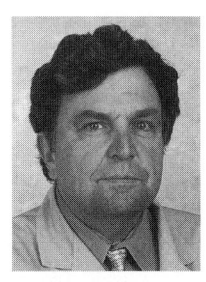

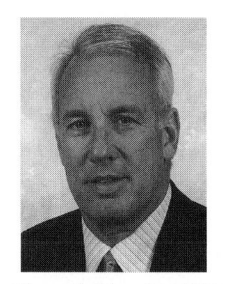

The literature is replete with activities, monographs, and texts focused on the topic of monitoring. The term *monitor* is derived from the word *monere*, "to warn or remind." Many investigators have extended this definition to include diagnostic tests (eg, troponin, electrolytes, hemoglobin) as methods for "monitoring" various organ functions. For the purpose of this monograph, we have elected to assess the topic in the context of the generation of data (diagnostic or monitoring) for the pathophysiologic assessment of the individual patient. In some articles, the focus is on specific monitoring tools, whereas other articles apply more generally to the assessment of specific organ functions.

The appropriate application of monitors or interpretation of diagnostic tests necessitates an understanding of the indications as well as the limitations of the tool. The sensitivity and specificity of the information will impact the clinical relevance, applicability, and value of the data. There remains a need for high-quality technological assessment that is uniformly and consistently defined and applied. What should be the determinant for the use of a new monitor or diagnostic test? Numerous metrics are applied in an attempt to ascertain the "value" of the new technology. Is a noninvasive test with less risk but less-reliable data a benefit? Should mortality be the metric for defining the generation of data?

For the past three decades, numerous investigators have tried to determine the value of pulmonary artery catheter (PAC) monitoring. Many of them have concluded that the PAC is of limited value in the patient populations studied and that there is limited benefit to warrant its use. A recent editorial has called into question the conclusions of these studies relating to the methodologies and the metric used to determine PAC benefit, ie, mortality [1]. Monitors are not therapeutic agents! Antibiotics, antihypertensives, chemotherapy, and thrombolytics are employed to change mortality outcome. Mortality should not be the primary metric for technology assessment. The first level of assessment should be related to the data generated. Accuracy, precision, bias, specificity, and sensitivity are some of the metrics. Ease and ability to measure and interpret the data are important. Application and integration of the data in the management of the patient is key. If the cardiac output generated from a PAC doesn't change mortality, why should the same data derived from a noninvasive cardiac output technology impact outcome? Data are information to be used to generate knowledge. Knowledge, if appropriately interpreted and applied, is used to alter morbidity and mortality. Articles have continuously demonstrated deficiencies in the knowledge of clinicians in the understanding and application of information attained from various monitors or diagnostic tests.

Although not discussed in this issue, there is limited high-grade evidence-based medicine (EBM) supporting the role for pulse oximetry, yet expert opinion and clinical experience (not mortality measurements) have strongly supported its routine use and application as a standard of care in operating room anesthesia. Its limitations in not measuring fractional saturation are understood and compensated for in the interpretation of the data. Similarly, the growing use of transesophageal echocardiography as a diagnostic and monitoring tool in cardiac surgery is strongly supported by expert opinion but not by high-grade EBM demonstrating mortality benefit. Finally, even if there are appropriate understanding and reasonable EBM for a technology, they must be coupled with effective therapeutic interventions for the management of the pathophysiologic problem.

In this issue, we have attempted to assess several categories of monitoring. Space limitations, however, preclude addressing many of the technologies or diagnostics employed in clinical practice. We have selected topics of common applications (ECG, temperature), growing use (noninvasive cardiac function), clinical controversy (awareness), organ function (central nervous system, spine, renal, hepatic, coagulation), and value determination (technology assessment). Many of the articles reflect the opinions of the individual authors and referenced representation of the available information.

The inconsistencies of technology assessment and application, and the variability in the definition of value continue to be significant clinical dilemmas. It is our hope that with a continued effort at education, the more uniform use of EBM, and better guidelines/protocols for care, this problem can be reduced in the future. We must seek to define value as more than just acquisition cost or level of invasiveness. No matter how inexpensive, simple, or noninvasive a test or monitor is, if the information generated is not understood or appropriately applied, we cannot expect to derive a clinical benefit. The management of an arrhythmia necessitates the correct electrocardiographic interpretation and therapeutic intervention. The diagnosis of a sinus-bradycardia secondary to hypoxemia is not necessarily an indication for atropine. We must continually strive to address the competency of the "carpenter" as well as the quality of the tool.

We would like to thank each of the contributing authors for their expertise and for their efforts at presenting the available information and providing perspective on their topics. A special thank you to Rachel Glover from Elsevier for her assistance and patience, to Anna Crawford for her diligence and efforts on our behalf, and to our colleagues in health care, who participate in the life-long learning process. We believe our patients will be the beneficiaries. Finally to our families, Bobbie, Todd, Kim, Pam, Kimberly, Elizabeth, William and Debbie, Lauren and Olivia, thank you. Your love, support, and understanding inspire us, enable us, and make it all worth doing.

Jeffrey S. Vender, MD
Feinberg School of Medicine
Northwestern University
2650 Ridge Avenue
Evanston, IL 60201, USA

E-mail address: jvender@enh.org

Joseph W. Szokol, MD
Feinberg School of Medicine
Northwestern University
2650 Ridge Avenue
Evanston, IL 60201, USA

E-mail address: jszokol@enh.org

Glenn S. Murphy, MD
Feinberg School of Medicine
Northwestern University
2650 Ridge Avenue
Evanston, IL 60201, USA

E-mail address: gmurphy@enh.org

Reference

[1] Vender JS. Pulmonary artery catheter utilization: the use, misuse, or abuse. J Cardiothorac Vasc Anesth 2006;20(3):295–9.

Technology Assessment for the Anesthesiologist

J.P. Abenstein, MSEE, MD

Mayo Clinic College of Medicine, 200 First Street, Southwest, Rochester, MN 55905, USA

Health care costs have increased in the United States much faster than the gross domestic product (GDP) for more than four decades [1]. In 1960, about 5% of the United States GDP was spent on medical care. It is now estimated that US health care expenditures are in excess of 15% of GDP. In comparison, the United Kingdom and Japan only spent 7.6% of their GDP on health care in 2001, and Germany expended on 10.7% of GDP on health care [2]. There are many reasons for the rise in health care costs, such as an aging population, violence, and poor life style choices. Much of the analysis, though, has focused on the impact of medical technology, defined as all drugs, devices, procedures, and organizational systems (eg, electronic medical records) [3]. It is currently the consensus view that technology acquisition and application are primarily responsible for the rapidly rising cost of health care in the United States [4].

This issue is particularly important to anesthesiologists, because procedural suites, including operating rooms and intensive care units, are some of the most cost-intensive environments in a medical facility. Technology is a major cost driver within these locations, and the practice of anesthesiology, like much of procedure-based medicine, is highly dependent on advanced technology. As medical reimbursement continues to decline, the capital available to purchase new equipment decreases. Every dollar spent on technology that is overpriced, does not work, or is not needed is a dollar that cannot be spent on effective patient care. Therefore, it is vital that the evaluation process be thought out carefully, be consistent with the process within the medical center, and have the support of institutional leadership and department members. Strategies may differ from department to department, but those with a defined evaluation process will be able to hold down costs and avoid purchasing technologies that do not meet practice needs.

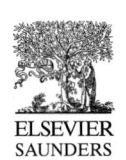

E-mail address: abenstein.john@mayo.edu

Health care technology assessment is a process for examining the medical, economic, and societal implications of purchasing and using health care technology [4–6]. Health care technology assessment is a comprehensive research methodology that explores the short- and long-term consequences of the introduction of new medical technology. When done incorrectly, it can be short sighted by being overly concentrated on cost control, short-term efficacy, and risks, while underemphasizing issues associated with indirect, delayed, and unintended impact on the patient and society. Well-done assessments include information about direct medical costs and downstream nonmedical expenses (eg, lost wages and decreased quality of life) [7].

This article discusses new and interesting technologies. When considering whether to incorporate a new medical technology into one's practice both the health care-related and economic consequences of that decision should be evaluated. In this article, the basic principles of health care technology assessment are discussed. It is unlikely that a practicing anesthesiologist or even a large academic department will have all the tools or data to conduct a formal technology assessment before purchase. Still, these principles can be applied to most new technologies and can assist anesthesiologists in making sound decisions grounded on the available science.

Cost effectiveness

When a technology is chosen to be reviewed, by what criteria should it be evaluated? The fundamental goal of medical care is to improve the treatment of disease, improve the patient's quality of life, and to balance the interest of the individual with that of the broader society. The criteria for evaluation include:

- Safety
- Improvement in health outcomes.
- Degree to which a technology is clinically effective and cost-effective
- Other factors, including social good (vulnerable and underserved populations) and public health impact

Cost effectiveness is a controversial and misunderstood term. It is used interchangeably with cost–benefit and cost minimizing. A working definition of a cost-effective technology is one of the following:

- At least as effective and less costly than alternative technologies
- More effective and more costly than alternative technologies, but resultant patient health outcomes justify additional expenditures
- Less effective and less costly than alternative technologies, but resultant patient health outcomes from the use of the alternative does not justify additional expenditures

A straightforward, although somewhat simplistic, way to categorize the introduction of a new technology is to determine the expected patient and economic outcomes. A new technology can be expected to improve, worsen, or not change clinical outcomes as compared with existing treatments. The technology will increase, decrease, or not change net resource expenditures, (ie, cost, efficiency or personnel). If the new practice improves outcomes for the same or less expense, the change is considered to be cost-effective. Conversely, if the new technology worsens outcomes for the same or greater cost, it is not cost-effective. This relationship is seen in Table 1.

In this example, there are three instances where the practice change (ie, new technology) is cost-effective and therefore, should be embraced. There are also three categories where the change is not cost-effective and should not be introduced. What is seen most commonly in medicine is that a new technology will increase costs, and, at times, improve outcomes. If new technology is expected to improve patient outcomes, but at an increased cost, the next step is to decide whether the clinical improvement is worth the cost.

A cost-effectiveness analysis is used to evaluate whether the benefits of a new health care technology, whether therapeutic or diagnostic, justify the total cost of that technology. When determining whether a new technology is cost-effective, one must determine the impact it will have on eventual patient outcomes, often measured as the difference in mortality rate over a certain time frame as compared with the current treatment. The incremental cost of treatment also must be determined, and this includes not only the capital cost of purchasing the technology, but also the operational costs (eg, supplies, maintenance, upgrades), the fiscal costs (eg, time value of money, depreciation, opportunity costs), and, if available, the down-stream costs (eg, lost wages, lost productivity, long-term health care costs). This information can be used to produce an incremental cost-effectiveness ratio (ICER):

$$ICER = (C_1 - C_0)/(E_1 - E_0) < TH$$

where C_0 is the cost of the standard intervention (control); C_1 is the cost of the new intervention; E_0 is the health benefit of the control; E_1 is the health benefit of the new intervention, and TH is the threshold of cost effectiveness [8].

Table 1
Cost-effectiveness of a practice change

Costs	Patient outcomes		
	Better	Same	Worse
Higher	Maybe	No	No
Same	Yes	Maybe	No
Lower	Yes	Yes	Maybe

Cost-effectiveness matrix showing the relationship of patient outcomes and cost implications of a practice change. This relationship holds true whether the change is a new drug, procedure, diagnostic strategy, or technology. Cells identify whether a practice change should be embraced (ie, yes, no, or maybe).

If the analysis includes the expected length of life of those patients who benefited from the new technology, these data can be used to calculate a metric of cost effectiveness, dollars per life year saved (DLYS). If the incremental decrement to a patient's quality of life (eg, 0 is dead and 1 is perfectly healthy), secondary to disease or to the treatment, is determined, then the dollars per quality-adjusted life year saved (QALYS) also can be calculated. These two metrics are the standard by which the value of medical treatments and technologies are determined in the context of a cost-effectiveness analysis [9,10]. Simply put, dollars/life year saved is the ratio of incremental costs associated with a practice change relative to the estimated incremental life expectancy gains. For example, if a new monitor is being considered that offers improved ischemia monitoring (eg, 12-lead electrocardiogram [ECG]), then the analysis would focus on how many patients would need to be monitored to avoid a myocardial infarction and death, and how long these patients would be expected to live. With these data, the DLYS can be determined.

The orthodox medical ethic in the United States, which developed after World War II, is that everything medicine has to offer must be done for a patient regardless of cost. This is the bedrock conviction of many, if not most, American physicians, that they have the moral and legal responsibility to their patients to advocate on their behalf, no matter what the cost [11]. As attractive as this viewpoint is to many medical professionals, it is not shared by other stakeholders in health care, such as payers, administrators, and particularly those in legislative and regulatory bodies, who have the responsibility to consider the broader issues of affordability, access, and quality.

It is also important not to ignore the bottom right cell in Table 1, the instance where outcomes are worse and costs are reduced. Most physicians would reject this concept out of hand, but payers, administrators, and others do not. It is not inconceivable that a new technology, or denial of a new technology, which generates significant cost saving, whose outcomes are reduced modestly for a small number of patients, and for which the saved resources could be applied elsewhere to improve outcomes in the larger population would be viewed favorably. In fact, in a 2003 article, Noyes explicitly states that a technology should be adopted if "greater than $100,000 saved per quality-adjusted life year lost" [8]. As one considers the task of technology assessment, this perspective (ie, acceptability of lower costs in exchange for worse outcomes) must not be forgotten.

Tissue plasminogen activator as a template for technology assessment

Thrombolytic therapy is an emergency medical treatment for acute myocardial infarction (MI). The purpose of the therapy is to dissolve the clots blocking coronary arteries, causing the infarction. Technology assessments on thrombolytic therapy have been done because:

- Significant controversy existed as to whether tissue plasminogen activator (tPA) is better than the standard therapy (streptokinase [SK]).

- If tPA produces better patient outcomes, is it worth the difference in price ($2750 versus $320)? [12]

An in-depth technology assessment of thrombolytic therapy is possible, because very large prospective, randomized outcome studies have been published, which more-or-less make the analysis of the data straightforward. The data are summarized in Table 2 [13–23].

As can be seen, both SK and tPA are very effective in reducing mortality after an acute MI, (ie, mortality rates of untreated patients are as high as 25%). In the 1993, Global Utilization of Streptokinase and t-PA for Occluded Coronary Arteries [GUSTO-1, tPA] was given in an accelerated regimen, (higher infusion rate at the beginning of therapy, loading dose), followed by heparin. This study also received a tremendous amount of interest because:

- Results with tPA were different from previous studies, GUSTO-1 showing a statistically significant difference in outcome in patients who were treated with tPA.
- tPA was administered differently in GUSTO, making comparisons with the previous studies difficult.
- Subgroup analysis showed even greater differences between groups.
- Improved outcomes in the United States with tPA, no difference in Europe
- Better outcomes in younger patients, those with anterior MIs, and earlier treatment (ie, less than 4 hrs since onset of symptoms)
- Higher nonfatal stroke rate with tPA
- More difficult to equilibrate with mortality statistics
- Costs associated with these strokes not forthcoming

The GUSTO study was well designed and had enrolled a large number of patients. Therefore, its results are well suited for a cost-effectiveness analysis. For patients suffering from an acute MI, treatment with accelerated tPA

Table 2
Mortality and stroke data for postmyocardial infarction thrombolytic studies

Study	Year	Number of patients randomized	Aspirin only	SK + aspirin	tPA + aspirin
ISIS-2	1988	17,187	10.7 (0.5)	8.0 (0.6)*	NA
GISSI-2	1990	20,891	NA	8.5 (0.9)	8.9 (1 .3)**
ISIS-3	1992	41,299	NA	10.6 (1.0)	10.3 (1.4)**
GUSTO-1	1993	41,021	NA	7.3 (1.3)	6.3 (1.55)***

Outcomes expressed as % of treated patients.
* Statistically significant difference in mortality rate in patients treated with SK + aspirin as compared to those treated with aspirin only.
** Statistically significant difference in stroke rate in patients treated with t-PA + aspirin as compared to those treated with SK + aspirin.
*** Statistically significant difference in mortality and stroke rate in patients treated with t-PA + aspirin as compared to those treated with SK + aspirin.

and aspirin, as compared with SK and aspirin, results in a 1% decreased mortality rate (ie, for every 100 patients treated with tPA, one additional patient will be alive 30 days later as compared with SK). On the down side, use of tPA will increase the nonfatal stroke rate by 2.5 per 1000 treated patients.

The estimated mean 1 year total health care cost (ie, physicians' fee and hospital costs), excluding thrombolytics, was $24,575 for patients who were treated with SK compared with $24,990 for patients who were treated with tPA. When the pharmacologic costs between tPA and SK are included, the incremental cost of treating with tPA was $2845 [12]. Because it takes 100 treated patients to save one incremental life (ie, 30-day survival of 92.7% and 93.7% for SK and tPA, respectively), the cost is:

$$\$2845 \times 100 = \$284,500 \text{ per life saved}$$

The actuarial life expectancy of a successfully treated acute MI patient is 14 years. The per-year cost of saving a life is:

$$(\$2845 \times 100)/14 \text{ y} = \$20,321 \text{ per life year saved}$$

Generalizing the above relationship:

$$((C_1 - C_0) \times P)/L = DLYS$$

where C_0 is the cost of the established therapy (control state); C_1 is the cost of the new therapy; P is the number of patients treated with the new therapy to generate an incremental saved life; L is the actuarial life expectancy of those treated successfully with the new therapy, expressed as years, and DLYS is dollars per life year saved.

The question then with treating an acute MI patient with tPA is whether a cost of about $20,000 per life year saved is an acceptable expense from a societal perspective. To answer that question, one must review the history of renal dialysis in the United States [24].

Although, rudimentary renal dialysis was first developed in 1944 in German-occupied Holland, this technology did not take hold in the United States until the 1960s. Immediately, there were significant concerns regarding the cost of dialysis. There were far fewer dialysis centers than there were patients to be treated. Financial constraints meant only a few dialysis centers offered treatment. Too many patients, vying for too few beds, created one of the first medical ethics crises in the United States. In Seattle, four committees determined who had access to the limited dialysis resources. The medical committee ensured patients were otherwise healthy; the psychological committee evaluated their ability to handle the emotional stresses, and the financial committee confirmed that patients had at least $30,000 to cover 3 years of treatment. The admissions advisory committee, sometimes referred to as the "Life or Death Committee," was the last to review the patient. The committee consisted of a banker, surgeon, lawyer, minister, labor leader, housewife, and government official. It examined the personal lives and community involvement of the remaining applicants and essentially determined who was worth saving. An exposé in Life Magazine generated widespread outrage that anonymous committees were choosing who would live and who would die.

An intense lobbying effort was generated to achieve federal funding for dialysis. This effort engaged physicians and patients. This culminated with the 1971 testimony of Shep Glazer, then vice president of the National Association of Patients on Hemodialysis, before the US House Ways and Means Committee while attached to a dialysis machine. Soon after these hearings, Congress approved the legislation that led to the implementation of the Medicare End-Stage Renal Dialysis Program. It provided federal funding for virtually all patients who required dialysis because of end-stage renal disease.

By this action, the US government made a policy decision that it was unacceptable to allow patients to die from a treatable disease, in this case end-stage renal failure. From an ethical perspective, it really does not matter what an individual dies from. Based on this reasoning, with the federal government as a proxy for society, from a societal perspective medical care that costs less, in dollars-per-year-of-life-saved, than the average annual cost of keeping a dialysis patient alive is cost-effective. Today, a year of dialysis costs about $50,000, and therefore technologies are considered to be cost-effective if they cost less than $50,000 to 80,000 per year of life-saved [25].

In spite of what appears to be a very high cost of $284,500 to save just one life, for a disease (ie, coronary artery disease) that affects the lives of millions of people, the treatment of acute MI with tPA is cost-effective. This holds true, even though the total incremental cost to society is substantial. It is estimated that if tPA is substituted routinely for SK in the treatment of acute MI, there would be about 250,000 patients treated with tPA per year. This would increase annual health care costs in the United States by over $500 million, but in exchange for this expense, there would be an additional 2500 Americans alive each year [12].

Left ventricular assist devices—cost-effectiveness analysis at the extreme

Chronic heart failure is a common disease responsible for high mortality and morbidity. Heart failure represents a complex clinical syndrome caused by many different etiologies whose clinical manifestations reflect a fundamental abnormality—a decrease in the myocardial contractile state so that cardiac output delivers insufficient blood flow and oxygen to meet the metabolic requirements of the tissues and organs. There are about 4 to 5 million patients with heart failure in the United States. About 400,000 new diagnosis of heart failure are made per year [26]. The mortality rate is estimated to be 70,000 deaths per year from heart failure [27].

Medical management is the predominant treatment for patients with chronic heart failure. Although medical therapies (eg, angiotensin-converting enzyme [ACE] inhibitors and beta blockers) have decreased morbidity and mortality for patients with heart failure [28,29], irreversible end-stage cardiac disease, unresponsive to pharmacologic therapy, afflicts about 60,000 patients per year [30]. Inotropic drugs and mechanical support with intra-aortic balloon pump are the maximum available nonsurgical therapy for patients with end-stage heart failure.

Cardiac transplantation is the most effective intervention for end-stage cardiac failure, with 1- and 5-year survival rates of 85.6% and 79.5%, respectively [31]. Without a transplant, patients with New York Heart Association (NYHA) class IV heart failure have only a 20% to 30% survival rate [30]. The limited supply of donor hearts prevents heart transplantation from being a treatment option for many patients with end-stage heart failure. Patients who have very poor functional status, advanced age, and severe comorbidities, such as diabetes, chronic obstructive pulmonary disease (COPD), or liver cirrhosis, are less likely to survive a heart transplant and have poor long-term survival. Such patients are often not transplant candidates.

Left ventricular assist devices (LVADs) can augment native left ventricular function. LVADs can lend short-term support to patients recovering from postcardiotomy shock. They also can be used as a bridge to heart transplantation. They are now seen, by some, as a potential destination therapy for patients who are not heart transplant candidates. This is a source of significant controversy because of the expense and its reported limited success. A cost-effectiveness analysis can help understand the economic and health consequences of using an LVAD as destination therapy.

Oz reported on the outcomes and costs associated with 68 patients who received a LVAD in the Randomized Evaluation of Mechanical Assistance for the Treatment of Congestive Heart failure (REMATCH) trial [32]. There were 17 in-hospital deaths and 51 hospital survivors. Hospital survivors had inpatient costs of $159,271 plus or minus 106,423. Those who did not survive had inpatient costs of $315,015 plus or minus 278,713. The average cost of the implantation, excluding professional fees, was $210,187 (plus or minus 193,295), the cost of the device itself was about $60,000, and the Center for Medicare and Medicaid Services (CMS) sets its DRG reimbursement at $70,000 for LVAD therapy. For initial hospitalization, the average length of stay is 43.5 days. Professional fees were estimated from a 2001 study of 12 bridge-to-transplant patients [33]. Oz reported that the average annual readmission cost was $105,326. Outpatient costs were estimated from studies by Moskowitz and colleagues [33] and Gelijns and colleagues [34], which analyzed costs associated with long-term LVAD implantation in bridge-to-transplant patients. The average weekly outpatient cost was $352, yielding a full month cost of $1531. When these costs were put together, the average one-year cost for placing an LVAD, as destination therapy, was estimated to be $505,373, while the average 1-year cost for optimal medical management was $178,693.

Survival data for these two groups are seen in Table 3.

Based on these data a cost-effectiveness calculation can be made using the mean data:

(LVAD cost − Med Rx cost)/(LVAD survial − Med Rx survial)

= DLYS($505,373 − $178,693)/(1.07 − 0.61) year

= $816,700 per life year saved

Even if median survival is used instead of mean survival, the DLYS only decreases to $526,903 per life year saved. This is 10 times the long-established inflation adjusted cost-effectiveness threshold of $50,000 to 80,000 per life year saved. It is reasonable to expect that increased surgical and medical experience in caring for these patients, coupled with improved and less expensive devices, may bring the effective costs down by reducing implantation costs, hospital length of stay, and rehospitalization. It appears impractical, however, to expect these costs to recede to the accepted cost-effectiveness threshold. If the outcomes in patients with these devices substantially improve, then, because of the large patient population that suffers from end-stage cardiac failure, there could be a new lobbying effort to guarantee adequate payment for this therapy from the federal government. If this occurs, then the cost-effectiveness threshold would be raised substantially, leading to considerable rippling effects throughout the US health care economy.

Cost-effective analysis and the anesthesiologist

Although a cost-effectiveness analysis can be a powerful tool to determine whether a new medical technology should be embraced, its applicability has limitations. The most obvious is that this tool is dependent on the availability of detailed patient outcomes and cost data. As is seen in the previous two examples, technology that is considered to be disruptive, either because of its

Table 3
Survival data in patients receiving a left-ventricular assist device (LVAD) versus those receiving optimal medical management (Med Rx) for end-stage cardiac failure

	LVAD	Med Rx	Difference
Median survival			
Days	405	180	
Months	13.30	5.90	7.40
Years	1.11	0.49	
Mean survival			
Days	392	221	
Months	12.87	7.26	5.61
Years	1.07	0.61	

absolute cost (eg, LVAD), or because of its impact on large populations (eg, tPA), can be expected to generate the data necessary to carry out a cost-effectiveness analysis. The availability of this kind of analysis is infrequent, because population-based studies, economic analysis, and technology assessment research is time-consuming and expensive. Major technology assessments that use existing data generally cost between $40,000 and 50,000. Prospective research (eg, prospective, randomized clinical studies) can cost more than $500,000. Because of the expense and complexity, formal technology assessment research is done infrequently by institutions, even those that will use the results as part of their decision-making process.

Organizations often look to the medical literature as the initial source of economic and outcomes data. Unfortunately, even by accessing the literature do groups find the information they need, in a format that they can rarely use for their internal technology assessment. Numerous organizations do their own technology assessments, which are available by subscription. The Emergency Care Research Institute (ECRI, www.ecri.org) is one such organization. Subscribing to these services can be useful, not only for the technology reports, but also to gain an understanding of how new medical technologies and therapies are evaluated. These reports have their limitations, however. They can be expensive, and they commonly analyze new medical technologies from a societal perspective. This can be problematic to a medical organization, because they may be paying the bulk of the expense for the new technology, particularly if they are not in a fee-for-service environment, while the offsetting economic benefit is seen by patients (eg, less pain, return to work earlier) or employers (eg, less disability payments). A simple example within anesthesiology can illustrate why the boundaries of an analysis matter.

If an anesthesiology department is instructed to get their drug costs as low as possible, the initial response could be to eliminate all but the oldest and least expensive medications. The anesthesiologists could have their practice limited to only halothane, morphine, pancuronium, succinylcholine, and so on. From the perspective of the department of anesthesiology, this would be a very economical change with little if any patient outcome consequence, particularly if the time frame for outcomes is only the period from operating room (OR) entry to the OR to exit. If the patients are slow to wake up in the OR, they can be transported intubated (and ventilated) to the recovery room, where it becomes that department's problem and expense. If the broader perspective is examined, however, these choices may not be the best. Shorter-acting agents may be better, because their increased expense may be offset by the cost savings of shorter stays in the recovery room or outpatient area. A decreased nausea and vomiting rate is also associated with shorter recovery room time, decreased hospital admissions, and lower total costs. A better patient experience may bring patients back to the institution for further medical care and possibly improve the reputation of the facility, bringing in even more patients. This example is very limited, but it is important to understand that where one draws the boundaries of a cost-effectiveness analysis can have significant effects on the results and what conclusions will be drawn.

A technology assessment produced from the perspective of a medical center or physician group will look different than that seen in the literature. Such an assessment would:

- Occur earlier in the technologic development and distribution life cycle
- Be responsive to the medical knowledge, experience, and practice patterns in the organization
- Be sensitive to the needs of the local community and its medical conditions
- Place less emphasis on nonhospital outcomes or long-term costs
- Examine liability issues
- Give less consideration to impacts on the broader health care system

Assuming that the medical center has access to the appropriate information and has the expertise to carry out a technology assessment, making use of the basic principles as discussed previously, and having a clear understanding of the perspective the assessment is speaking to, such an assessment can make a real difference in assisting a facility in making rational and defensible decisions on the acquisition of new technologies. Although a formal technology assessment is impractical at the departmental level, the basic principles of this process can be a useful guide for decision making.

Unfortunately, this level of detail is infrequently available for emerging technologies in anesthesia or even critical care. Even when there are available outcomes data, they often are not presented in a prospective randomized study that compares the new technology to standard therapy. Cost data are commonly lacking, outside of the cost of purchasing the technology and possibly any supply costs. Longer-term consequences, such as 30- or more day mortality, rehospitalization, patient functional status, much less nonmedical costs, are infrequently available. Therefore, other strategies often must be applied when evaluating new anesthesia and critical care technologies.

Technology assessment—application of blue cross criteria

At the institutional and particularly the departmental level, where the available data are limited, a refinement of the technology assessment process should be used. A good example of such a process is the technology assessment criteria used by the Blue Cross Blue Shield Association [35]. In order for a new technology to adopted, it must be shown that:

- The technology has final approval from the appropriate government regulatory bodies.
- The scientific evidence permits conclusions concerning the effect of the technology on health outcomes.

- The technology improves health outcomes.
- The technology is beneficial as any established alternatives.
- The improvement is attainable outside the investigational setting.

The different state Blue Cross Blue Shield Insurance Companies have medical advisory committees, which are made up of physicians and community members who make recommendations to Blue Cross, as to whether a medical intervention is accepted medical practice and should be reimbursed. They use these criteria as the basis for their recommendations. The committees do not make the decision, nor do they recommend a reimbursement level. The Blue Cross technology assessment criteria should be considered by other organizations. These criteria are somewhat flexible, in that sound institutional judgment can be used to fill what voids exist in the data set. The criteria are designed to be a step-wise progression that can lead the technology assessment team toward the decision on whether to adopt a new medical technology.

Technology must have final regulatory approval

As discussed previously, the term "medical technology" applies to all drugs, procedures, and organizational systems. The first criteria that a new technology must meet is that is has final approval from the US Food and Drug Administration (FDA) or other governmental body that regulates the technology (eg, Nuclear Regulatory Agency). Any provisional approval that is given as an interim step by the regulatory body is not sufficient. Surgical procedures, such as transplants, generally involve no regulatory approval. The off-label use of approved drugs is eligible for further review, because the medication itself has been approved.

These criteria must be absolute. Not only is using unapproved medications and devices legally questionable, it is ethically unsupportable. An unapproved technology may be used only if a protocol has received prospective review, approval, and ongoing oversight by an institutional review board (IRB). Informed consent also must be obtained from each patient enrolled in such protocols.

To assure that such approval has been granted, it is recommended that the technology assessment group directly access the documentation of the technology approval. Unfortunately, proponents or manufacturer representatives may claim that their device has received such approval when in fact it is pending, believing, for example, that by the time the device or drug shows up it will have received approval. This hope is not always manifested. If an unapproved device or drug is mistakenly used, it could put both the patient and the institution at considerable risk. Therefore, it is imperative that the assessment group insist on seeing evidence of regulatory approval themselves and not settle for assurances. Most often, a straightforward Internet search can answer this question.

Scientific evidence must permit conclusions regarding health outcomes

The scientific evidence should consist of well-designed studies published in peer-reviewed journals. The quality of the various studies and consistency of results are considered in evaluating the evidence. Ideally, the results of these published investigations will be from prospective, randomized, comparative studies. As the scientific evidence diverges from this high standard, the ability of the technology assessment group to draw firm conclusion diminishes. If all that is available are short case series reports (eg, "I did so many cases, and these were my results"), it would be inappropriate to give much if any weight to such results or to conclude that the scientific evidence allows for conclusions regarding health outcomes.

Systems to stratify evidence by quality have been developed, such as this one by the US Preventive Services Task Force [36]:

- Level I—evidence obtained from at least one properly designed randomized controlled trial
- Level II-1—evidence obtained from well-designed controlled trials without randomization
- Level II-2—evidence obtained from well-designed cohort or case-control analytic studies, preferably from more than one center or research group
- Level II-3—evidence obtained from multiple time series with or without the intervention. Dramatic results in uncontrolled trials might also be regarded as this type of evidence.
- Level III—opinions of respected authorities, based on clinical experience, descriptive studies, or reports of expert committees

The scientific evidence should demonstrate that the technology can measure or alter the physiological changes related to a disease, injury, illness, or condition. In addition, there should be evidence or a convincing argument based on established medical facts that such measurement or alteration affects health outcomes. Opinions and evaluations by national medical associations, consensus panels, or other technology evaluation bodies are evaluated according to the scientific quality of the supporting evidence and rationale.

The technology must improve net health outcomes

Using the same basic evidence criteria discussed previously, the technology assessment group also must determine whether the proposed technology makes a difference in eventual patient outcome. The technology's beneficial effects should outweigh any of its harmful effects. There are many incidences in the literature where a medication or device can be shown to work (eg, an MRI scan produces an accurate image of the anatomy, or a medication lowers blood pressure as intended), but not make any difference in eventual outcomes (eg, swan-ganz catheters [37,38]). This can be seen when investigations focus on intermediate health metrics such as blood pressure or temperature on recovery room admission. The science can be clear that there is a difference between groups with the use of a new technology, but extrapolations of these differences to improved outcomes does not constitute scientific evidence.

Another, and possibly more important, consideration is whether the reported improved net outcomes are clinically relevant. The literature may demonstrate a statistically significant improvement in health outcomes with use of a technology, but that improvement may be so small as not to be clinically relevant. This is where medical judgment must come into play.

The technology must be at least as beneficial as existing alternatives

The scientific studies must show that the technology works and that impact on outcomes is clinically relevantly, but the technology still must be compared with existing medical care. Showing that something works as compared with a placebo is not adequate. Further analysis is required to compare the patient outcomes with the new technology to current accepted medical practice. In addition, it should be determined for how long the benefits of the new technology last. Is it a transient improvement, only to recede over time, to eventually be of less benefit than the standard treatment?

The benefit must be achievable outside of an investigational environment

The new technology must be useable in routine practice environments. The fact that an academic medical center is able to report success with the support of research fellows, scientists, and other support personnel may not be reproducible in a private practice environment. Preferably the evidence, but a least the judgment of the assessment group, must conclude that the results seen in the literature can be replicated in other medical institutions.

Unless a new technology, or a new use for an accepted technology, meets all five criteria, it is not deemed accepted medical practice. In the context of an institutional or departmental technology assessment process, unless the criteria are met, the new technology should not be adopted by the practice. Physician preference, enthusiasm, or some educational benefit is not an adequate justification for adopting a new medical technology.

Fiscal analysis

Although a full-fledged cost-effectiveness analysis may not be feasible, the assessment group must work through the fiscal implications of introducing a new technology. To the extent possible they should determine the:

- Capital expense—the cost of purchasing, installing, and in the case of information technology, configuring and interfacing the technology. Is there associated space and remodeling expense?

- Operational cost—the annual expense of supplies, maintenance, upgrades, and personnel.
- Depreciation schedule—how long will the technology last? When will it need to be replaced? What is the expected inflation rate that will devalue the technology as it depreciates?
- Time value of money—what would have been the return on investment if the expense was deferred?
- Down-stream expenses—what impact will the new technology have on productivity? Will it increase demands for personnel, bed space, supplies, and so on after its use? Will patients be required to stay in the hospital longer, or will their stay decrease? What is the complication profile?
- Reimbursement—will use of the technology be reimbursed by third party payers? If so, based on what information and by how much? What is the difference between government and private payers?
- Patient volumes—what is the expected impact on patient volumes? What is the expected payer mix of the targeted patient population?
- Access—what impact will the new technology have on access to care? Will it consume disproportionate resources making access to other health care services more difficult for patients, or will it open access?

The tools needed to produce a fiscal analysis are often beyond that of a technology assessment group, but these questions need to be answered. The purchasing and accounting departments will have the tools to produce a financial effect analysis. This report can predict the net fiscal impact the proposed technology will have on the institution. It can predict whether total expenses will be met by the expected reimbursement. Such a report also should include a sensitivity analysis to examine what impact there will be if the assumptions prove incorrect. For example, what would be the consequence if twice or half as many patients are treated with the device? What would happen if the government to private payer mix is 60:40 instead of 40:60?

With the answers to the five technology criteria and a well-formulated financial effect analysis, the technology assessment group can make a recommendation built on a foundation of scientific facts, sound medical judgment, and fiscal reasoning. Even if a new technology does not bring in more revenue, even if it is a net expense, it still may be worth adopting if the health outcomes are worth the expense, or if the down-stream consequences are favorable (eg, increases access for services that offer positive fiscal return).

In today's medical reimbursement environment, it is inevitable that some services will lose money, but it is the mission of all health care organizations to provide needed health care. It is also a reality that some services are reimbursed at a significantly greater rate than their expense. Therefore, such services can make up for the negative return seen elsewhere. At the end of a technology assessment process, these conclusions will have to be drawn:

- Is one confident that the technology has been shown to work?

- Can one conclude that use of the technology will be associated with relevant improved outcomes?
- Can one adapt to the disruptions the new technology will bring to the medical institution?
- Is the negative margin acceptable?

Such a process allows medical institutions to make informed decisions that are consistent with their fundamental mission of providing quality health care, while remaining in business to be able to continue to provide quality health care (ie, "no money, no mission").

Closing the loop

A common error many institutions make is to never re-examine a project after it has been approved. The decision to embrace a new technology, whether it is very expensive, such as a new multi-slice CT scanner, or something mundane, such as a new anesthesia machine, is based on many different criteria. A well-done assessment will have looked at the science, conferred with local, and, at times, national experts, and will have gathered as much fiscal information as possible. Unfortunately, despite the hard work, the decision to purchase still is built upon assumptions and incomplete information. The scientific literature may show much different results after approval. The fiscal projections may turn out to have been incorrect. The expected patient volumes may not have materialized. Any number of things may turn out differently than anticipated during the evaluation process.

Therefore, it is critical that the organization carries out a postimplementation review. This should be just as detailed as the technology assessment that was done before the purchase. The technology assessment group should look at any new papers that may have been published subsequent to adoption. The local experience should be examined, particularly the patient outcomes seen with the new technology, as used by the medical center's staff caring for its own patients. Were these results consistent with what was expected? Along the same line, the various fiscal issues also should be reviewed. How did the patient volumes, mix, reimbursement and so on compare with what had been anticipated? If the results are the same as projected, then the group made the correct decision. If not, where did the analysis go wrong, and what can be done differently in future assessments to improve the decision-making process? Finally, based on how the new technology has worked out within the organization, the hard question needs to be asked whether to continue use of the technology.

Applicability to anesthesiology

The process of formal technology assessment with a cost-effectiveness analysis, or even the Blue Cross process, may seem like overkill for the kind of decisions an anesthesiology department may make. It is in fact critical that the same discipline be applied to medical technology decisions made by anesthesiologists as in any other part of the medical facility. The total costs associated with anesthesia and the down-stream consequences can be substantial.

For example, anesthesiology decides to introduce a new invasive line catheter, such as a central line that continuously measures venous oxygen saturation. Initially, the thinking may be that the decision is no big deal. The cost of the surgical procedure is in excess of $5,000, as is the facility fee, not to mention the cost of the hospital stay. The incremental cost of the catheter is only $200, so why worry about it? In fact, the consequences of this decision can be substantial. First, although the cost to the payer is measured in many thousands of dollars, the margin (ie, the difference between the cost of care and the reimbursement for care) can be very small. The addition of just a few hundred dollars of additional, nonreimbursable expense can substantially decrease that margin. In addition, the catheter will continue to be used after the patient leaves the operating suite. When the patient arrives in the ICU, the catheter will need to be attached to another monitor; the nurses and technicians will have to be trained to use the device. The nondisposable cables and connectors will have a finite life and therefore will have to be purchased and replaced. The rippling effect within the institution can be substantial. The catheter will need to be replaced after a few days; other services will begin to use them based on anesthesia's decision, and medical therapy will be based on the displayed values. Each ripple has associated health care and fiscal consequences. There is the question of what benefit does the patient receive? The medical literature can answer part of that question, but it also must be considered whether the patient population the catheter will be put into is the same that the studies have investigated. It is possible, that now that a new physiologic parameter is available, that the decisions made based on that parameter will not be correct with patients now doing worse than they previously were without the benefit of the advanced technology.

As can be seen, even a decision as minor as deciding on purchasing a new central line can have nontrivial consequences to the medical facility and one's patients. Other decisions (eg, which kind of physiologic monitor, anesthesia machine, or electronic medical record product) will have even greater implications. Therefore, it is imperative that anesthesiologists take the process of technology assessment seriously. Given the specialty's historic leadership in medical technology, patient safety, and organizational management, it should be expected that a facility's department of anesthesiology should take a leading role in any technology assessment process.

Summary

The expense associated with modern heath care in the United States is very high, in excess of 15% of the GDP, continues to grow and has become a significant public policy issue. New technologies, defined as all drugs, devices, procedures, and organizational systems, are major contributors to rising health care costs. The use of health technology assessment tools can assist those in leadership positions in making rational decisions as to which new technologies to adopt.

The classical approach is to use data from prospective, randomized, clinical trials that compare the outcomes of those treated with the new technology and the accepted therapy. Using this information and detailed economic data, the cost-effectiveness ratio can be determined. The accepted metrics are either dollars per life year saved or dollars per quality-adjusted life year saved. If the new medical intervention costs less than $50,000 to $80,000 per life year saved, it is considered to be cost-effective and worthy of adoption. This kind of analysis is complex and expensive. In addition, the required information is not always available, limiting the applicability of this approach. Finally, the economic analysis often includes down-stream expense and benefit not relevant from a medical center perspective.

Another approach is to focus the analysis to what impacts the medical center. This includes determining whether the technology has received the necessary approvals and has been shown to be effective, to improve health outcomes, to be at least as effective as standard therapy, and to be achievable outside the investigative setting. A fiscal analysis also must be done to determine what will it cost to acquire and operate the technology, what are the anticipated patient volumes and payer mix, and what will be the down-stream consequences to the medical center. If the process concludes that the technology works, makes a positive difference to patient care, and is fiscally and operationally acceptable, it should be purchased.

After the technology has been installed and has been used, a postimplementation review should be done. This review should go over the same attributes that led to the decision to purchase. It should be determined whether the expected patient volumes, outcomes, income, and expenses were seen. If not, the technology assessment process should be refined to make better decisions in the future. Finally, if the results are at a substantial negative variance from what was anticipated, abandoning the technology should be considered.

Anesthesiology either directly controls or indirectly influences a significant portion of medical technology in every medical center. Therefore, the processes that have been discussed in this article should be used by the department of anesthesiology to assure optimal patient care and the fiscal stability of the organization.

References

[1] Tuman KJ, Ivankovich AD. High-cost, high-tech medicine: are we getting our money's worth? J Clin Anesth 1993;5:168–77.

[2] Clarke RCE. OECD in figures: statistics on the member countries, in 2003 health expenditures and resources. Paris: Organization for Economic Cooperation and Development, Health Expenditures and Resources; 2003. p. 8.
[3] Greer AL. Medical technology: assessment, adoption, and utilization. J Med Syst 1981;5: 129–45.
[4] Veluchamy S, Saver CL. Clinical technology assessment, cost-effective adoption, and quality management by hospitals in the 1990s. QRB Qual Rev Bull 1990;16(6):223–8.
[5] Jacoby I, Pauker SG. Technology assessment in health care: group process and decision theory. Isr J Med Sci 1986;22:183–90.
[6] Stevens C. Guidelines spread, but how much impact will they have? Med Econ 1993;70(13): 66–76.
[7] Shepard DS. Cost-effectiveness in health and medicine. J Ment Health Policy Econ 1999; 2(2):91–2.
[8] Noyes K, Holloway RG. Evidence from cost-effectiveness research. NeuroRx 2004;1(3): 348–55.
[9] Garber AM, Phelps CE. Economic foundations of cost-effectiveness analysis. J Health Econ 1997;16(1):1–31.
[10] Laupacis A, Feeny D, Detsky AS, et al. How attractive does a new technology have to be to warrant adoption and utilization? Tentative guidelines for using clinical and economic evaluations. CMAJ 1992;146(4):473–81.
[11] Perry S, Pillar B. A national policy for health care technology assessment. Med Care Rev 1990;47(4):401–17.
[12] Mark DB, Hlatky MA, Califf RM, et al. Cost effectiveness of thrombolytic therapy with tissue plasminogen activator as compared with streptokinase for acute myocardial infarction. N Engl J Med 1995;332(21):1418–24.
[13] Boissel JP. The ISIS-2 study. International Study of Infarction Survival. Rev Prat 1988; 38(19):1285–8.
[14] Fresco C, Franzosi MG, Maggioni AP, et al. The GISSI-2 trial: premises, results, epidemiological (and other) implications. Gruppo Italiano per lo Studio delia Sopravvivenza nell'Infarto Miocardico. Clin Cardiol 1990;13(Suppl 8):VIII32–6.
[15] Maggioni AP, Franzosi MG, Fresco C, et al. GISSI trials in acute myocardial infarction. Rationale, design, and results. Chest 1990;97(Suppl 4):146S–50S.
[16] Sleight P. Survival following thrombolytic therapy. Eur Heart J 1990;11:1–4.
[17] Gulba DC, Claus G. Thrombolytic therapy of myocardial infarct. Status after GISSI-2 and ISIS-3. Internist (Berl) 1992;33(4):206–15.
[18] The GUSTO Angiographic Investigators. The effects of tissue plasminogen activator, streptokinase, or both on coronary artery patency, ventricular function, and survival after acute myocardial infarction. N Engl J Med 1993;329(22):1615–22.
[19] The GUSTO Investigators. An international randomized trial comparing four thrombolytic strategies for acute myocardial infarction. N Engl J Med 1993;329(10):673–82.
[20] Madhani J, Movsowitz H, Kotler MN. Tissue plasminogen activator (t-PA). Ther Drug Monit 1993;15(6):546–51.
[21] Gruppo Italiano per lo Studio della Sopravvivenza nell'Infarto Miocardico.GISSI-2. A factorial randomized trial of alteplase versus streptokinase and heparin versus no heparin among 12,490 patients with acute myocardial infarction. Lancet 1990;336(8707):65–71.
[22] In-hospital mortality and clinical course of 20,891 patients with suspected acute myocardial infarction randomized between alteplase and streptokinase with or without heparin. The International Study Group. Lancet 1990;336(8707):71–5.
[23] ISIS-3. A randomised comparison of streptokinase vs tissue plasminogen activator vs anistreplase and of aspirin plus heparin vs aspirin alone among 41,299 cases of suspected acute myocardial infarction. ISIS-3 (Third International Study of Infarct Survival) Collaborative Group. Lancet 1992;339(8796):753–70.
[24] Hanna K, editor. Biomedical politics. Washington: National Academy Press; 1991.

[25] Weinstein, MC, Fineberg HV, AS E. Clinical decision analysis. WB Saunders; 1980.
[26] Eichhorn EJ. Prognosis determination in heart failure. Am J Med 2001;110:14S–36S.
[27] Zeltsman D, Acker MA. Surgical management of heart failure: an overview. Annu Rev Med 2002;53:383–91.
[28] Greenberg B. The medical management of chronic congestive heart failure. In: Hosenpud JD, editor. Congestive heart failure. Philadelphia: Lippincott, Williams and Wilkins; 2000. p. 673–95.
[29] Cohn JN. Pathophysiology and clinical recognition of heart failure. In: Willerson JT, Cohn JT, editors. Cardiovascular medicine. Philadelphia: Churchill Livingstone; 2000. p. 1147–64.
[30] Oz MC, Rose EA, Levin HR. Selection criteria for placement of left ventricular assist devices. Am Heart J 1995;129(1):173–7.
[31] Miniati DN, Robbins RC. Heart transplantation: a thirty-year perspective. Annu Rev Med 2002;53:189–205.
[32] Oz MC, Gelijns AC, Miller L, et al. Left ventricular assist devices as permanent heart failure therapy: the price of progress. Ann Surg 2003;238(4):577–83.
[33] Moskowitz AJ, Rose EA, Gelijns AC. The cost of long-term LVAD implantation. Ann Thorac Surg 2001;71(Suppl 3):S195–8.
[34] Gelijns AC, Richards AF, Williams DL, et al. Evolving costs of long-term left ventricular assist device implantation. Ann Thorac Surg 1997;64(5):1312–9.
[35] Anonymous. Technology evaluation center criteria. Chicago: Blue Cross Blue Shield Association; 2006.
[36] Roman SH, Silberzweig SB, Siu AL. Grading the evidence for diabetes performance measures. Eff Clin Pract 2000;3(2):85–91.
[37] Murphy GS, Nitsun M, Vender JS. Is the pulmonary artery catheter useful? Best Pract Res Clin Anaesthesiol 2005;19(1):97–110.
[38] Dalen JE, Bone RC. Is it time to pull the pulmonary artery catheter? JAMA 1996;276(11):916–8.

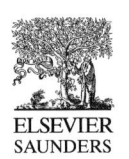

Electrocardiography: The ECG

A.D. John, MD[a],*, Lee A. Fleisher, MD[b]

[a]*Department of Anesthesia and Critical Care, Johns Hopkins University School of Medicine, 600 North Wolfe Street, Baltimore, MD 21287-4904, USA*
[b]*Department of Anesthesiology and Critical Care, The University of Pennsylvania School of Medicine, 3400 Spruce Street, Philadelphia, PA, USA*

The electrocardiogram (ECG) is a standard American Society of Anesthesiologists monitor and should be continuously displayed during an operative procedure. In addition to providing a wealth of physiological information, including information on the electrical activity of the heart, the ECG assists in monitoring and detecting a variety of changes, such as cardiac arrhythmias, electrolyte changes, and ischemia.

Myocardial cells are dynamic, undergoing depolarization and repolarization. The result of this activity is the contraction and relaxation of the heart and the maintenance of cardiovascular function. The depolarization and repolarization of the myocardial cell generates electrical dipoles, which can be pictorially represented as vectors. Vectors have mathematical properties that allow summation. Einthoven was the first to visualize the electrical activity of the heart as a summation of vectors with the resultant vector representing a single dipole within an equilateral triangle. The six standard leads (I, II, III, aVR, aVL, aVF) give a frontal-plane view of the heart. The combination of these leads gives a biplanar or two-dimensional view of a dynamic three-dimensional structure. The ECG represents the surface recording of the instantaneous electrical activity of the heart.

Components of ECG analysis

The normal ECG consists of P waves, PR interval, QRS complex, ST segment, T wave, QT interval, and, at times, a U wave (Fig. 1). Atrial activity is represented in the P wave and PR interval while the QRS wave, ST segment, T wave, and QT segment provide information on ventricular activity. ECG analysis provides information on atrial size, atrial activity, ventricular size,

---

* Corresponding author.
E-mail address: ajohn1@jhmi.edu (A.D. John).

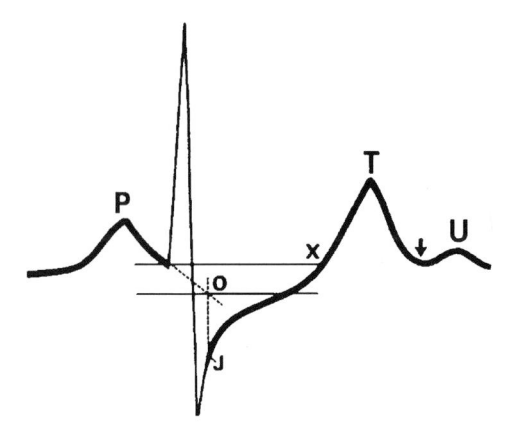

Fig. 1. Basic ECG. Arrow indicates. J, J wave; P, P wave; T, T wave; U, U wave.

ventricular activity, rate of cardiac activity, the synchronization of atrial and ventricular conduction, and the presence of damaged or ischemic myocardium. Through a detailed and systematic approach to analysis, the clinician can extract precise information provided in the ECG. However, the clinician should always bear in mind potential sources of error in the analysis.

Normal electrical activity begins in the sinoatrial node, spreads to the right atrium, then to the interatrial septum and left atrium on the way toward the atrioventricular node. The P wave represents this atrial electrical activity as the electrical impulse moves through the right atrium anteriorly and inferiorly, the interatrial Bachman bundle, and the left atrium posteriorly and inferiorly to the atrioventricular node via anterior, middle, and posterior Purkinje pathways with the left atrial appendage being the last atrial component to contract. A biphasic P wave in lead V1 and V2 often represents the transition of right atrial contraction anteriorly and inferiorly and the left atrial contraction posteriorly and inferiorly, but this is not seen in the other leads because of the sequential spread of electrical activity from the right to the left atrium. A negative deflection of the P wave is normal in aVR and may also be seen in lead III [1]. The width of the impulse represents the time duration for the impulse to spread, while the height of the impulse or amplitude represents the strength of the signal received by the sensing electrode. The normal duration of a P wave is <0.12 seconds and presents with an amplitude of <0.2 mV [2].

The PR interval measures the time for an impulse through atrioventricular conduction to travel from the sinoatrial node, through the atria and the atrioventricular node, down the bundle branches, and through the Purkinje network until the onset of ventricular contraction. The PR interval includes the time for atrial depolarization, as revealed in the P wave, and the time for atrial repolarization, as measured by the PR segment—the time from the P wave to the onset of the QRS complex—and thus the PR interval assesses the period of atrial activity. To accurately measure this period, the lead with the widest P wave, the longest QRS wave, and shortest PR interval should be chosen for measurement. As revealed in the PR segment, the period of atrial repolarization, which is usually in an opposite direction to the P wave, is usually flat or horizontal, but during periods of increased heart rate may be sloping downward with sloping steeper in leads with P waves of larger amplitude. The normal PR interval varies and increases with age. Children tend to have shorter PR intervals and older individuals longer PR intervals, but the normal PR interval should remain <0.20 second [1].

The QRS complex encompasses the period of ventricular activation, depolarization, and contraction. This is the time when most of the heart's musculature engages in a smooth, synchronized, concerted effort to propel the blood to both the pulmonic and systemic circulations to maintain life processes. The morphology, duration, axis, and amplitude of the QRS complex represents the summation of this electrical activity, which results in the twisting, wringing contractions of the heart and forward propulsion of the blood. Electrical activation, which begins in the high left portion of the middle septal region, spreads downward toward the apex. Out of this initial wave, two waves emerge. One travels from the lower left septum spreading toward the right. The other travels from the right lower septum spreading to the left. Both waves follow anterior and posterior pathways. The apical anterior aspects of the heart are initially activated with electrical activity spreading finally to the posterior basilar portion of the heart [1].

The QRS complex in its entirety represents this electrical activity with the component elements of the QRS complex including the Q wave, the R wave, the S wave, and, at times, a QS wave and an R^1 wave. The Q wave is the first negative or downward deflection after the P wave and represents ventricular vectors moving away from the sensing electrode. A small Q wave may be present in normal adults in the inferior leads (II, III, and aVF); the left lateral precordial leads (V6, V5 > V4 > >V3), and occasionally in leads I and VL. The greater the amplitude and the longer the duration, the greater the likelihood that the Q wave is indicative of a myocardial infarction, especially when it was not present on a prior ECG. A significant Q wave is taken to be >40 ms with an amplitude greater than one quarter to one third the height of the QRS complex. The R wave is the first positive deflection after the P wave and increases in amplitude from the right to the left precordium, indicating a greater proximity of the heart to the electrode. The S wave is a negative or downward deflection following the R wave. The S wave tends to be most prominent in the right precordial leads, especially V2 and also somewhat prominent in aVR. The QS wave represents a single downward or negative deflection after the P wave, which is not followed by an R wave. This downward deflection may be seen in obese patients with a horizontal heart position in lead III, whereas in thin patients with a vertical heart problem, it may be seen in lead aVL. In rare cases, the QS wave may represent a normal variant if present in leads III, aVL, and aVF [1]. The R^1 wave is another positive deflection after the R wave and may represent the late depolarization of the right ventricular outflow tract or the late depolarization of the basilar aspect of the septum. When seen in lead V1, the R^1 wave may be indicative of a right bundle branch block [1].

The morphology of the QRS complex must sum a variety of three-dimensional vectoral representations of a dynamic process occurring in a large mass of cardiac tissue, accounting for the vectoral representation of the initial septal and paraseptal depolarization, followed by the ventricular free-wall activation, and finally the vectoral representation of basilar ventricular activity. The morphology of the QRS complex with its constituent elements helps to define ventricular electrical activity and also reveals the presence of abnormal conduction, ischemia, and hypertrophy, as well as the presence of pacing devices. The amplitude of the QRS complex reflects not only the proximity and size of the heart, but also the presence of disease processes, such as emphysema, pneumothorax, cardiac tamponade, constrictive pericarditis, and scleroderma, which presents with low voltage. The electrical axis represents the direction of the mean QRS complex vector in the frontal plane. This axis may be determined in one of two ways:

- Find the lead with the most isoelectric QRS complex. The axis will be perpendicular to this lead in the direction of the limb lead with the most positive deflection; or
- Determine the vectoral sum of the QRS complex in leads I and AVF.

These two methods do not always produce the same result. The normal QRS axis lies between −30° and +90°, usually +60° in the direction of lead II. Left axis deviation begins to occur as the axis moves toward 0° and −30° and becomes markedly pronounced when it extends beyond −30° toward −90° with the QRS positive in lead I and negative in lead II. With aging, the electrical axis gradually moves leftward and, with obesity, the heart shifts to a more horizontal plane, also resulting in leftward movement. In addition, left axis deviation is also associated with atrioventricular canal defects; ostium primum atrial septal defects; left anterior hemiblock; right bundle branch block; a combination of right bundle branch block and left anterior hemiblock; intraventricular conduction disturbance, such as hyperkalemia; and a periinfarction block [1]. Right axis deviation occurs as the electrical axis moves toward +90° and +180° with a negative QRS in lead I and, in cases of extreme right axis deviation, the QRS is negative in both leads I and aVF. A rightward axis is normal in infants and children, and may also be present in thin adults whose hearts lie in a more vertical plane. Medical conditions associated with right axis deviation include right ventricular hypertrophy; a left posterior fascicular block, which may also be associated with other signs of inferior or posterior ischemia; chronic obstructive pulmonary disease, especially when presenting with an S1, S2, or S3; and lateral myocardial infarction [1]. The QRS duration is indicative of the time it takes for ventricular activation and should be measured in the lead with the clearest and widest QRS complex in the frontal plane with normal being defined as <0.12 second [2].

The J point in an ECG represents the transition from ventricular activation and depolarization to the period preceding ventricular repolarization. The ST segment encompasses this period between ventricular depolarization and ventricular repolarization. The analysis of the ST segment of this specific aspect and time period of electrical activity plays a preeminent role in the analysis, definition, and detection of myocardial ischemia.

ST segment changes may reveal depression, which indicates endocardial ischemia and subendocardial injury, or they may reveal elevation, which indicates transmural ischemia, transmural injury, and infarction (Box 1). ST segment changes are reflective of local currents of injury, which may result in cells having a lower resting membrane potential, causing partial depolarization. Early repolarization may also occur from these local currents of injury and result in ST segment changes [3]. The significance of ST segment changes is defined by a change from baseline of >0.1 mV, where baseline is defined by a line connecting the beginning of the QRS complex of one beat with the beginning QRS complex of the subsequent beat for three consecutive beats on a line that is isoelectric and free of tachycardia [1]. Other causes of ST-segment changes are discussed throughout this article.

The T wave represents the period of ventricular repolarization with ventricular recovery as repolarization procedes in the same direction as depolarization, represented by the QRS complex. Certain areas of the ventricle take longer to repolarize than to depolarize and this time differential encompasses the concept of ventricular gradient. A normal T wave has a slower ascent and a more rapid descent and, in the right precordium, a biphasic T wave that is initially positive and then negative may be seen. However, a negative initial deflection followed by a positive deflection is usually abnormal. Since the normal T-wave vector is directed leftward, anteriorly and inferiorly the T wave is usually negative in aVR and may be inverted in the right precordial leads as part of a juvenile pattern, but should be upright in the lateral precordium with upright T waves in leads I, II, V5, and V6 [1]. Since repolarization is a highly energy-dependent process, T-wave

---

Box 1. Causes of ST segment changes

- Myocardial ischemia
- Myocardial infarction
- Conduction changes
- Drug effects (eg. digitalis)
- Autonomic effects
- Left ventricular hypertrophy
- Measurement artifacts

changes or abnormalities reflect changes in ventricular repolarization and, as such, may be indicative of myocardial ischemia. There are other causes of T-wave changes. Cerebrovascular accidents, especially subarachnoid hemorrhage, may present with diffuse T-wave inversion putatively from a hypothalamic-mediated vagal activation. A neurogenic T-wave pattern may also be seen after vagotomy, bilateral carotid endarterectomy, or radial neck dissection. Altered ventricular activation, such as bundle branch block, Wolff–Parkinson–White, strain patterns, apical hypertrophic cardiomyopathy, preexcitation, post-tachycardia, pacing, or, in certain patients, an idiopathic global T-wave inversion, may result in T-wave changes [3].

Electrical systole is represented by the QT interval, which should be measured in the lead with most clearly defined T waves from the beginning of the QRS complex to the end of the T wave (Fig. 2). The QT interval varies with heart rate as well as the location of the heart with respect to the recording electrode, which results in the phenomenon of QT dispersal. To correct for heart rate variation, a corrected QT interval (QTc) is most commonly defined by the QT interval in seconds divided by the square root of the

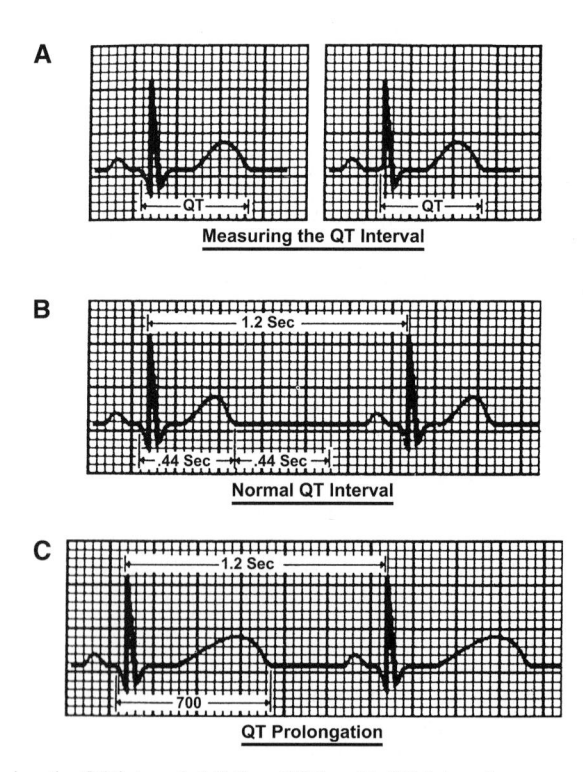

Fig. 2. Measuring the QT interval. (*A*) Two ECGs with QT interval measurements. (*B*) ECG with normal QT interval. (*C*) ECG showing prolonged QT interval (*From* Grauer K, Curry RW Jr. Clinical electrocardiography. 2nd edition. Cambridge (MA): Blackwell Scientific Publications; 1992; with permission.)

R–R interval in seconds with normal considered below 0.44 to 0.46 second [1]. The QT interval may be shortened in the presence of certain conditions, such as acidosis, hyperkalemia, and hypercalcemia, and with the use of medication, such as digoxin. A prolonged QT interval is often taken as a precursor to the onset of malignant ventricular arrhythmias and the presence of ischemia. Other causes include congenital prolonged QT syndrome, such as Jervell–Lange–Nielsen, which is associated with deafness, and Romano–Ward, which has no association with deafness. Organophosphate poisoning can produce a prolonged QT syndrome similar to congenital prolonged QT syndrome. Other causes of QT prolongation include hypokalemia, hypocalcemia, hypomagnesemia, class-1A antiarrhythmics, class-III antiarrhythmics, psychotropic medications, central nervous disorders (eg, subarachnoid hemorrhage, ruptured berry aneurysms, and cryptococcal meningitis), hypothermia, and even fad diets [1,4].

The U wave occurs in diastole in the same direction as the T wave, but with a fraction of its amplitude and is best seen in leads V2 and V3. The cause of the U wave is not certain and at times may even represent a second notching of the T wave. A large positive U wave may be due to hypokalemia or antiarrhythmic medication, whereas a negative U wave may represent ischemia, hypertension, or right ventricular hypertrophy [1,4].

Once the components of the normal ECG with the information that they convey are understood, an analysis of the ECG can be undertaken. The ECG should be analyzed in a consistent and systematic manner. The first step is to assess if all the component elements of the ECG as described above are present and, if not, to determine which components are missing. Second, the rate of ventricular conduction should be determined with the adult normal being defined as a heart rate between 60 to 100 beats per minute. Tachycardia represents a heart rate >100 beats per minute and bradycardia represents a heart rate <60 beats per minute. After the rate has been determined, the rhythm should be determined. Does a P wave precede every QRS complex? Is the patient in sinus rhythm? If not, what is the rhythm? Clinical correlation with assessment of cardiovascular perfusion should be immediately undertaken. Is there a pulse? What is the blood pressure? What is the oxygen saturation? Hemodynamically unstable rhythms should be treated emergently according to the protocols of advanced cardiac life support and with cardiopulmonary resuscitation. If the patient is hemodynamically stable, then further analysis should determine electrical axis, conduction delays and blocks, atrial and ventricular size, electrolyte abnormalities, and the presence or absence of ischemia. The most common sources of error continue to be incorrect analysis, misplaced leads, loss of leads, motion artifacts, and shivering, all of which can contribute to the misinterpretation of data and suboptimal care. Lead placement and filters have a significant impact on intraoperative echocardiography. Although 12-lead systems are available for continuous intraoperative monitoring, most systems are restricted to 5 leads (with only 1 precordial lead). The surgical incision may also influence lead placement, which affects sensitivity and specificity required for detecting and interpreting the aforementioned abnormalities. Finally, filtering systems may be used to decrease the effects of electrocautery and movement, but may lead to distortion and incorrect interpretation of the ECG.

Conduction defects and blocks

Conduction defects or blocks may occur anywhere within the cardiac conducting pathways from the sinoatrial node to the atrioventricular node, the bundle of His, down the bundle branches, fascicle, and Purkinje system to the ventricular myocardium. The blocks commonly encountered include right and left bundle branch blocks; left anterior and posterior fascicular block; first, second, and third heart block; and atrioventricular dissociation. Conduction defects may be due to various causes with varying degrees of significance. They may also require treatment and intervention.

In first-degree (1°) atrioventricular block, there is sequential conduction from the sinoatrial node to the atrioventricular node to the ventricles, but the time required for conduction is prolonged with the PR interval being > 0.20 second. First-degree atrioventricular block may be caused by an increased vagal tone; medications, such as β-blockers, calcium channel blockers, propafenone, flecainide, and amiodarone; differing diseases, including myocardial ischemia, myocardial infarction, congenital heart disease (eg, atrial septal defect), Ebstein's anomaly, infectious diseases (eg, streptococcal infection and rheumatic fever), myocarditis, infiltrative myocardial disease; and adrenal insufficiency [5]. Patients with 1° atrioventricular block usually do not require any treatment for their conduction defect. Possible exceptions are patients with heart failure and a markedly prolonged 1° block > 0.30 second who may benefit from atrioventricular sequential pacing [4].

In second-degree (2°) atrioventricular block, certain atrial impulses are not conducted to the ventricles. This is designated by a ratio of P wave to QRS complexes. If there are four P waves but only three QRS complexes, this is designated as 4:3 conduction and also 4:1 block, where conduction refers to the P waves followed by QRS complexes and block refers to the number of QRS complexes that fail to follow a P wave [1]. There are two types of 2° atrioventricular block: Mobitz type I (Wenckebach) and Mobitz type II. In Mobitz type-I 2° block, there is usually a progressive lengthening of the PR interval until there is a nonconducted P wave. The QRS morphology is not widened, but remains normal and this block most commonly occurs at the level of the atrioventricular node. Mobitz type-I block may be seen with intense vagal stimulation in normal individuals during sleep and in well-conditioned athletes. It may also be seen in hyperkalemia, acute rheumatic fever, degenerative conduction disease, and calcium deposition in the conducting system, as well as in myocardial disease. Digitalis, lithium, clonidine, methyldopa, flecainide, and propafenone, as well as calcium channel and β-blockers are associated with Mobitz type-I conduction block and should be discontinued if this block occurs. Inferior ischemia or infarction may result in type-I 2° block, which tends to resolve within hours or may last up to a week. If there is associated bradycardia and hypoperfusion, a right ventricular infarction should be excluded and appropriate antivagal therapy and resuscitation, including, on occasion, temporary pacing, may be required [4,5]. In Mobitz type-II 2° block, the PR interval tends to be constant and accompanied by a nonconducted impulse with a widened QRS complex. This is a more ominous block because the site of the conduction defect tends to be infranodal with an increased tendency to progress to complete heart block. When there is a 2:1 block, it may be hard to differentiate a Mobitz type-I block from a Mobitz type-II block. Mobitz type-I block in this situation may have an increased PR interval and narrow QRS complex and tends to decrease with increased heart rate or atropine. On the other hand, a Mobitz type-II block would be favored by a widened QRS complex and a tendency to decrease with carotid sinus massage. A Mobitz type-II block indicates significant disease of the conduction system and is associated with infiltrative diseases, such as amyloidosis, hemochromatosis; connective tissue diseases, such as lupus and scleroderma; cardiac disease; cardiomyopathy; and Chagas' disease. Also, Mobitz type-II block, when associated with an anterior myocardial infarction, signifies a large amount of myocardial damage. A Mobitz type-II block requires prompt recognition and treatment with pacemaker placement [1,3–5].

Third-degree (3°) atrioventricular block or complete heart block represents the failure of atrial impulses to activate the ventricles. The location of this block may be at the atrioventricular node or infranodal. The P–P interval and R–R interval may be regular, but atrial impulses are not conducted to the ventricle. If the conduction defect occurs at the atrioventricular node, the QRS complex tends to be narrow and the ventricular escape rhythm occurs at a rate of 40 to 60 beats per minute. If the escape rhythm is <40 beats and the QRS complex is widened, then the block tends to be infranodal. On physical examination, an S1 may vary in intensity and occasional canon *a* waves may be seen on central venous pressure examination. Medications, such as digitalis, lithium, propafenone, flecainide, methyldopa, clonidine, calcium channel blockers, and β-blockers, may cause complete heart block. Third-degree atrioventricular block may be caused by infiltrative diseases, such as amyloidosis and hemochromatosis; calcium and fibrous deposition; granulomatous diseases, such as sarcoidosis; collagen vascular disease, such as lupus and rheumatoid arthritis; infectious diseases, such as Lyme disease, Chagas' disease, endocarditis, diphtheria and syphilis; hyperkalemia; hypo- and hyperthyroidism; and valvular diseases, such as calcific aortic stenosis and mitral annular calcification. Third-degree atrioventricular block may also follow cardiac surgery. Complete 3° heart block associated with an inferior myocardial infarction is more likely to be transient, but may take 1 or 2 weeks to resolve. By comparison, complete 3° atrioventricular block associated with an anterior myocardial infarction tends to be permanent with a worse prognosis, and requires permanent pacing. Complete heart block is often unresponsive to treatment with medications atropine and isoproterenol, and requires pacing, especially if hemodynamically unstable [1,3–5].

Atrioventricular dissociation is not synonymous with complete heart block. Rather, it is a manifestation of a primary rhythm disturbance whereby the atria are activated by one pacemaker and the ventricles are activated by a separate pacemaker. Default represents the failure or slowing of the primary pacemaker and the replacement or control of the ventricular rate by a secondary or latent pacemaker. Usurpation represents the acceleration of a secondary or latent pacemaker to take control over ventricular rate and may manifest as an accelerate idioventricular rhythm, accelerate junctional rhythm, or ventricular tachycardia. Usurpation may occur in addition to or as well as atrioventricular block. Treatment is dependent on identification of the primary rhythm disturbance and assessment of hemodynamic stability [1,3,4].

Fascicular and bundle branch blocks

The conduction system to the left ventricle consists of the left anterior fascicle, which lies anteriorly and superiorly and is supplied by the left anterior descending artery; and the left posterior fascicle, which lies posteriorly and inferiorly and is supplied by branches of both the left and right coronary arteries. A left anterior fascicular block (LAFB) is characterized by (1) a left axis deviation of the QRS complex from $-30°$ to $-90°$, (2) a narrow QRS complex ≤ 0.12 second, (3) small Q waves in I, aVL or the left precordium, and (4) RS complexes in II, III, and aVF (* 1, 3, 5). It is important to exclude other causes of left axis deviation, such as Wolff–Parkinson–White syndrome, hyperkalemia, emphysema, and inferior myocardial infarction, before making the diagnosis of LAFB. The most common causes of LAFB are coronary artery disease, hypertensive heart disease, cardiomyopathy, and valvular heart disease, especially aortic valvular disease. Other causes include congenital heart disease, such as primum atrial septal defects, atrioventricular canal defects, and ventricular septal defects. Prognosis of LAFB depends on the severity of the underlying heart disease. A left posterior fascicular block (LPFB) is a rarer finding and is characterized by (1) right axis deviation of the QRS complex to $+90°$ to $+140°$, (2) a narrow QRS complex ≤ 0.12 second, (3) Q waves or QR pattern in inferior leads II, III, and aVF, and (4) RS pattern in the lateral leads I and aVL. Other causes of right axis deviation, such as a lateral myocardial infarction, chronic obstructive pulmonary disease, and right ventricular hypertrophy, must first be excluded. The most common cause of LPFB is coronary artery disease with hypertensive heart disease. Cardiomyopathy and aortic valvular disease are other common causes of LPFB. As with LAFB, the prognosis of LPFB depends on the underlying heart condition and no specific treatment is required for either LAFB or LPFB [1,3–5].

Right bundle branch block (RBBB) occurs when the right bundle is blocked and the left ventricle is depolarized normally with the electrical impulses to depolarize the right ventricle spreading from the left ventricle. RBBB is characterized by (1) a wide QRS complex ≥ 0.12 second, (2) an RSR′ pattern in the right precordium leads V1 and V2, , (3) a wide S wave in the left lateral precordium V5, V6, I, and aVL [1,3–5]. RBBB sometimes occurs in patients without heart disease and, for these patients, there is no adverse prognosis. Most patients with RBBB, however, have heart disease, including coronary artery disease, hypertensive heart disease, cor pulmonale, myocarditis, Chagas' disease, cardiomyopathies, degenerative disease of the conduction system, and sclerosis of the cardiac skeleton. For those patients with RBBB presenting with an acute myocardial infarction, there is a markedly increased mortality. Patients with the Brugada syndrome—RBBB with ST segment elevation in the right precordium—have an increased risk of ventricular tachycardia and sudden death [3]. RBBB usually requires no specific therapy.

Left bundle branch block (LBBB) is usually indicative of significant cardiac disease and, in the setting of an acute myocardial infarction, is associated with a significantly increased risk of mortality. LBBB is characterized by (1) widened QRS complex ≥ 0.12 second, (2) broad, notched and slurred R waves in the lateral precordium V5 and V6 as well as I and aVL, (3) small or absent R waves in the right precordium V1 and V2 with deep S waves, (4) absent septal Q waves in the left-sided leads, and (5) delayed intrinsicoid deflection in V5 and V6 [1,3–5]. The presence of LBBB makes the diagnosis of an acute myocardial infarction, especially lateral and inferior myocardial infarction, more difficult. LBBB is usually the result of structural heart disease due to ischemia, cardiomyopathy, advanced valvular disease, inflammation, or degeneration. In the presence of significant structural disease or bilateral bundle branch block, pacing is warranted [1,3–5]. Dorman and colleagues [6] evaluated the prognostic significance of bundle branch block and found that it is associated with co-existing cardiovascular disease, such as hypertension, coronary artery disease, and heart failure. The investigators also found that LBBB may be associated with a decreased response to stress, but that bundle branch block alone is not an independent risk factor for cardiac complication. Rather, bundle branch block should alert to the possibility of co-existing cardiovascular conditions.

The gold standard for the determination of atrial and ventricular size is the echocardiogram. Nevertheless, the ECG still provides useful information on atrial and ventricular size. Right atrial enlargement or abnormality is characterized by (1) a peaked P wave in lead II >0.25 mV, (2) P wave in leads V1 or V2 >0.15 mV, and (3) a rightward shift of the P-wave vector to more than $+75°$. The right atrium contributes to the early component of the P wave, which manifests as an increase in amplitude. Signs of right atrial enlargement are often found in association with signs of right ventricular enlargement. P pulmonale is usually described as a rightward shift of the P-wave vector and peaked P waves in leads II, III, and aVF. P pulmonale is often seen in congenital heart lesions, such as tetralogy of Fallot, Eisenmenger syndrome, tricuspid atresia and pulmonic stenosis, and has a stronger correlation with decreased arterial saturation than right atrial enlargement. P pulmonale may also be found in association with left atrial enlargement, tachycardia, and angina [1,3]. Left atrial enlargement is characterized by (1) a broad notched P wave with a duration of >0.12 second in lead II (resembling an M), (2) a leftward shift of the P-wave vector to $+15°$ to $-30°$, (3) an increased terminal negative portion of the P wave in lead V1, resulting in a biphasic P wave in lead V1 that is negative for >1 mm in depth, with a duration of >0.04 second. An enlarged left atrium manifests with an increase in the duration of the P wave, which correlates with an increase in left atrial volume. Valvular heart disease, especially mitral stenosis, is associated with this pattern of left atrial enlargement, and patients with increased left atrial size have a higher likelihood of developing paroxysmal atrial tachycardia [1,3].

The right ventricle has much less mass than the left ventricle and even with right ventricular hypertrophy (RVH) the electrical manifestations on the ECG may not be as apparent. RVH may present with (1) significant right axis deviation of $>90°$, as long as other causes, such as RBBB, lateral myocardial infarction, and left posterior fascicular block, can be excluded, (2) tall R wave, small S wave, and increased R/S ratio in lead V1 with R >0.7 mV in V1, and R/S in V1 >1, as long as Wolff–Parkinson–White, posterior infarction, normal young-adult variation, and isolated left ventricular hypertrophy can be excluded, (3) QR pattern in V1, which may be present only in severe RVH, (4) deep S wave, small R wave, R/S ratio <1 in leads V5 and V6 (However, deep S wave, small R wave, R/S ratio <1 in leads V5 and V6 may also be present in patients with LAFB, anterior myocardial infarction, or chronic obstructive pulmonary disease), (5) ST segment depression and T-wave inversion in the right precordium and also II, III, and aVF (A negative–positive biphasic T wave may also be seen with RVH.), and (6) S1, S2, and S3, which also may be seen in emphysema and occasionally in normal individuals [1,3].

Even though an echocardiogram allows better visualization of the myocardium, the presence of left ventricular hypertrophy on the ECG identifies a subset of the general population at a significantly increased risk for myocardial morbidity and mortality, especially if there are any ST-T–wave abnormalities and particularly for women [3]. Although many criteria are available for determining left ventricular hypertrophy, including the

Sokolow–Lyon index, the Romhilt–Estes point system, and the Cornell voltage criteria, currently cited voltage criteria include the following:

Largest R wave + largest S wave in the precordial leads >4.5 mV
S in V1 + R in V6 >3.5 mV
S in V2 + R in V6 >4.3 mV
S in V1 >2.5 mV
R in aVL >1.3 mV [1,3].

Noordzij and colleagues [7] hypothesized that, in the presence of multiple cardiac-risk indices, the routine use of electrocardiography may not be of value in providing prognostic information. Rather, electrocardiography may be redundant. In a retrospective examination of a 10-year period (1991–2000) encompassing over 23,000 patients and 28,000 surgical procedures where patients had been classified by type of surgery, cardiovascular risk factors, and preoperative electrocardiography, the prognostic value of electrocardiography was assessed. Abnormal ECG changes were defined as atrial fibrillation, bundle branch block (left or right), left ventricular hypertrophy, premature ventricular complexes, paced rhythms, Q waves, or ST changes. The investigators determined that those patients with an abnormal ECG, compared with those patients with a normal ECG, had an increase risk of cardiovascular death (1.8% versus 0.3%), and the addition of ECG findings to cardiovascular risk indices improved the predictive value of the index. The prognostic value of the ECG was more beneficial for patients undergoing intermediate and high-risk procedures than for those undergoing low-risk procedures [7].

Electrolyte, thyroid, temperature effects

Although sodium plays an important role in electrical activity, it does not produce consistent or significant effects on the ECG. Hypernatremia does prolong the cardiac action potential. In the setting of hyperkalemic conduction disturbances, hypernatremia shortens the duration of the QRS complex, while hyponatremia prolongs the duration of the QRS complex [1,3,4].

Potassium is the electrolyte most often associated with distinctive ECG changes. Hyperkalemia may be mild, moderate, or severe with varying or progressive ECG changes. Mild to moderate hyperkalemia is characterized by a narrowing and peaking of the T wave, while the QRS complex remains normal. Moderate to severe hyperkalemia is characterized by a flattening of the P wave or even loss of the P wave; the widening of the QRS complex, which becomes less distinct; the possible elevation of the ST segment, especially in the right precordium V1 and V2; an increasing PR interval; and the possible development of 1° and 2° blocks. Severe hyperkalemia may present with a nondiagnostic ECG, or may show the progressive widening of the QRS complex, which may resemble wide complex ventricular tachycardia or even a sine wave before the onset of ventricular fibrillation or asystole. Failure to appreciate the significance of hyperkalemia may lead to inadequate treatment, inappropriate treatment, and loss of life [1,3,4]. Hypokalemia promotes the development of both ventricular and supraventricular ectopy, which may lead to ventricular tachycardia, torsades de pointes, or ventricular fibrillation. Rapid onset of hypokalemia may occur with intense sympathetic stimulation from epinephrine and may also occur with the administration of non–potassium-sparing diuretics or sodium bicarbonate. ECG manifestations of hypokalemia are due to abnormal and delayed repolarization and are manifested by (1) ST segment depression ≥ 0.5 mm, (2) an increasing U-wave amplitude, (3) a decreasing T-wave amplitude with the U-wave amplitude being greater than the T wave, and (4) an unchanging QRS duration [1,3,4].

Calcium affects the duration of the plateau phase of the action potential (ie, phase two of the action potential) and manifests as changes in the duration of the ST segment and the QT interval. Hypercalcemia shortens the duration of the action potential. The ST segment becomes shorter or may even disappear. The QTc also shortens and occasionally the QRS duration may increase. The morphology of the P wave, T wave, and U waves remains the same, but occasionally the U-wave amplitude may slightly increase. Hypercalcemia may cause 2° and 3° atrioventicular block and severe hypercalcemia may cause sudden death from ventricular fibrillation. However, for the most part, arrhythmias tend to be uncommon with hypercalcemia [1,3,4]. Hypocalcemia manifests when ST segments and the QTc also become prolonged. With severe hypocalcemia, the T wave may become flat or inverted [1,3,4].

Magnesium blocks the calcium channel and modulates the effects of potassium currents. Severe hypermagnesemia depresses the atriventricular node and causes intraventricular conduction delays that may lead to complete heart block and cardiac arrest. Hypomagnesemia is associated with hypokalemia and hypocalcemia and may be associated with ventricular arrhythmias, reduced T-wave amplitude, and ST depression. Whether these associations stem from magnesium or a deficiency of other electrolytes remains uncertain [1,3,4].

Thyroid disorders present with ECG changes. Hyperthyroidism often manifests with sinus tachycardia or atrial fibrillation before other clinical signs and diagnoses. The P wave and QRS complex often have increased amplitude and may simulate left ventricular hypertrophy. Nonspecific ST-T–wave changes, which are fluctuating, may be seen. The fleeting nature and day-to-day variations of the hyperthyroid state cause these fluctuations, which are more extreme than those seen in pericarditis or myocarditis. The PR interval tends to be prolonged and 1° atrioventricular block may be present, but 2° and 3° atrioventricular block are much less common [1,3,4]. Successful treatment of the hyperthyroid state tends to resolve these ECG changes. Hypothyroidism, especially myxedema, may present with sinus brachycardia; low P-, QRS-, T-wave voltage; QT prolongation; flat or inverted T waves, ST-T–wave changes similar to those associated with pericarditis; and a high incidence of atrioventricular and intraventricular conduction defects, leading to torsades de pointes. These changes respond to treatment of the hypothyroid state [1,3,4].

Temperature changes are also associated ECG changes. Hyperthermia produces a hypermetabolic state with increased catecholamine stimulation, tachycardia, and, possibly, an increased risk for ventricular fibrillation and ventricular tachycardia [1]. As hypothermia develops, the duration of the action potential lengthens with profound hypothermia affecting both depolarization and repolarization. The J-Osborn wave represents an elevation of the J point and early ST segment. The lower the temperature, the more prominent the J-Osborn wave. As the temperature drops and hypothermia becomes more pronounced, atrial fibrillation develops, J-Osborn waves may be seen, with ventricular fibrillation and cardiac standstill occurring with profound hypothermia [1,3,4].

Alternans represents the regular alternating of the electrical pattern as noted on the ECG. Sinus tachycardia and total electrical alternans is often seen with pericardial effusion and cardiac tamponade. Sinus rhythm with heart rate alternans (R-R alternans) may be seen in congestive heart failure. ST segment alternans is associated with vasospastic angina, ischemia, and subarachnoid hemorrhage. P-wave alternans, though rare, may be noted with pulmonary embolism. QRS alternans with tachycardia usually represent reentrant atrioventricular nodal rhythms. T-wave alternans with QT prolongation may precede torsades de pointes [1,3].

Ischemia

The ECG is a key component in the diagnosis of ischemia. Changes in the ST segment caused by ischemia may result from currents of injury, which can lower resting-membrane potential, decrease the velocity and amplitude of the action potential, and cause early repolarization by decreasing the duration of the action potential. ECG changes that are considered significant are ST segment elevations or depression >1 mm from baseline. Other ECG abnormalities, such as LBBB, left ventricular hypertrophy with strain, and conduction abnormalities may obscure ST segment changes. ST segment changes may present with reciprocal changes. That is, ST segment elevation with reciprocal ST depression and ST segment depression with reciprocal ST elevation. Ischemic changes to specific areas may present ECG changes in specific leads: extensive anterior I, aVL, V1 through V6; anterior septal V1 through V3; anterior apical V3 and V4; anterior lateral V4 through V6; high lateral I, aVL, V5 and V6; posterior reciprocal changes in V1; and right ventricular V4R, V1, V2, and V3 [1,3,4].

The accuracy as well as the sensitivity and specificity of the information obtained from intraoperative ECG monitors depends on a variety of factors, including mode, filters, template and lead selection. The work of Mangano and colleagues [8,9] showed that visual detection of ST segment changes is poor, below 50%. Leung and colleagues [10] demonstrated that ST segment trend analysis available in intraoperative monitors has an average sensitivity of up to 78% and specificity of almost 90%. The narrowing of the bandwidth in the monitoring mode and the use of filters to minimize artifact from poor electrode contact and mechanical ventilation may adversely affect the accuracy of ST segment trend analysis [11,12] Each monitor manufacturer has a proprietary algorithm for determining elevations and depression and these vary despite recommendations from the American Heart Association for standardization. The computer sets the isoelectric and J-points by default and if the computer-chosen set points are inaccurate, then the calculated ST segment analysis will be inaccurate. Fleisher [11], therefore, recommends that the computer-chosen template be displayed and reviewed before the start of each procedure to ensure the accuracy of ST segment analysis, and, if these are significant ST segment changes, to print the ECG strip for detailed analysis. The work of London and colleagues [13] verified that the combination of leads II and V5 detected 80% of significant ST segment changes and, with the addition of V4, sensitivity was increased to 96%. Recently, Landesberg and colleagues [14] reexamined optimum lead selection and found that lead V4 had 83% sensitivity versus 76% sensitivity for lead V5 in detecting significant prolonged ischemia, and, when two precordial leads were used, there was a 95% sensitivity in detecting significant perioperative ischemia (Fig. 3).

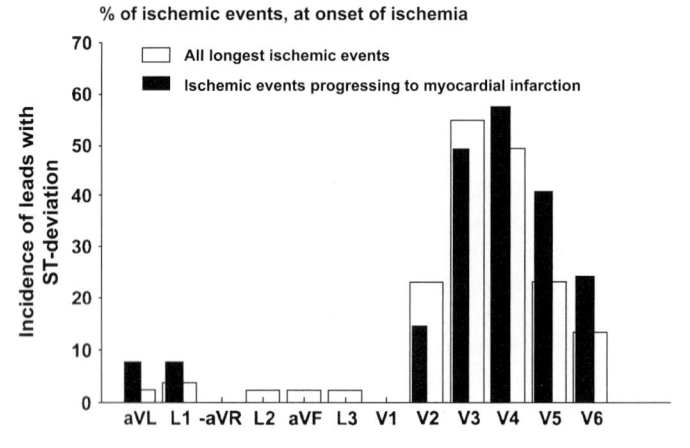

Fig. 3. The incidence of ST segment deviation by ECG lead in patients undergoing vascular surgery. Lead V4 is the strongest predictor of perioperative myocardial infarction. (*From* Landesberg G, Mosseri M, Wolf Y, et al. Perioperative myocardial ischemia and infarction: identification by continuous 12-lead electrocardiogram with online ST-segment monitoring. Anesthesiology 2002;96:264–70; with permission.)

With the advent and widespread use of echocardiography, many have questioned the need for ECG analysis. When using trained, skilled, and experienced cardiac anesthesiologists, Berquist and colleagues [15] found that real-time echocardiographic detection of myocardial ischemia had a sensitivity and specificity of approximately 76%. According to the American College of Cardiology/American Heart Association Task Force on Practice Guidelines, perioperative transesophageal echocardiography is still considered only a category-II indication for the detection of myocardial ischemia [16]. Even now echocardiography requires advanced training and expensive equipment not always routinely available. Also, because probe insertion occurs after the induction of anesthesia, echocardiography is often not available during the crucial period for ischemic detection. By comparison, the ECG is a routine monitor that provides a wealth of information and a high degree of sensitivity and specificity in ischemic detection.

Since the duration of ST segment changes correlates with the incidence of perioperative myocardial infarction in those at risk, prompt verification by obtaining a printed ECG recording and institution of therapy are warranted for optimal patient care.

The relationship between ST segment changes and perioperative myocardial ischemia developed from the work of Slogoff and Keats in 1985. This work noted the relationship between ST segment changes and perioperative myocardial infarction [17]. Using Bayes theorem, which states that the posttest probability is a function of pretest probability, Fleisher [11] notes that, in patients at risk for cardiac ischemia, the likelihood that significant ST segment changes correlate with ischemia is high. Cardiac-risk indexes continue to be validated as demonstrated by multiple studies, including the recent work by Boersma and colleagues [18]. The appropriate use of cardiac-risk indexes aids in the determination of patient risk in the perioperative setting, assessment of ECG information, and optimal patient care.

Implications

The ECG is a valuable tool in monitoring the patient. Information presented on an ECG should be analyzed systematically with an understanding of the constituent elements of an ECG, the rate, the rhythm, the morphology, the axis, the presence of conduction abnormalities, electrolyte changes, and ischemic changes. To accurately assess the information presented, hemodynamic information and cardiac-risk analysis should be integrated to have a complete picture. An RBBB is associated with a higher mortality and increased risk of cardiac events in those with a prior myocardial infarction or abnormal dobutamine stress echocardiogram [19]. Biagini and colleagues [19] found that a complete RBBB was as equally predictive as an LBBB for increased mortality. The presence of an LAFB is an independent predictor of mortality in those at risk for coronary artery disease, even if they have not had a prior myocardial infarction [20]. In patients with coronary artery disease and ischemic cardiomyopathy, analysis of QT depression helps determine the amount of viable hibernating myocardium. That is, those with preserved QT depression have viable myocardium available, but those with high QT dispersion have nonviable scar tissue [21]. For patients with heart failure and an LBBB who have biventricular pacing, an analysis of the ECG can reveal, with a sensitivity and specificity of over 90%, if there is loss of resynchronization therapy. Lead V1 is analyzed and if the R/S ratio ≥ 1, then there is left ventricular capture and biventricular pacing. If this is not the case, then lead I is assessed and if the R/S ratio is <1, then there is left ventricular capture. If the R/S ratio >1 in lead I, then there is right ventricular capture and loss of biventricular pacing. The algorithm allows physicians to analyze an ECG and evaluate the presence of biventricular pacing with a high degree of sensitivity and specificity even without a programming device [22]. Thus the wealth of information available through a thorough and accurate ECG analysis is enormous.

References

[1] Surawicz B, Knilans TK. Chou's electrocardiography in clinical practice: adult and pediatric. 5th edition. Philadelphia: LUB Saunders; 2001.
[2] Wagner GS. Marriott's practical electrocardiography. 10th edition. Philadelphia: Lippincott Williams & Wilkins; 2001.
[3] Zipes DP, Libby P, Bonow RO, et al. Braunwald's heart disease: a textbook of cardiovascular medicine. 7th edition. Philadelphia: Elsevier Saunders; 2005.
[4] Fuster V, Alexander RW, O'Rourke RA, et al, editors. Hurst's the heart. 11th edition. New York: McGraw-Hill; 2004.
[5] Hillis LD, Lange RA, Winiford MD, et al. Manual of clinical problems in cardiology. 6th edition. Philadelphia: Lippincott Williams & Wilkins; 2003.
[6] Dorman T, Breslow MJ, Pronovost PJ, et al. Bundle-branch block as a risk factor in noncardiac surgery. Arch Intern Med 2000;160:1149–52.
[7] Noordzij PG, Boersma E, Bax JJ, et al. Prognostic value of routine preoperative electrocardiography in patients undergoing noncardiac surgery. Am J Cardiol 2006;97:1103–6.
[8] Mangano DT, Hollenberg M, Fegert G, et al. Perioperative myocardial ischemia in patients undergoing noncardiac surgery—I: incidence and severity during the 4-day perioperative period. The Study of Perioperative Ischemia (SPI) Research Group. J Am Coll Cardio 1991;17: 843–50.
[9] Mangano DT, Wong MG, London MS, et al. Perioperative myocardial ischemia in patients undergoing noncardiac surgery—II: incidence and severity during the 1st week after surgery. The Study of Perioperative Ischemia (SPI) Research Group. J Am Coll Cardio 1991;17: 851–7.
[10] Leung JM, Voskanian A, Bellows WH, et al. Automated electrocardiogram ST segment trending monitors: accuracy in detecting myocardial ischemia. Anesth Analg 1998;87:4–10.
[11] Fleisher LA. Real-time intraoperative monitoring of myocardial ischemia in noncardiac surgery. Anesthesiology 2000;92:1183–8.
[12] Slogoff S, Keats AS, David Y, et al. Incidence of perioperative myocardial ischemia detected by different electrocardiographic systems. Anesthesiology 1990;73:1074–81.
[13] London MJ, Hollenberg M, Wong MG, et al. Intraoperative myocardial ischemia: localizations by continuous 12-lead electrocardiography. Anesthesiology 1988;69:232–41.
[14] Landesburg G, Mosseri M, Wolf Y, et al. Perioperative myocardial ischemia and infarction: identification by continuous 12-lead electrocardiogram with online ST-segment monitoring. Anesthesiology 2002;96:264–70.

[15] Bergquist BD, Leung JM, Bellows WH. Transesophageal echocardiography in myocardial revascularization: I. Accuracy of Intraoperative real time interpretation. Anesth Analg 1996;83:1132–8.
[16] Cheitlin MD, Armstrong WF, Aurigemma GP, et al. ACC/AHA/ASE 2003. Guideline update for the clinical application of echocardiography—summary article: a report of the American College of Cardiology/American Heart Association Task Force on Practice Guidelines (ACC/AHA/ASE Committee to Update the 1997 Practice Guidelines on the Clinical Application of Echocardiography). J Am Coll Cardiol 2003;42:954–70.
[17] Slogoff S, Keats AS. Does perioperative myocardial ischemia lead to postoperative myocardial infarction? Anesthesiology 1985;62:107–14.
[18] Boersma E, Kertai MD, Schouten O, et al. Perioperative cardiovascular mortality in noncardiac surgery: validation of the Lee cardiac risk index. Am J Med 2005;118:1134–41.
[19] Biagini E, Shinkel AFL, Rizzello V, et al. Prognostic stratification of patients with right bundle branch block using dobutamine stress echocardiography. Am J Cardiol 2004;94:954–7.
[20] Biagini E, Elhendy A, Schinkel AF, et al. Prognostic significance of left anterior hemiblock in patients with suspected coronary artery disease. J Am Coll Cardiol 2005;46:858–63.
[21] Schinkel AF, Bax JJ, Poldermans D. Clinical assessment of myocardial hibernation. Heart 2005;91:111–7.
[22] Ammann P, Sticherling C, Kalusche D, et al. An electrocardiogram-based algorithm to detect loss of left ventricular capture during cardiac resynchronization therapy. Ann Intern Med 2005;142:968–73.

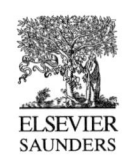

Arterial and Central Venous Pressure Monitoring

Atilio Barbeito, MD[a,b], Jonathan B. Mark, MD[a,b],*

[a]*Department of Anesthesiology, Duke University Medical Center, Box 3094, Durham, NC 27710, USA*
[b]*Anesthesiology Service (112C), Veterans Affairs Medical Center, 508 Fulton Street, Durham, NC 27705, USA*

"The same old Watson! You never learn that the gravest issues may depend upon the smallest things." — Sherlock Holmes in *The Adventure of the Creeping Man* by Sir Arthur Conan Doyle

Vigilance is the motto of the American Society of Anesthesiologists, and no other single word best describes the task of the anesthesiologist. In this regard, monitoring is paramount. Monitors allow us to ascertain whether physiologic homeostasis is present, alert us to undesirable changes in patient condition, and allow us to assess the response to therapeutic interventions. The information in the arterial pressure and central venous pressure (CVP) waveforms is abundant, but it shows itself only to the educated eye. One cannot see what one does not know exists.

In this article, we begin by identifying some technical aspects of invasive pressure monitoring that will allow the physician to assess intelligently the quality of the data gathered. We will then focus on the arterial pressure and CVP waveforms and how additional, clinically important information can be obtained from their detailed analysis.

Technical aspects of direct pressure measurement

The catheter transducer system

The arterial pressure pulse is a complex wave that may be reconstructed by summing individual sine waves of successively higher frequencies. The sine wave occurring at the rate of the pulse is called the first harmonic, or

---

* Corresponding author.
E-mail address: mark0003@mc.duke.edu (J.B. Mark).

fundamental, frequency. Each subsequent harmonic is a simple multiple of the previous one, much like octaves in the musical scale. Faithful display of arterial pressure waveforms requires accurate reproduction of the first six to ten harmonics of the fundamental frequency by the monitoring system [1].

The system most commonly used in current clinical practice to monitor invasively arterial blood pressure consists of an intravascular catheter connected to an electronic transducer via low-compliance, saline-filled tubing. This device contains a deformable diaphragm connected to a Wheatstone bridge, which converts the mechanical energy of the pressure waves into electric signals. The signals are then amplified, displayed, or recorded.

Ideally, the pressure waves recorded through the intravascular catheter should be transmitted undistorted to the transducer and then to the amplifier, display, or recording system. Unfortunately, the mechanical transmission system oscillates (rings or resonates) after being set in motion by the arterial pressure wave. These oscillations produce small pressure waves that are superimposed on those caused by the pressure pulse itself, thereby introducing artifacts that distort the measured pressure. The amount of distortion introduced depends on the natural resonant frequency of the monitoring system and the frequencies of the multiple sine waves that constitute the monitored pressure waveform.

If any of the frequencies in the arterial waveform are in the same range as the natural frequency of the monitoring system, the amplitudes of these wave components will be augmented. Clinically, augmentation will cause artifactual increases in systolic pressure, (also called pressure overshoot, ringing, or resonance), and artifactual decreases in diastolic pressure. In these cases, the systolic pressures may be artifactually increased by as much as 30% [2]. Diastolic blood pressure and CVP waveforms have lower frequency components and tend to be distorted less. Resonance is generally encountered when the monitoring system used has a low natural frequency and the heart rate is high. Stated another way, to ensure accurate measurement of an arterial pressure waveform, the natural frequency of the measurement system needs to be at least six to ten times higher than the fundamental frequency of the pressure wave, which is equal to the heart rate. For example, the natural frequency of the pressure monitoring system should be ≥ 20 Hz to provide accurate blood pressure measurement when the heart rate is 120 beats per minute (2 cycles per second or 2 Hz).

While it might seem optimal to use a system with a high natural frequency, this is difficult to achieve in clinical practice. Most disposable transducers have natural frequencies of several hundred hertz, but the addition of saline-filled tubing and stopcocks that may trap tiny air bubbles results in a monitoring system with a markedly reduced natural frequency. For example, increasing the length of tubing to 150 cm from 30 cm decreases natural frequency by over 50% [3]. To maximize its natural frequency, a pressure monitoring system should be constructed of short lengths of stiff tubing that are free of air bubbles and blood clots.

Catheter transducer systems with low natural frequency can still be useful clinically because another mechanical property, damping, has additional influence on the monitored waveforms. Damping describes the absorption of oscillatory energy by frictional forces. A monitoring system is optimally damped if it dissipates the energy produced by the components of the measuring system, conducting only the oscillations that correspond to the monitored pressure waveform. Optimal damping is difficult to achieve. Most monitoring systems are underdamped, but have a natural frequency high enough so that the effect on the monitored waveform is limited [4]. Fig. 1 shows the relationship between damping and natural frequency of pressure monitoring systems, and describes the characteristics of typical transducer systems in clinical use.

When systolic pressure overshoot is observed, it is common practice to incorporate a small air bubble into the system to increase damping. However, while air bubbles increase damping, they simultaneously lower the natural frequency of the system and, paradoxically, can cause artifactual increases in systolic pressure and artifactual decreases (but much less so) in diastolic pressure.

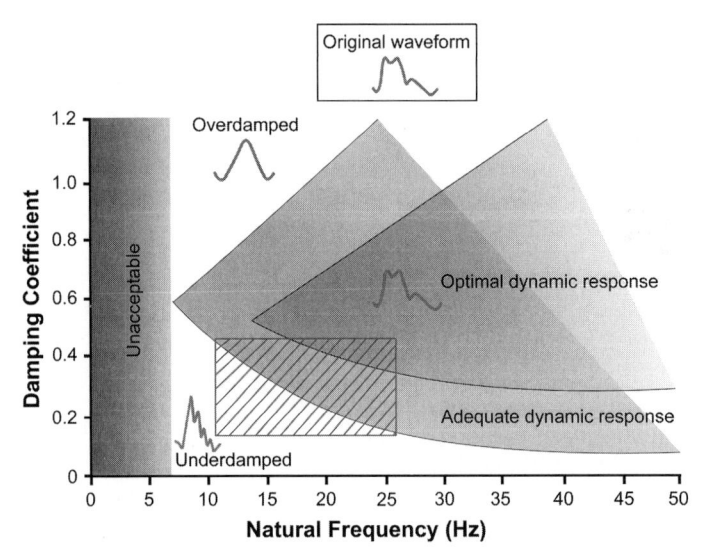

Fig. 1. Influence of natural frequency and damping coefficient on the dynamic response of pressure monitoring systems. Catheter–tubing–transducer systems in the optimal dynamic response area will record accurately a wide range of arterial pressure waveforms. Those falling within the adequate dynamic response range will faithfully reproduce most pressure waveforms, while those in the overdamped or underdamped regions will have waveform distortions that are characteristic of those technical limitations. Monitoring systems with natural frequencies in the unacceptable range should be adjusted to improve performance. Typical clinical monitoring systems reside in the hatched area, some showing optimal dynamic response, but many being underdamped. (*Adapted from* Mark JB. Atlas of cardiovascular monitoring. New York: Churchill Livingstone; 1998. p. 111; with permission.)

For the reasons stated above, it is important to know the natural frequency and damping coefficients of the monitoring system in use. Although not completely accurate in vivo [5], the "fast flush test" is a clinically useful method that allows the determination of these values through examination of the artifact that follows a pressurized flush of the monitoring catheter [6,7]. From this flush artifact, one can calculate with reasonable accuracy the natural frequency and damping coefficient of the monitoring system.

Pressure transducer setup

Before invasive arterial or venous pressure monitoring, the pressure transducer must be zeroed and placed in the appropriate position relative to the patient. Intravascular pressures are referenced against ambient atmospheric pressure by exposing the pressure transducer to air through an open stopcock and pressing the zero-pressure button on the monitor. Zeroing refers to adjustment of the Wheatstone bridge in the transducer so that zero current flows to the detector at zero pressure.

Positioning of the pressure transducer is crucial and represents the part of the transducer setup process most prone to error. The transducer must be horizontally aligned with a specific position on the patient's body that represents the upper fluid level in the chamber or vessel from which pressure is to be measured. It is important to recognize that when fluid-filled catheter systems are used for pressure measurement, this horizontal level is the only factor that contributes to the measured pressure, not the position of the catheter tip within the chamber or vessel [8].

Proper positioning of the pressure transducer is critical for measurement of CVP and other central vascular pressures because seemingly small errors in transducer height amplify errors in measuring cardiac filling pressure. In view of these considerations, CVP transducers should be positioned approximately 5 cm posterior to the left sternal border at the fourth intercostal space, since this point better represents the upper fluid level of the right atrium compared with the more commonly used transducer alignment at the mid-axillary line. In the typical patient, transducer alignment at the mid-axillary line will result in a CVP overestimation of approximately 5 mm Hg. While these same considerations are relevant to the measurement of arterial blood pressure, the precise location of the arterial pressure transducer is less important, owing to the relatively large pressures being measured relative to the magnitude of the potential error in pressure measurement from an improperly positioned transducer.

When a patient is being monitored in the sitting position, transducer height takes on additional considerations. If the transducer is placed at the standard thoracic level, the arterial pressure at the level of the heart will be recorded. However, monitoring of cerebral perfusion pressure requires that the transducer be placed at the level of the brain, approximating the position of the circle of Willis. As expected, the arterial pressure at the level of the brain will be considerably lower than the pressure at the level of the heart in the sitting patient and will be exactly equal to the pressure measured at heart level minus the hydrostatic pressure difference between the heart and brain [9].

Arterial blood pressure measurement

Indications for direct arterial pressure monitoring

Indications for direct arterial pressure monitoring can be grouped into three main categories [10]:

- Inability to obtain noninvasive blood-pressure measurements (eg, for burned patient with all extremities affected)
- Need for beat-to-beat monitoring of blood pressure, because of (1) a concurrent disease that necessitates close hemodynamic observation (eg, severe aortic stenosis); (2) the anticipated hemodynamic change resulting from the operative procedure is sudden or large in magnitude (eg, cardiac or major vascular surgery); or (3) pharmacologic or mechanical manipulation of the cardiovascular system is planned (eg, deliberate hypotension or intraaortic balloon counterpulsation)
- Need for multiple arterial blood gas or other laboratory analyses (eg, bilateral lung lavage)

A noninvasive blood-pressure monitor should always be available to corroborate direct blood-pressure readings and to serve as backup in case of equipment failure.

Complications of direct arterial pressure monitoring

The most frequent complication of arterial catheterization is equipment misuse and misinterpretation [11]. Such events as distal ischemia, thrombosis with sequelae, nerve injury, infection and bleeding are rare (<0.1%) [12]. Factors associated with an increased risk of complications include prolonged cannulation, preexisting vasculopathy, extracorporeal circulation, use of vasopressors, female gender, and multiple insertion attempts [13]. Although the Allen test is often used to identify patients at high risk for ischemic complications from radial artery catheterization, its use cannot be relied upon to avoid this adverse outcome [14,15]. Lines and stopcocks must be clearly labeled and manipulated with care to avoid unintentional intra-arterial injection of drugs or air. Routine replacement of peripheral arterial catheters as a technique to reduce nosocomial infection in the intensive care unit is not recommended for catheters that are functioning and have no evidence of causing local or systemic complications [16]. Prolonged hyperextension of the wrist can cause transient median nerve conduction deficits, so prompt return of the wrist to a neutral position after arterial cannulation is recommended to minimize the chances of nerve injury [17].

Normal arterial waveform morphology

The normal arterial waveform recorded in the radial artery should follow the ECG R wave by approximately 120 to 180 ms and consists of a steep systolic upstroke, peak, and decline that correspond to left ventricular ejection. The down slope is interrupted by the dicrotic notch, which is sharp when pressure is recorded in the aorta and undoubtedly represents aortic valve closure, but is delayed and slurred when pressure is recorded more peripherally and is related to arterial wall properties instead. The arterial pressure wave continues to decline following the dicrotic notch and the ECG T wave, reaching it lowest point at end diastole (Fig. 2).

Digital readouts of systolic and diastolic pressures are derived from the highest and lowest values on the arterial pressure trace, which are then displayed as a running average over a certain time interval. The mean arterial pressure is measured by the monitor as the integrated area under the pressure curve.

In recent years a renewed interest has emerged for detailed analysis of the arterial pressure waveform morphology. This trend should expand clinical monitoring and research capabilities. Modern devices allow measurement of left ventricular function by analysis of the pulse contour and provide a true continuous beat-to-beat minimally invasive measurement of cardiac output. Several studies have shown clinically acceptable agreement between pulse contour and thermodilution cardiac-output monitoring [18–21]. Other devices allow acquisition of pressure waveforms from peripheral sites and the reconstruction of central aortic pressure by various transfer functions [22]. Several indices describing left ventricular systolic function and arterial

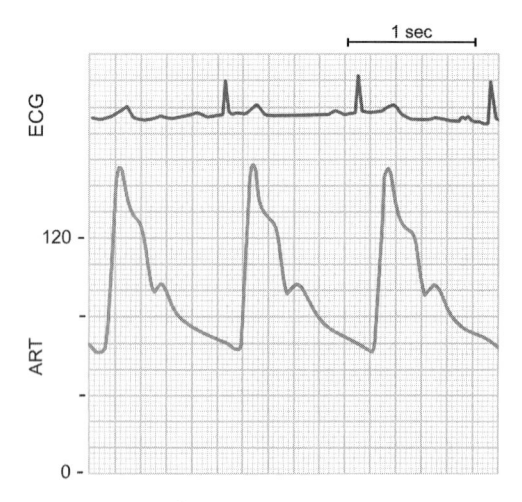

Fig. 2. Normal arterial pressure (ART) waveform. (*Adapted from* Mark JB. Atlas of cardiovascular monitoring. New York: Churchill Livingstone; 1998. p. 94; with permission.)

properties can then be calculated by quantitative analysis of the reconstructed aortic pressure waveform.

Differences between central and peripheral arterial pressure

The most common site used to monitor arterial pressure invasively is the radial artery. Waveform morphology and both systolic and diastolic arterial pressure values for central arteries are different from those for peripheral arteries. Indeed, the pulse is amplified as it moves toward the periphery owing to an increase in systolic pressure and a decrease in diastolic pressure. In contrast, mean arterial pressure in the radial artery closely approximates mean aortic pressure. Therefore, clinical therapy is often better guided using radial artery mean arterial pressure than radial artery systolic blood pressure. These collective changes in the arterial pressure waveform as it travels to the periphery are termed distal pulse amplification and are the result of wave reflection and the nonuniform elasticity of the arterial tree, with stiffness increasing as the distance from the aortic valve increases.

Apart from the obvious mechanical obstruction to flow from atherosclerosis, arterial dissection, or arterial embolism, several physiologic changes, pathologic conditions, and pharmacologic interventions alter the relationship between central and peripheral arterial pressures. For example, aging and hypertension decrease arterial distensibility and augment pulse pressure. However, these effects are more pronounced in central than in peripheral arteries [23,24]. Caffeine, a blood-pressure–elevating agent, increases wave reflection in hypertensive patients and affects central systolic and pulse pressures to a greater extent than peripheral pressure values [25]. Patients in septic shock requiring high-dose vasopressor therapy exhibit significant differences between radial and femoral systolic and mean arterial pressures. In contrast to the common situation of patients with peripheral pressures greater than central pressures, patients in septic shock show higher central arterial pressures, although the mechanism is not completely understood [26]. A similar situation can be observed in patients undergoing cardiopulmonary bypass. Soon after initiation of bypass, mean radial arterial pressure underestimates mean femoral arterial pressure, and the gradient persists at least through the initial minutes after bypass [27].

In summary, compared with central arterial blood pressures, peripheral arterial pressures have steeper systolic upstrokes, higher systolic peaks, slurring (femoral) or loss (dorsalis pedis) of the dicrotic notch, and a lower end-diastolic pressures [28]. Additionally, changes that occur with aging, various disease states, and in response to drugs or extracorporeal circulation affect central and peripheral pressures differently. As a corollary to this, central systolic pressure is the pressure that the left ventricle "confronts" as afterload, and central pressure through diastole determines coronary flow. Hence, reliance on peripheral pressures alone for monitoring and intervention may have shortcomings.

Influence of the respiratory cycle on the arterial pressure waveform

One additional clinically important application of arterial pressure monitoring is the assessment of cardiac preload through analysis of the cyclic variation in arterial pressure that occurs during positive-pressure mechanical ventilation. These variations demonstrate cardiopulmonary interactions that result from changes in intrathoracic pressure and lung volume. These are briefly described below.

With the onset of positive-pressure inspiration, the rise in lung volume effectively "squeezes" the pulmonary venous bed, increases drainage of blood from the pulmonary veins into the left atrium, and augments left ventricular preload. Concurrently, left ventricular afterload falls because of the increased intrathoracic pressure. The increase in left ventricular preload and decrease in afterload produce an increase in left ventricular stroke volume and an increase in systemic arterial pressure. At the same time, the increase in intrathoracic pressure seen in early inspiration reduces systemic venous return and decreases right ventricular preload and right ventricular stroke volume. Toward the end of inspiration or during early expiration, the reduced right ventricular stroke volume that occurred during inspiration leads to reduced left ventricular filling and, as a result, left ventricular stroke volume falls and systemic arterial blood pressure decreases. This cyclic variation in systemic arterial pressure may be measured and quantified as the systolic pressure variation (SPV).

SPV may be further subdivided into inspiratory and expiratory components by measuring the increase (Δup) and decrease (Δdown) in systolic pressure as compared with the end-expiratory, apneic baseline pressure (Fig. 3). Normally a mechanically ventilated patient will have a Δup and Δdown of about 5 mm Hg each and a total SPV of < 10 mm Hg. In animals and humans, increased SPVs (particularly Δdown) have been shown to be sensitive

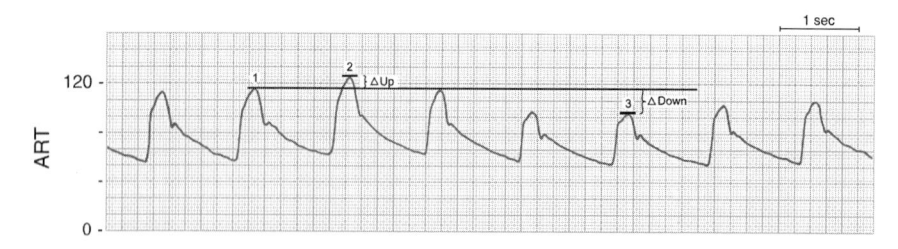

Fig. 3. Arterial pressure (ART) waveform showing systolic pressure variation during positive-pressure mechanical ventilation. End-expiratory systolic blood pressure (*1*) serves as a baseline from which an early inspiratory increase (*2*, Δup) can be measured, followed by a delayed decrease (*3*, Δdown). The large Δdown and total systolic pressure variation of nearly 30 mm Hg suggests the diagnosis of hypovolemia, even though tachycardia and hypotension are not present. (*Adapted from* Mark JB. Atlas of cardiovascular monitoring. New York: Churchill Livingstone; 1998. p. 282; with permission.)

indicators of hypovolemia and responsiveness to fluid administration [29,30]. Exaggerated SPV remains present in many hypovolemic patients, even when compensatory mechanisms maintain arterial blood pressure and central filling pressure values near normal [31].

SPV seen in clinical practice has to be interpreted with caution. While there is a cyclic change in arterial pressure during spontaneous ventilation, using SPV to predict hypovolemia has only been well validated in patients receiving positive-pressure mechanical ventilation. The magnitude of SPV is influenced by ventilatory parameters, including tidal volume and peak inspiratory pressure. Values are confounded further by the presence of arrhythmias, changes in chest wall and lung compliance, addition of positive end-expiratory pressure, or other pulmonary pathology [32].

Abnormal arterial pressure waveform morphology

Several disease states have characteristic arterial pressure waveforms. Pulsus alternans (congestive heart failure), pulsus bisferiens (aortic insufficiency), pulsus parvus and tardus (aortic stenosis), pulsus paradoxus (cardiac tamponade), and the "spike-and-dome" pattern seen in hypertrophic cardiomyopathy may be identified from direct recordings of the systemic arterial pressure [33] (Fig. 4). These abnormal arterial pressure waveforms, while characteristic of underlying cardiovascular pathology, are not absolutely diagnostic. Accurate clinical interpretation depends on attention to the previously described technical details of arterial pressure measurement and requires that the clinical context be considered.

Central venous pressure measurement

Estimation of CVP is an important tool in the assessment of a patient's cardiovascular status. A number of techniques have been used over the years to estimate CVP, including inspection of jugular venous pulsations in the neck, measurement of jugular venous height, and detection of hepatojugular reflux. These indirect methods are unreliable in surgical or critically ill patients and have largely been supplanted by direct measurement of CVP through catheters placed into the central vessels of the chest, most commonly through the internal jugular, subclavian, or femoral veins.

Indications for central venous cannulation

There are a number of indications for central venous cannulation:

- To monitor cardiac filling pressures
- To administer fluids or drugs that can cause peripheral vein sclerosis (eg, vasoactive drugs, hyperalimentation drugs, hypertonic solutions, and chemotherapeutic agents)

- To rapidly administer fluids or blood products in trauma or major surgery
- To aspirate air emboli
- To insert a temporary transvenous pacemaker or a pulmonary artery catheter
- To gain temporary or permanent venous access for hemodialysis or plasmapheresis
- To obtain venous access when peripheral venous access is not obtainable

Complications of central venous cannulation

More than 5 million central venous catheters are placed in the United States every year, and approximately 15% are associated with complications [34]. These are classically divided into mechanical, infectious, and thromboembolic.

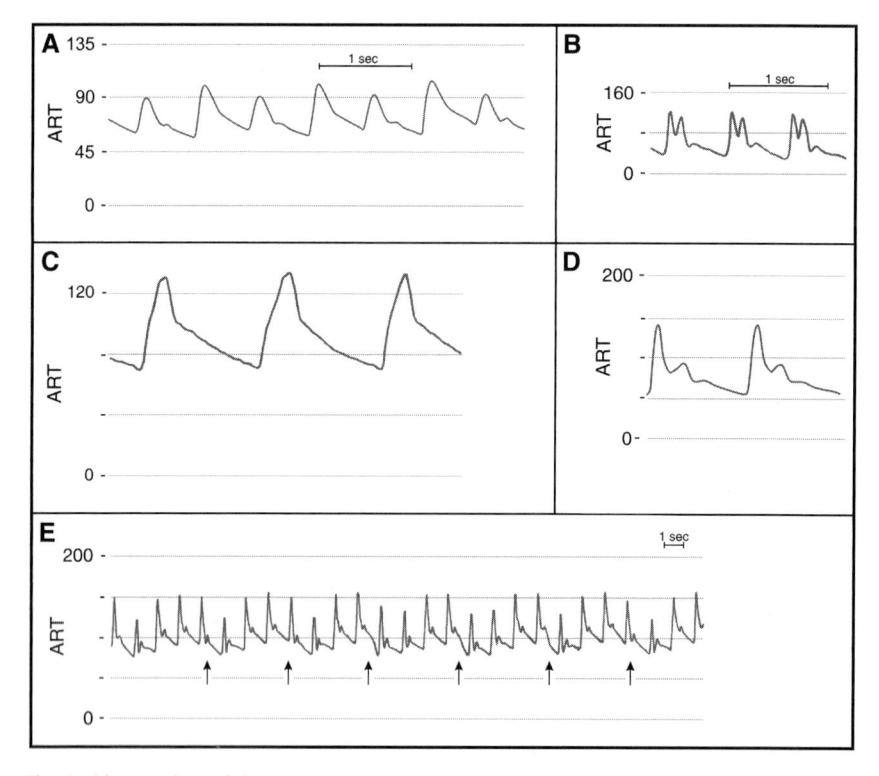

Fig. 4. Abnormal arterial pressure (ART) waveforms in various disease states. (*A*) Pulsus alternans (congestive heart failure). (*B*) Pulsus bisferiens (aortic insufficiency). (*C*) Pulsus parvus and tardus (aortic stenosis). (*D*) "Spike-and-dome" pattern (hypertrophic cardiomyopathy). (*E*) Pulsus paradoxus (cardiac tamponade). The *arrows* indicate the onset of spontaneous inspiration. (*Adapted from* Mark JB. Atlas of cardiovascular monitoring. New York: Churchill Livingstone; 1998. p. 311, 325; with permission.)

The majority of mechanical complications are vascular injuries and range from minor localized hematoma to uncommon but life-threatening vascular perforation into the pericardium, resulting in cardiac tamponade. Unintended arterial puncture with hematoma formation is the most frequent complication of both internal-jugular and subclavian-vein catheterization [11]. Delayed vascular complications, such as cardiac tamponade, can be prevented by radiographic confirmation of proper catheter-tip location in the proximal superior vena cava, above the pericardial reflection. On a posteroanterior chest radiograph, this position corresponds to the portion of the superior vena cava below the inferior border of the clavicles and above the level of the tracheal carina.

The risks of mechanical complications from central venous catheterization can be reduced by the use of ultrasound-guided cannulation techniques. Real-time ultrasound imaging, when compared with the standard landmark technique, has been shown to decrease complications and reduce the number of insertion attempts during internal jugular-vein cannulation [35,36]. While ultrasound-guided subclavian-vein catheterization has not been as clearly validated in clinical trials, imaging is likely helpful for this site as well [34]. The Agency for Healthcare Research and Quality has listed the use of real-time ultrasound guidance for central venous catheterization as 1 of 11 practices to improve health care [37]. The greatest benefit of ultrasound guidance may apply to trainees or inexperienced operators and when patient anatomy or clinical setting are unfavorable. As yet, no studies describe the impact of ultrasound-guided central venous catheter insertion on overall patient outcomes (eg, mortality, length of stay) [37]. Also unknown is whether the additional equipment and manipulation associated with real-time ultrasound guidance may increase the rate of catheter-related infections, or whether the increased dependence on this technology by trainees is potentially detrimental.

Infectious complications of central venous catheterization remain common, cause significant morbidity and mortality, and are costly to treat [38]. The impact of catheter-related bloodstream infections on overall health care quality and cost has generated some major initiatives. The Leapfrog Group, the Agency for Healthcare Research and Quality, and the Institute for Healthcare Improvement have all instituted campaigns aimed at improving overall health care quality in the United States. These campaigns include recommendations regarding the prevention of infections related to central venous catheters. These recommendations can be summarized as follows: (1) hand hygiene, (2) maximal barrier precautions, (3) chlorhexidine skin antisepsis, (4) optimal catheter site selection (the subclavian vein is the preferred site), (5) use of antibiotic-impregnated catheters, and (6) daily review of line necessity to allow prompt removal of unnecessary catheters [39,40]. As with peripheral arterial catheters, current guidelines from the Centers for Disease Control and Prevention do not support routine catheter site changes or scheduled changes over a guidewire to reduce the risk of infection [16].

Catheter-related venous thrombosis is a significant problem in critically ill patients [41]. Its incidence varies with insertion site, being highest with femoral catheter insertion and lowest with subclavian catheterization [42].

Interpretation of central venous pressure

Normal mean CVP is 5 ± 3 mm Hg. Clinicians often assume that low values indicate hypovolemia and high values indicate hypervolemia or heart failure. However, isolated single CVP measurements are of limited utility. Instead, trends in CVP measurement over time or changes in CVP in response to therapy are better indicators of a patient's intravascular volume status. For example, a rapid fluid bolus (eg, 500 mL) administered to a hypovolemic patient with good ventricular function will increase CVP minimally (<2 mm Hg), with a return to baseline within 10 to 15 minutes due to circulatory reflexes and stress relaxation of the vessels. The combination of a minimal rise in CVP and an associated increase in arterial blood pressure indicates a "volume-responsive" patient who may be hypovolemic. In contrast, the same fluid bolus given to a patient who responds with a large increase in CVP without an accompanying improvement in blood pressure, suggests that additional volume loading is not indicated. Therefore, under most clinical circumstances, a trend in CVP values or its change with therapeutic maneuvers is more reliable than a single measurement.

CVP is measured in the superior vena cava close to the right atrium, and for clinical purposes is assumed to equal right atrial pressure and right ventricular end-diastolic pressure. This pressure is monitored as a surrogate for right ventricular filling volume, which is proportional to muscle fiber length or preload, the major determinant of stroke output of the right ventricle for any given level of contractility.

When using a filling pressure, such as CVP, as a surrogate for estimating cardiac volume, one must take into consideration several points:

- The diastolic-pressure–volume relationship in cardiac muscle is not linear, but rather curvilinear, with a progressively steeper slope at higher volumes.
- Ventricular compliance may change independent of end-diastolic volume (eg, as a consequence of ischemia). The same effective preload may be represented by two different CVP values if ventricular compliance changes Fig. 5.
- CVP measurements are referenced to atmospheric pressure, but physiologically, it is transmural pressure (the difference between intracardiac and intrathoracic-extracardiac pressure) that determines ventricular preload. Increased intrathoracic or high intrapericardial pressure (eg, high positive end-expiratory pressure levels, cardiac tamponade, large pleural effusion) may attenuate venous return but, at the same time, paradoxically increase measured CVP (Fig. 6).

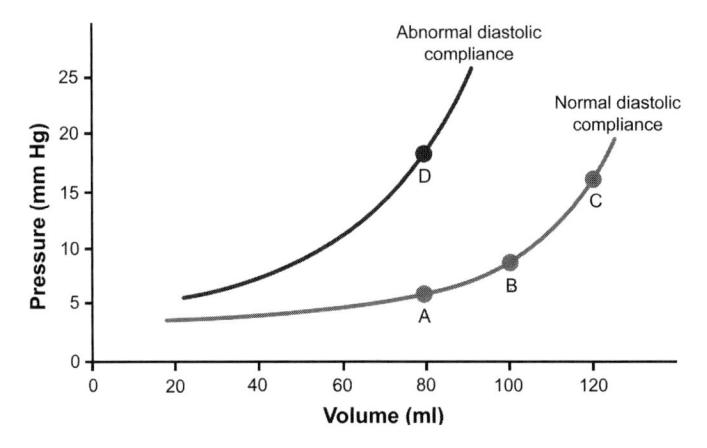

Fig. 5. Pressure–volume relationship in a ventricle with normal or abnormal compliance. When ventricular compliance is normal (*grey curve*), a 20-mL increase in right ventricular end-diastolic volume (RVEDV) produces a 2-mm-Hg rise in CVP (point *A* to point *B*) when RVEDV is 80 mL, but an 8-mm-Hg rise in CVP (point *B* to point *C*) when RVEDV is 100 mL. When ventricular compliance changes (*black curve*), as with ischemia or ventricular hypertrophy, higher filling pressures are required to generate the same RVEDV (point *A* to point *D*). *Abbreviation:* RVEDV = right ventricular end-diastolic volume (*Adapted from* Mark JB. Atlas of cardiovascular monitoring. New York: Churchill Livingstone; 1998. p. 252; with permission.)

In summary, changes in CVP over time or in response to fluid administration are more useful clinically than reliance on absolute numeric values. Central venous pressure must be considered to be the result of the complex interaction between intravascular volume status, ventricular compliance, and intrathoracic pressure.

Normal central venous pressure waveform morphology

Fig. 7 illustrates a typical CVP trace and its relationship to the ECG. With onset of ventricular systole, the tricuspid valve closes and the tricuspid

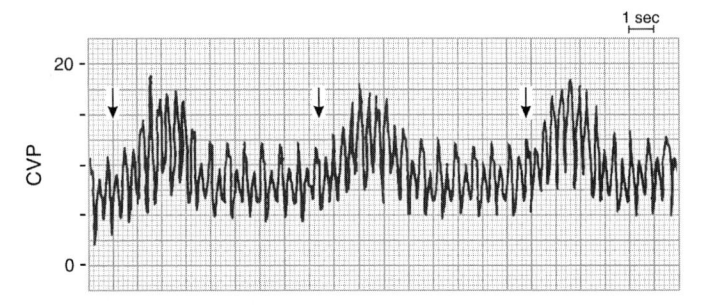

Fig. 6. CVP changes during positive-pressure mechanical ventilation. Mean CVP increases at onset of each positive-pressure breath (*arrows*), but venous return decreases when the measured CVP increases. (*Adapted from* Mark JB. Atlas of cardiovascular monitoring. New York: Churchill Livingstone; 1998. p. 269; with permission.)

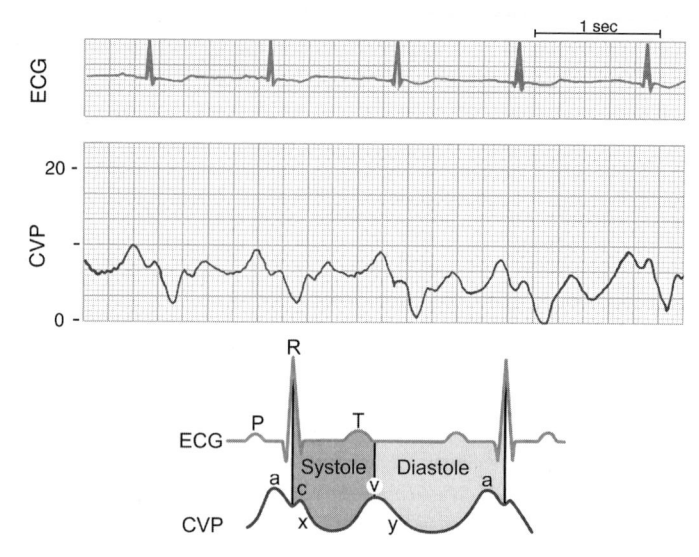

Fig. 7. Normal CVP and its temporal relationship to the ECG. a, *a* wave; c, *c* wave; P, P wave; R, R wave; T, T wave; v, *v* wave; x, x descent; y, y descent. (*Adapted from* Mark JB. Atlas of cardiovascular monitoring. New York: Churchill Livingstone; 1998. p. 20; with permission.)

annulus moves toward the cardiac apex. The former produces the *c* wave, which is small and inconsistent, while the latter generates a drop in pressure in the right atrium, producing the *x* descent. Ventricular ejection drives venous return through the vena cavae, which increases right atrial volume and pressure in mid- to late systole, thereby inscribing the CVP *v* wave. Ventricular diastole then begins with the opening of the tricuspid valve, and blood fills the right ventricle, producing the *y* descent in CVP. Finally, the last part of diastole is marked by atrial contraction, which raises atrial pressure to its highest value and produces the *a* wave.

Abnormal CVP waveform morphology

The characteristics and amplitude of the CVP waveform components change significantly with arrhythmias and tricuspid valve pathology. During junctional rhythm, delayed retrograde atrial depolarization causes atrial contraction to occur during ventricular systole, when the tricuspid valve is already closed. A tall *a* wave, termed a cannon *a* wave, is observed, and its timing and amplitude vary according to the precise timing of right atrial contraction (Fig. 8). Since the "atrial kick" is lost during junctional rhythm, stroke volume, cardiac output, and systemic blood pressure are markedly decreased in patients dependent on this booster pump for adequate ventricular filling. In patients with atrial fibrillation, the CVP *a* wave is absent and, as in junctional rhythm, ventricular filling may be impaired.

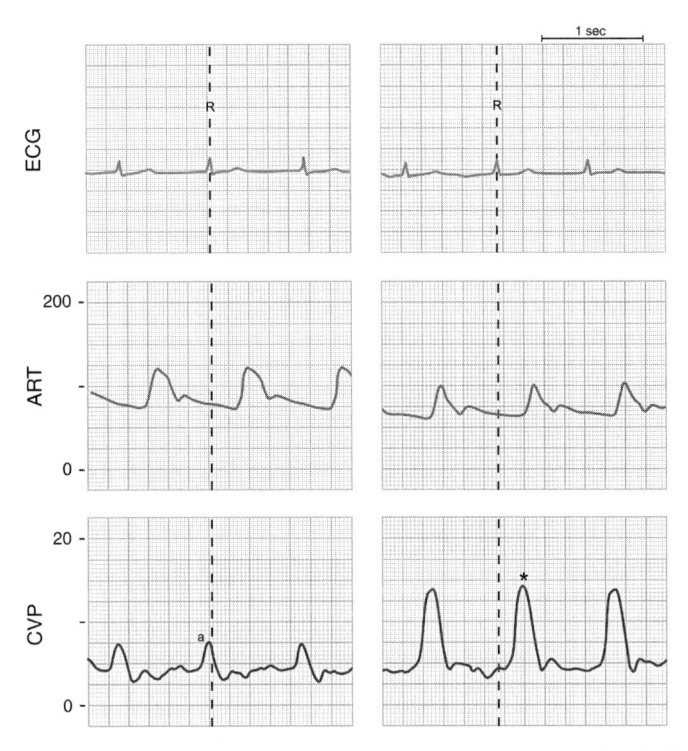

Fig. 8. Junctional rhythm (*right panels*) causes retrograde atrial depolarization during ventricular systole. Atrial contraction against the closed tricuspid valve inscribes a tall early systolic cannon *a* wave in the CVP trace (*asterisk*). Loss of atrioventricular synchrony reduces ventricular preload, leading to arterial hypotension. Note that the ECG does not clearly reveal the rhythm change because the P-wave amplitude is very small. *Abbreviations:* ART, arterial pressure. R, ECG R wave. (*Adapted from* Mark JB. Atlas of cardiovascular monitoring. New York: Churchill Livingstone; 1998. p. 228; with permission.)

Tricuspid valve stenosis produces a CVP trace that displays a prominent *a* wave and an attenuated *y* descent that reflect the obstruction to right atrial emptying. A tall *a* wave may also be present in patients with right ventricular diastolic dysfunction. With tricuspid regurgitation, retrograde filling of the right atrium causes the *c* and *v* waves to merge, eliminating the *x* descent and resulting in a large holosystolic regurgitant *cv* wave (Fig. 9). It is important to recognize that the digital value for CVP displayed on the electronic monitor is influenced by these tall regurgitant *v* waves and does not necessarily reflect the end-diastolic pressure indicative of right ventricular preload.

Other less common conditions can have a striking influence on the shape of the CVP waveform. In pericardial constriction, the mean CVP is increased, the *a* and *v* waves are prominent, and the *x* and *y* descents are steep (Fig. 10). In contrast, cardiac tamponade also results in a marked elevation of CVP, but

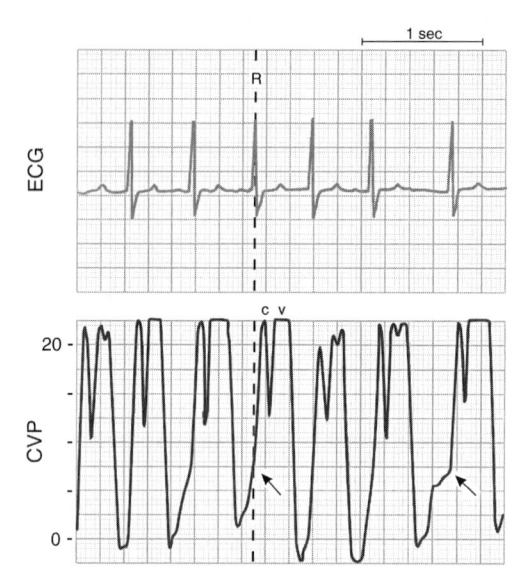

Fig. 9. Tricuspid regurgitation inscribes a tall regurgitant c-v wave in the CVP trace with obliteration of the x descent. Mean CVP is markedly increased in TR, and right ventricular end-diastolic pressure is lower than mean CVP and best estimated before onset of the c-v wave (*arrows*). *Abbreviations:* R, ECG R wave. (*Adapted from* Mark JB. Atlas of cardiovascular monitoring. New York: Churchill Livingstone; 1998. p. 294; with permission.)

the y descent is characteristically attenuated. Note that the increased CVP seen in both constriction and tamponade reflects the extramural compressive effect of the restrictive pericardium or effusion, and cardiac filling is reduced in both conditions.

Summary

Pressure monitoring systems influence the contour of the displayed waveforms and, on occasion, can introduce significant artifact in the pressure traces. It is important to understand the technical details of invasive pressure monitoring to interpret better the information presented.

Careful observation of the arterial pressure waveform can provide information about ventricular function, the arterial system, and ventricular preload. In particular, systolic pressure variation during the respiratory cycle in mechanically ventilated patients is a clinically useful indicator of volume status.

CVP monitoring is also used to assess intravascular volume, but this measurement is significantly influenced by ventricular compliance and intrathoracic pressure. Under most clinical circumstances, a trend in CVP values or its change with therapeutic maneuvers is more reliable than a single

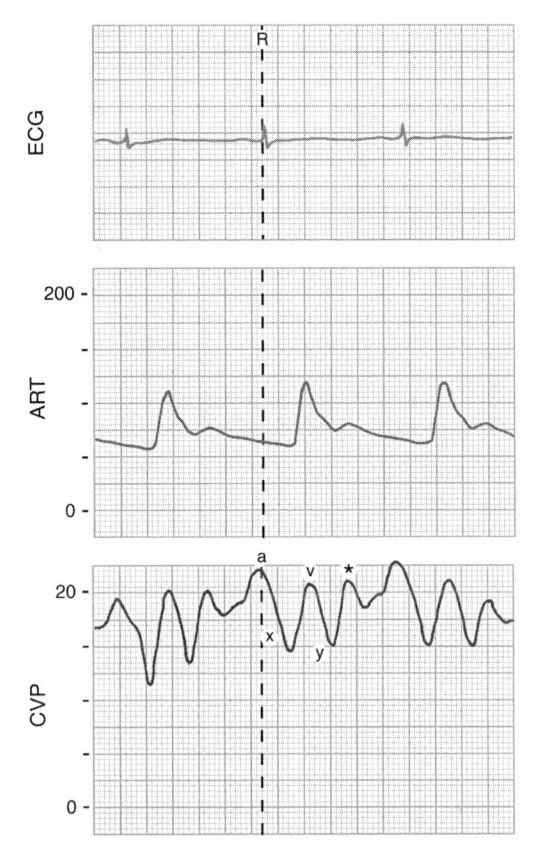

Fig. 10. Pericardial constriction increases right- and left-sided cardiac filling pressures. The CVP shows an M or W pattern, with tall a and v waves and steep x and y descents. A mid-diastolic plateau wave or h wave (*asterisk*) may also be seen when the heart rate is slow. *Abbreviations:* ART, arterial pressure; R, ECG R wave. (*Adapted from* Mark JB. Atlas of cardiovascular monitoring. New York: Churchill Livingstone; 1998. p. 318; with permission.)

measurement. Like arterial pressure waveforms, CVP waveform morphology can provide important information about clinical pathophysiology.

References

[1] Kleinman B. Understanding natural frequency and damping and how they relate to the measurement of blood pressure. J Clin Monit 1989;5(2):137–47.
[2] Gardner RM. Direct blood pressure measurement—dynamic response requirements. Anesthesiology 1981;54(3):227–36.
[3] Hunziker P. Accuracy and dynamic response of disposable pressure transducer-tubing systems. Can J Anaesth 1987;34(4):409–14.
[4] Pittman JA, Sum Ping J, Mark JB. Arterial and central venous pressure monitoring. Int Anesthesiol Clin 2004;42(1):13–30.
[5] Hipkins SF, Rutten AJ, Runciman WB. Experimental analysis of catheter-manometer systems in vitro and in vivo. Anesthesiology 1989;71(6):893–906.

[6] Kleinman B, Powell S, Gardner RM. Equivalence of fast flush and square wave testing of blood pressure monitoring systems. J Clin Monit 1996;12(2):149–54.
[7] Kleinman B, Powell S, Kumar P, et al. The fast flush test measures the dynamic response of the entire blood pressure monitoring system. Anesthesiology 1992;77(6):1215–20.
[8] Courtois M, Fattal PG, Kovacs SJ Jr, et al. Anatomically and physiologically based reference level for measurement of intracardiac pressures. Circulation 1995;92(7):1994–2000.
[9] Mark JB. Technical requirements for direct blood pressure measurement. In: Mark JB, editor. Atlas of cardiovascular monitoring. New York: Churchill Livingstone; 1998. p. 99–126.
[10] Tegtmeyer K, Brady G, Lai S, et al. Videos in clinical medicine. Placement of an arterial line. N Engl J Med 2006;354(15):e13.
[11] Singleton RJ, Webb RK, Ludbrook GL, et al. The Australian Incident Monitoring Study. Problems associated with vascular access: an analysis of 2000 incident reports. Anaesth Intensive Care 1993;21(5):664–9.
[12] Mandel MA, Dauchot PJ. Radial artery cannulation in 1,000 patients: precautions and complications. J Hand Surg [Am] 1977;2(6):482–5.
[13] Wilkins RG. Radial artery cannulation and ischaemic damage: a review. Anaesthesia 1985;40(9):896–9.
[14] Mangano DT, Hickey RF. Ischemic injury following uncomplicated radial artery catheterization. Anesth Analg 1979;58(1):55–7.
[15] Slogoff S, Keats AS, Arlund C. On the safety of radial artery cannulation. Anesthesiology 1983;59(1):42–7.
[16] O'Grady NP, Alexander M, Dellinger EP, et al. Guidelines for the prevention of intravascular catheter-related infections. Infect Control Hosp Epidemiol 2002;23(12):759–69.
[17] Chowet AL, Lopez JR, Brock-Utne JG, et al. Wrist hyperextension leads to median nerve conduction block: implications for intra-arterial catheter placement. Anesthesiology 2004;100(2):287–91.
[18] Goedje O, Hoeke K, Lichtwarck-Aschoff M, et al. Continuous cardiac output by femoral arterial thermodilution calibrated pulse contour analysis: comparison with pulmonary arterial thermodilution. Crit Care Med 1999;27(11):2407–12.
[19] Linton NW, Linton RA. Estimation of changes in cardiac output from the arterial blood pressure waveform in the upper limb. Br J Anaesth 2001;86(4):486–96.
[20] Zollner C, Haller M, Weis M, et al. Beat-to-beat measurement of cardiac output by intravascular pulse contour analysis: a prospective criterion standard study in patients after cardiac surgery. J Cardiothorac Vasc Anesth 2000;14(2):125–9.
[21] Pittman J, Bar-Yosef S, SumPing J, et al. Continuous cardiac output monitoring with pulse contour analysis: a comparison with lithium indicator dilution cardiac output measurement. Crit Care Med 2005;33(9):2015–21.
[22] Karamanoglu M. A system for analysis of arterial blood pressure waveforms in humans. Comput Biomed Res 1997;30(3):244–55.
[23] Benetos A, Laurent S, Hoeks AP, et al. Arterial alterations with aging and high blood pressure. A noninvasive study of carotid and femoral arteries. Arterioscler Thromb 1993;13(1):90–7.
[24] London GM, Guerin AP. Influence of arterial pulse and reflected waves on blood pressure and cardiac function. Am Heart J 1999;138(3 Pt 2):220–4.
[25] Vlachopoulos C, Hirata K, O'Rourke MF. Pressure-altering agents affect central aortic pressures more than is apparent from upper limb measurements in hypertensive patients: the role of arterial wave reflections. Hypertension 2001;38(6):1456–60.
[26] Dorman T, Breslow MJ, Lipsett PA, et al. Radial artery pressure monitoring underestimates central arterial pressure during vasopressor therapy in critically ill surgical patients. Crit Care Med 1998;26(10):1646–9.

[27] Chauhan S, Saxena N, Mehrotra S, et al. Femoral artery pressures are more reliable than radial artery pressures on initiation of cardiopulmonary bypass. J Cardiothorac Vasc Anesth 2000;14(3):274–6.
[28] O'Rourke MF, Yaginuma T. Wave reflections and the arterial pulse. Arch Intern Med 1984; 144(2):366–71.
[29] Perel A, Pizov R, Cotev S. Systolic blood pressure variation is a sensitive indicator of hypovolemia in ventilated dogs subjected to graded hemorrhage. Anesthesiology 1987;67(4): 498–502.
[30] Rooke GA, Schwid HA, Shapira Y. The effect of graded hemorrhage and intravascular volume replacement on systolic pressure variation in humans during mechanical and spontaneous ventilation. Anesth Analg 1995;80(5):925–32.
[31] Michard F, Teboul JL. Predicting fluid responsiveness in ICU patients: a critical analysis of the evidence. Chest 2002;121(6):2000–8.
[32] Pizov R, Cohen M, Weiss Y, et al. Positive end-expiratory pressure-induced hemodynamic changes are reflected in the arterial pressure waveform. Crit Care Med 1996;24(8):1381–7.
[33] Mark JB, Slaughter TF. Cardiovascular monitoring. In: Miller R, editor. Miller's anesthesia. 6th edition. Philadelphia: Elsevier Churchill Livingstone; 2005. p. 1265–362.
[34] McGee DC, Gould MK. Preventing complications of central venous catheterization. N Engl J Med 2003;348(12):1123–33.
[35] Randolph AG, Cook DJ, Gonzales CA, et al. Ultrasound guidance for placement of central venous catheters: a meta-analysis of the literature. Crit Care Med 1996;24(12):2053–8.
[36] Mansfield PF, Hohn DC, Fornage BD, et al. Complications and failures of subclavian-vein catheterization. N Engl J Med 1994;331(26):1735–8.
[37] Rothschild J. Chapter 21. Ultrasound guidance of central vein catheterization. In: Making health care safer: a critical analysis of patient safety practices. Rockville (MD): Agency for Healthcare Research and Quality; 2001. p. 253–61.
[38] Pittet D, Tarara D, Wenzel RP. Nosocomial bloodstream infection in critically ill patients. Excess length of stay, extra costs, and attributable mortality. JAMA 1994;271(20):1598–601.
[39] Saint S. Chapter 16. Prevention of intravascular catheter-associated infections. In: Making health care safer: a critical analysis of patient safety practices. Rockville (MD): Agency for Healthcare Research and Quality; 2001. p. 169–89.
[40] Maki DG, Stolz SM, Wheeler S, et al. Prevention of central venous catheter-related bloodstream infection by use of an antiseptic-impregnated catheter. A randomized, controlled trial. Ann Intern Med 1997;127(4):257–66.
[41] Hirsch DR, Ingenito EP, Goldhaber SZ. Prevalence of deep venous thrombosis among patients in medical intensive care. JAMA 1995;274(4):335–7.
[42] Timsit JF, Farkas JC, Boyer JM, et al. Central vein catheter-related thrombosis in intensive care patients: incidence, risks factors, and relationship with catheter-related sepsis. Chest 1998;114(1):207–13.

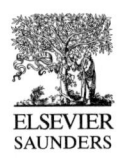

Intraoperative Monitoring with Transesophageal Echocardiography: Indications, Risks, and Training

Jesse Marymont, MD*, Glenn S. Murphy, MD

Evanston Northwestern Healthcare, Northwestern University, Feinberg School of Medicine, 2650 Ridge Avenue Evanston, IL 60201, USA

The use of transesophageal echocardiography (TEE) by anesthesiologists has been steadily increasing. This article is divided into three areas of intraoperative TEE: indications, risks, and training. The discussion incorporates four of the current guidelines for use of TEE in the perioperative period.

A first set of guidelines, "Practice Guidelines for Perioperative Transesophageal Echocardiography," was published in 1996 [1]. These guidelines were presented as a report by the American Society of Anesthesiologists (ASA) and the Society of Cardiovascular Anesthesiologists (SCA) Task Force on TEE. Ten years have passed since these ASA–SCA guidelines were published, and the ASA and the SCA are in the process of updating them.

A second set of guidelines, published in 2003, addresses transthoracic and transesophageal echocardiography [2]. These recent guidelines originate from the American College of Cardiology (ACC), the American Heart Association (AHA), and the American Society of Echocardiography (ASE). The ACC–AHA–ASE guidelines do not compete with the ASA–SCA guidelines. The ACC–AHA–ASE guidelines have added to the existing ASA–SCA guidelines, without any significant deletions. Thus, at the present time, the ACC–AHA–ASE indications for TEE are the state of the art for anesthesiologists.

A third set of guidelines, put forth by the ASE and SCA, describes the training requirements for anesthesiologists performing perioperative echocardiography [3].

A fourth set of guidelines, put forth by the ASE and SCA, describes how to perform an intraoperative multiplane transesophageal examination [4].

---

* Corresponding author.
 E-mail address: JMarymont@enh.org (J. Marymont).

The technical aspects of how to perform a perioperative TEE examination are beyond the scope of this article.

Intraoperative echocardiography: indications

When the routine perioperative evaluation of a patient (history, physical examination, laboratory, ECG, chest radiography) is insufficient, the TEE may deliver additional information. TEE is not a treatment modality. Rather, TEE is a monitoring and a diagnostic tool. TEE equipment is portable. Thus, one TEE probe and machine can provide coverage for multiple hospital units.

The ASA has published a statement on TEE [5]. According to this document, "TEE is a special tool and not a standard intraoperative technique. It provides unique information that no other diagnostic procedure can provide. TEE permits ongoing assessment of cardiovascular function and immediate treatment of abnormalities related to surgical interventions, anesthesia effects, and changing patient conditions." In this same document, the ASA states that "any physicians using TEE should be specifically credentialed by their institution to do so."

The intraoperative use of TEE during cardiac surgery may alter the anesthetic or surgical management [6–12].

The ACC, AHA, and ASE have provided a guideline for the clinical use of echocardiography [2]. Guidelines are important, as they present scientific evidence to support the use of TEE. The classification system used by the ACC, AHA, and ASE divides the scientific evidence into three classes (Box 1). Published guidelines may help the anesthesiologist to determine when intraoperative echocardiography is appropriate for a particular patient.

Intraoperative TEE is commonly used in hospitals that perform cardiac surgery. Depending upon the institution, anesthesiologists or cardiologists are usually responsible for placement of the TEE probe, the performance of the TEE examination, or both. The ASA–SCA guidelines of 1996 have been updated by the ACC–AHA–ASE guidelines of 2003. The ACC–AHA–ASE class-I recommendations for intraoperative echocardiography are useful and effective in the care of the patient (Box 2). Each of these class-I recommendations is discussed below.

Intraoperative echocardiography: class-I recommendations

Evaluation of acute, persistent, and life threatening hemodynamic disturbances in which ventricular function and its determinants are uncertain and have not responded to treatment

Usually, the history, physical examination and laboratory findings for a hypotensive patient lead the anesthesiologist to the correct diagnosis and plan of treatment. However, on rare occasions, significant hypotension continues despite the best efforts to diagnosis and treat the underlying cause

> **Box 1. ACC–AHA–ASE guidelines (2003) for the use of echocardiography**
>
> Class I: Conditions for which there is evidence or general agreement that a given procedure or treatment is useful and effective.
>
> Class II: Conditions for which there is conflicting evidence or a divergence of opinion about the usefulness or efficacy of a procedure or treatment.
>
> Class III: Conditions for which there is evidence or general agreement that the procedure or treatment is not useful or effective and in some cases may be harmful.
>
> ---
>
> *Adapted from* Cheitlin MD, Armstrong WF, Aurigemma GP, et al. ACC/AHA/ASE 2003 guideline update for the clinical application of echocardiography—summary article: a report of the American College of Cardiology/American Heart Association Task Force on Practice Guidelines (ACC/AHA/ASE Committee to Update the 1997 Guidelines for the Clinical Application of Echocardiography). J Am Coll Cardiol 2003;42:954–70.

or causes. A typical clinical situation is that of an elderly patient undergoing a surgical procedure where significant third-space fluid loss and blood loss has occurred. The anesthesiologist has given what is believed to be a sufficient quantity of intravenous fluids and blood replacement, yet significant hypotension is present. In this case, the class-I recommendation supports placement of a TEE to determine the etiology of the hypotension.

Cahalan [13] has offered a useful method by which TEE is able to discriminate between common etiologies for hypotension (Table 1). It should be stressed that a complete TEE examination [4] may reveal more than one abnormality (Box 3). The anesthesiologist must determine the best plan of intervention (Figs. 1 and 2).

Clinical studies suggest that TEE is an accurate monitor of left ventricular end-diastolic volume. Clements and colleagues [14] have demonstrated the utility of TEE as a monitor of left ventricular preload and left ventricular function. The investigators observed a close association between TEE measurements of left ventricular areas and radionuclide determinants of left ventricular volumes. The investigators concluded that the two-dimensional TEE short-axis image at the midpapillary muscle level is generally adequate for monitoring left ventricular volume and left ventricular function intraoperatively. Cheung and colleagues [15] looked at left ventricular preload in adult patients with normal and abnormal ventricular function. Patients were subjected to graded hypovolemia produced by collecting six aliquots of blood, each equal to 2.5% percent of their estimated blood volume. The left ventricular end-diastolic area decreased linearly in response to acute blood-volume

> **Box 2. ACC–AHA–ASE class-I recommendations for intraoperative echocardiography**
>
> - Evaluation of acute, persistent, and life-threatening hemodynamic disturbances in which ventricular function and its determinants are uncertain and have not responded to treatment.
> - Surgical repair of valvular lesions, hypertrophic obstructive cardiomyopathy, and aortic dissection with possible aortic valve involvement.
> - Evaluation of complex valve replacements requiring homografts or coronary reimplantation, such as the Ross procedure.
> - Surgical repair of most congenital heart lesions that require cardiopulmonary bypass.
> - Surgical intervention for endocarditis when preoperative testing was inadequate or extension to perivalvular tissue is suspected.
> - Placement of intracardiac devices and monitoring of their position during port-access and other cardiac surgical interventions.
> - Evaluation of pericardial window procedures in patients with posterior or loculated pericardial effusions.
>
> ---
>
> *Adapted from* Cheitlin MD, Armstrong WF, Aurigemma GP, et al. ACC/AHA/ASE 2003 guideline update for the clinical application of echocardiography—summary article: a report of the American College of Cardiology/American Heart Association Task Force on Practice Guidelines (ACC/AHA/ASE Committee to Update the 1997 Guidelines for the Clinical Application of Echocardiography). J Am Coll Cardiol 2003;42:954–70.

deficits. Cheung concluded that TEE could be used to detect and monitor the effects of acute blood loss in anesthetized patients undergoing coronary artery bypass grafting.

TEE is a sensitive monitor for detecting myocardial ischemia. Smith and colleagues [16] determined that intraoperative TEE can successfully demonstrate myocardial ischemia by revealing acute segmental wall-motion abnormalities. He also found that when new segmental wall-motion abnormalities continued until the end of the operation, myocardial infarction was likely to have occurred. Smith used two factors to evaluate left ventricular systolic wall motion: endocardial movement toward the center of the left ventricular chamber and left ventricular wall thickening. Smith believed that TEE was superior to the ECG for the detection of intraoperative ischemia.

Table 1
TEE differential diagnosis of hypotension

Etiology	End-diastolic area	Fractional area of change[a]
Hypovolemia	Decreased	Increased >0.8
Left ventricular failure	Increased	Decreased <0.2
Decreased SVR, severe MR, severe AR, or VSD	Normal	Increased >0.8

Abbreviations: AR, aortic regurgitation; MR, mitral regurgitation; SVR, systemic vascular resistance; VSD, ventricular septal defect.

[a] Fractional area of change (FAC) = (end-diastolic area (EDA) − end-systolic area (ESA))/EDA = stroke volume/EDA.

Adapted from Cahalan MK. Assessment of global and regional left ventricular systolic function. Surgical Anatomy Wet Laboratory and Basic Transesophageal Echo 2002; February 18–20:146–9.

Hauser and colleagues [17] used transthoracic echocardiography for monitoring during coronary angioplasty. Balloon inflation produced frequent new or increased wall-motion abnormalities in the distribution of the occluded coronary artery. Wall motion began to normalize with balloon deflation and reperfusion. Hauser concluded that during ischemia, left ventricular wall-motion abnormalities preceded ECG changes.

Reichert and colleagues [18] evaluated hypotensive postoperative cardiac surgical patients. Sixty patients were hypotensive despite positive inotropic medication and, in some patients, mechanical support. No clear cause of the hypotension could be determined by routine clinical evaluation. TEE elucidated the cause of hypotension in 55 of 60 patients (Box 4). Reichert

---

Box 3. Etiologies of hypotension revealed by TEE

Common etiologies
Hypovolemia
Decreased left ventricular systolic function (myocardial ischemia or infarction, cardiomyopathy)
Decreased systemic vascular resistance (arterial vasodilation, sepsis)

Less common etiologies
Decreased right ventricular systolic function (pulmonary embolus, right ventricular infarction)
Pericardial tamponade (poor diastolic filling)
Aortic dissection (severe aortic regurgitation)
Papillary muscle rupture (severe mitral regurgitation)
Ventricular septal defect (complication of myocardial infarction)
Valvular disease
Left ventricular outflow tract obstruction

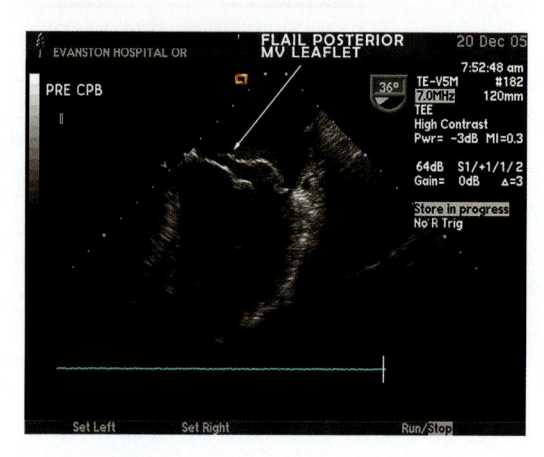

Fig. 1. TEE showing a flail posterior mitral valve (MV) leaflet (*arrow*). The patient presented with a sudden onset of hypotension. TEE revealed a normal left ventricular end-diastolic area and an increased left ventricular fractional area of change.

concluded that TEE, performed on patients after cardiac operations, can frequently determine the cause of hypotension.

Van der Wouw and colleagues [19] placed a TEE probe into 48 patients who had nonarrhythmogenic circulatory arrest beginning within or outside of the hospital. At least 5 minutes had transpired between the arrest and the placement of the TEE probe. All patients had been intubated, and all remained in circulatory arrest after initial resuscitative measures. Adequate images were obtained in all 48 patients (Box 5). Of these 48 patients, 31 later had a definite diagnosis available from a reference standard (eg, autopsy, surgery, and angioplasty). Of these 31 patients, 27 patients were given the correct diagnosis by TEE (87% correct). The investigators concluded that

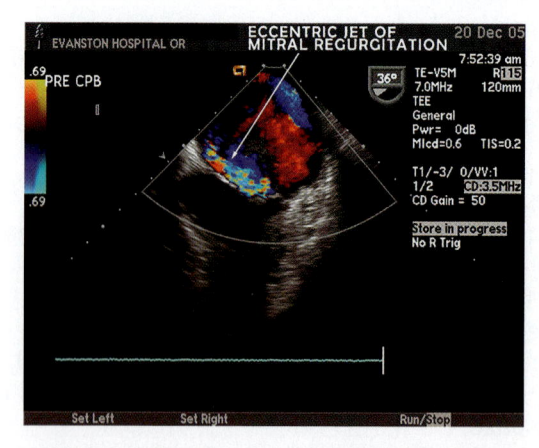

Fig. 2. A color flow Doppler image of the same patient as in Fig. 1. Due to the flail posterior mitral valve leaflet, a large eccentric jet of mitral regurgitation is present (*arrow*).

Box 4. TEE-determined etiology of hypotension after cardiac surgery in 60 patients

- 14 hypovolemia
- 6 tamponade
- 16 left ventricular failure
- 11 right ventricular failure
- 8 biventricular failure
- 5 inconclusive TEE exam

Data from Reichert CLA, Cees AV, Koolen JJ, et al. Transesophageal echocardiography in hypotensive patients after cardiac operations. J Thorac Cardiovasc Surg 1992;104:321–6.

TEE, performed during cardiopulmonary resuscitation, can reliably establish the cause of a circulatory arrest.

Surgical repair of valvular lesions, hypertrophic obstructive cardiomyopathy, and aortic dissection with possible aortic valve involvement

Mitral valve repair is a class-I indication for intraoperative TEE. The TEE examination performed before cardiopulmonary bypass is beneficial to help the surgeon define the abnormal mitral valve anatomy and the feasibility of mitral valve repair. After the repair, the anesthesiologist may

Box 5. TEE-based diagnoses in 48 patients undergoing cardiopulmonary resuscitation

- 21 myocardial infarction
- 6 cardiac tamponade
- 6 pulmonary embolism
- 1 traumatic aortic rupture
- 4 thoracic aortic dissection
- 1 papillary muscle rupture
- 1 end-stage pulmonary hypertension
- 1 supraventricular tachycardia
- 7 no structural cardiac abnormality

Data from Van der Wouw PA, Koster RW, Delemarre BJ, et al. Diagnostic accuracy of transesophageal echocardiography during cardiopulmonary resuscitation. J Am Coll Cardiol 1997;30:780–3.

assess the amount of residual mitral regurgitation as well as the extent of any systolic anterior motion of the anterior mitral valve leaflet into the left ventricular outflow tract.

The anesthesiologist must understand that general anesthesia may lessen the degree of mitral regurgitation (compared with the awake, sedated state). Grewal and colleagues [20] studied 43 patients with moderate or severe mitral regurgitation demonstrated by preoperative TEE (done with the patient awake and sedated). The preoperative TEE was performed with topical lidocaine and intravenous sedation. Then, within 30 days, the intraoperative TEE was performed after these same patients received a general anesthetic and intubation. Systolic blood pressure, mean arterial pressure, and left ventricular end-diastolic and end-systolic dimensions were significantly lower during the intraoperative study, reflecting altered loading conditions. Under general anesthesia, the mean color Doppler jet area and mean vena contracta decreased, and the mean pulmonary venous flow pattern changed from reversed to blunted, reflecting a significant reduction in the severity of mitral regurgitation. Overall, 22 of the 43 patients (51%) improved at least one mitral regurgitation severity grade when assessed under general anesthesia. Thus, Grewal concludes that intraoperative TEE may significantly underestimate the severity of mitral regurgitation. This decrease in mitral regurgitation severity with general anesthesia occurred in three specific groups of mitral valve pathology: (1) incomplete leaflet coaptation (due to left ventricular dilatation or dysfunction), (2) rheumatic valve disease, and (3) floppy mitral valve disease with valvular degeneration. Interestingly, patients with a flail mitral leaflet did not show improvement in parameters of mitral regurgitation. All patients with a flail leaflet had pulmonary venous flow reversal and severe mitral regurgitation in both the preoperative and intraoperative TEE.

Gisbert and colleagues [21] showed that the severity of organic and functional mitral regurgitation decreases from baseline with general anesthesia and increases after challenge with phenylephrine in the operating room. To more appropriately assess the mitral valve, Gisbert proposed that more studies are needed to evaluate the intraoperative use of phenylephrine in patients with mitral regurgitation.

Surgical repair of an aortic dissection is another class-I indication for intraoperative TEE. Simon and colleagues [22] evaluated TEE in the emergency surgical management of patients with aortic dissection. TEE was performed preoperatively in 32 patients with suspected aortic dissection. The preoperative TEE diagnosis and classification of dissection type was regarded as correct if it was confirmed by the surgeons during the operation. Preoperative TEE correctly identified 28 patients to have aortic dissection with an intimal flap; 4 patients had a nondissecting aneurysm of the ascending aorta. TEE was used in 20 of these patients for intraoperative monitoring and evaluation of the surgical repair. TEE may also be of value in the diagnosis of other pathology associated with aortic dissection (Figs. 3–5). Intraoperative TEE was able to identify these important secondary diagnoses (Box 6).

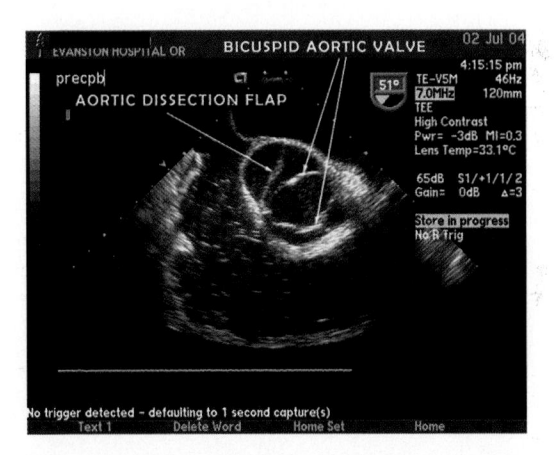

Fig. 3. TEE showing an ascending aortic dissection. Note the aortic dissection flap (*left arrow*) and the bicuspid aortic valve (*center* and *right arrows*).

Evaluation of complex valve replacements requiring homografts or coronary reimplantation, such as the Ross procedure

The Ross procedure involves replacing the abnormal aortic valve with a pulmonary autograft, reimplanting the coronaries, and replacing the pulmonic valve with a homograft [23]. Intraoperative TEE is useful to determine if the patient is a candidate for the Ross procedure. Once the procedure is completed, post–cardiopulmonary-bypass TEE is useful to determine the success of the Ross procedure. A substantial discrepancy in size between the aortic annulus and the pulmonary annulus must be avoided unless the aortic annulus is adjusted or sized to match the pulmonary annulus

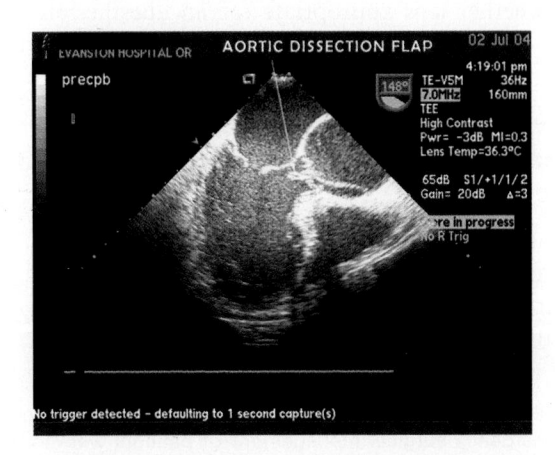

Fig. 4. TEE of the same patient as in Fig. 3. The aortic dissection flap is seen protruding through the aortic valve (*arrow*).

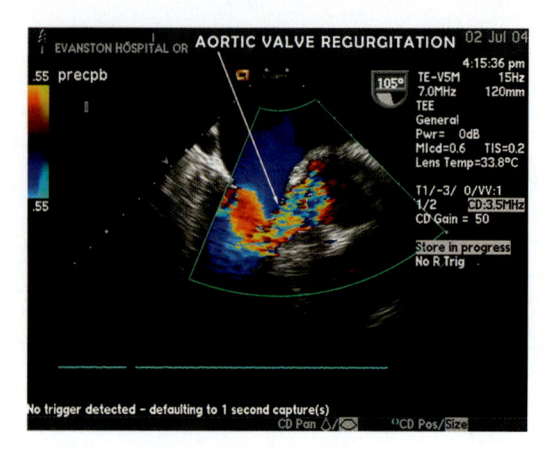

Fig. 5. TEE of the same patient as in Figs. 3 and 4. The patient with an ascending aortic dissection also has aortic valve regurgitation (*arrow*).

[24]. Before cardiopulmonary bypass, intraoperative TEE also is used to evaluate the structure of the pulmonary valve, although the value of the TEE in doing so is questionable [25]. A structurally normal pulmonary valve is needed for the patient to be a good candidate for the Ross procedure. After cardiopulmonary bypass, the intraoperative TEE is used to look for aortic insufficiency (from the pulmonary autograft). Evidence of ventricular wall-motion abnormalities may indicate possible intraoperative coronary artery damage.

Surgical repair of most congenital heart lesions that require cardiopulmonary bypass

Many ask whether it is appropriate for an anesthesiologist to perform and interpret intraoperative TEE during pediatric surgical repair of

---

Box 6. Secondary diagnoses associated with aortic dissection for 28 patients

- 16 aortic insufficiency
- 6 pericardial effusion
- 2 myocardial infarction
- 4 left ventricular ejection fraction <45%

Data from Simon P, Owen AN, Havel M, et al. Transesophageal echocardiography in the emergency surgical management of patients with aortic dissection. J Thorac Cardiovasc Surg 1992;103:1113–8.

congenital heart disease. The debate about this topic continues. Questions raised by numerous authors [25–34] include:

- What training and experience does the anesthesiologist–echocardiographer need?
- Should a distinction be made between TEE as a monitoring device (evaluation of volume status, ventricular function, presence of intracardiac air) and TEE as a diagnostic device (evaluation of anatomic abnormalities before and after surgical repair)?
- Is it acceptable for one anesthesiologist to be responsible for both complex anesthesia care and simultaneous TEE interpretation? For example, is it appropriate for one individual to simultaneously assist separation from cardiopulmonary bypass and evaluate the surgical repair?
- Should a pediatric cardiologist, with specific TEE expertise, be present in the operating room, or should he or she be present only if requested by the anesthesiologist or surgeon?

Surgical intervention for endocarditis when preoperative testing was inadequate or extension to perivalvular tissue is suspected

Daniel and colleagues [35] assessed the value of TEE in the detection of abscesses associated with endocarditis. An abscess was considered to be present when a definite region of reduced echocardiographic density was found on the TEE, or echolucent cavities within the valvular annulus or adjacent myocardial structures were found in the setting of valvular infection. Forty of the 46 abscesses documented by surgery or autopsy (87%) were correctly identified by TEE. Daniel states that patients with identified abscesses in the clinical setting of infective endocarditis are usually candidates for more aggressive therapy (including early surgery) than those without abscesses. All 44 patients with abscesses either required surgery (due to advanced heart failure or persistent infection) or died before operation (Fig. 6).

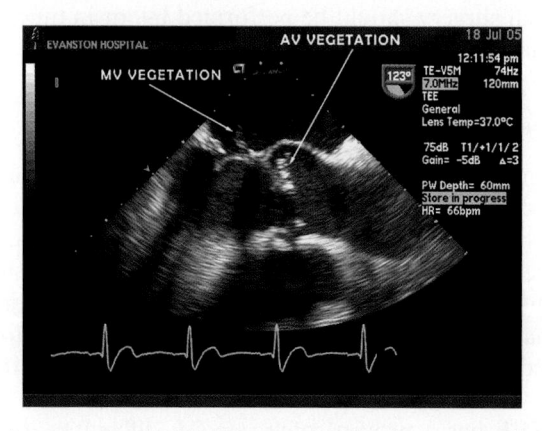

Fig. 6. TEE showing an aortic valve (AV) vegetation (*right arrow*) and a mitral valve (MV) vegetation (*left arrow*). No abscess is seen.

Placement of intracardiac devices and monitoring of their position during port-access and other cardiac surgical interventions

Applebaum and colleagues [36] evaluated TEE as the primary imaging technique to assist in the placement of endovascular catheters during minimally invasive, port-access cardiac surgery. Thirty-six patients were evaluated. TEE was used to visualize the coronary sinus os, right atrium and superior vena cava, and thoracic aorta to assist with placement of the coronary sinus catheter, venous cannula, and endoaortic clamp, respectively. TEE adequately visualized the cardiac structures and assisted in the placement of the endovascular catheters in all patients. Fluoroscopy was only helpful as an aid to TEE for placement of the coronary sinus catheter. Applebaum concluded that TEE is an excellent imaging modality for the proper placement of these endovascular catheters. The investigator states that fluoroscopy could be on standby for the placement of the coronary sinus catheter.

Evaluation of pericardial window procedures in patients with posterior or loculated pericardial effusions

Of all the class-I recommendations for intraoperative echocardiography put forth by the ACC, AHA, and ASE in 2003, the one least substantiated in the literature is the use of TEE during pericardial window procedures. There is little discussion in the ACC–AHA–ASE document about this recommendation. The "Practice Guidelines for Perioperative Transesophageal Echocardiography," published in 1996 by the ASA and SCA [1], states that "clinical experience suggests that posterior or loculated pericardial effusions that are easily missed by the surgeon may develop in patients receiving pericardial windows." The ASA–SCA guidelines list TEE as a class-I indication for pericardial window procedures to evaluate the adequacy of treatment. The ASA and SCA are very specific in their joint view that TEE "used to guide pericardial surgery should be performed by, or in timely consultation with, a physician with advanced TEE training" [1].

Intraoperative echocardiography: risks

The use of medical ultrasound, especially in the limited time period and low–ultrasound-power (intensity) setting of a TEE examination, is generally considered to be of minimal risk. With TEE, the ultrasound transducer is mounted at the end of a flexible endoscope. The TEE probe is then passed, with the patient awake, sedated, or under general anesthesia, into the esophagus and stomach. If awake or sedated, topical anesthesia onto the posterior pharynx is used for patient comfort. Lubrication applied to the TEE probe is beneficial.

Although TEE has a proven safety record, difficulties arising from the technique may occur [37] (Box 7). The insertion and manipulation of the

> **Box 7. Risks associated with TEE**
>
> *Probe insertion and manipulation*
> - Oral trauma
> - Pharyngeal, esophageal, gastric perforation
> - Esophageal and gastric bleeding
> - Swallowing dysfunction
> - Thermal injury
> - Transient bacteremia
> - Displacement of the endotracheal tube
> - Hemodynamic changes
>
> *Sedation or general anesthesia used to facilitate the TEE*
>
> *Incorrect interpretation of the echocardiogram*

TEE probe may result in anatomic damage to the patient. Swallowing dysfunction is possible. Hogue [38] found that intraoperative TEE, patient age, and duration of intubation after the operation were each independent predictors of swallowing dysfunction. This was important, because he noted that postoperative swallowing dysfunction was significantly associated with postoperative pneumonia, need for tracheostomy, and increased length of hospital admission in the intensive care unit and on the postoperative nursing ward. Damage to the pharynx, esophagus, and stomach are possible [39]. Gastrointestinal complications may present more than 24 hours postoperatively [40].

Placement of the TEE probe and the associated manipulation of the probe to perform a complete examination carry an infrequent but potentially significant risk. The decision to perform a perioperative TEE examination is based on weighing benefit against risk [41,42]. The guidelines listing TEE indications mentioned above may help an anesthesiologist evaluate the potential benefit. A preoperative discussion with the surgeon may be of benefit. Known oral, esophageal, or gastric pathology should be taken into consideration. A history of swallowing dysfunction may be important (Box 8). Proper maintenance and cleaning of the TEE probe are essential for patient safety.

Intraoperative echocardiography: training

Another risk of perioperative TEE is that of an incomplete examination or incorrect interpretation of the images. TEE may potentially be misused and lead to patient harm. Training opportunities in perioperative TEE begin at the resident level and extend through the attending level. By taking advantage of these educational opportunities, proficiency in perioperative TEE may be obtained.

> **Box 8. Potential contraindications to TEE**
>
> - Esophageal abnormalities
> - Cervical spine instability
> - Significant hiatal hernia
> - Previous esophageal or gastric surgery
> - Swallowing dysfunction
> - Previous radiation to the mediastinum
> - Abnormalities of the oral pharynx

The American Board of Anesthesiology and the ASA have put forth a content outline for the in-training examination [43] (Box 9).

The ASA–SCA guidelines [1,3] recognize two levels of training in perioperative TEE: basic training and advanced training. The ASA–SCA guidelines state: "Both basic and advanced TEE training refer to specialized training that extends beyond the minimum exposure to TEE during normal anesthesia residency training. Anesthesiologists with basic training are considered able to use TEE for indications that lie within the customary practice of anesthesiology. Anesthesiologists with advanced training are considered, in addition to the above, to be able to exploit the full diagnostic potential of perioperative TEE." Numerous websites provide reliable and up-to-date TEE information for the anesthesiologist (Table 2).

The National Board of Echocardiography offers the Examination of Special Competence in Perioperative Transesophageal Echocardiography (PTEeXAM). The title of testamur is designated to someone who successfully passes this examination. Once additional training and educational

> **Box 9. Anesthesiology in-training examination (TEE content)**
>
> - Principles of Doppler ultrasound
> - Echocardiography to monitor heart function
> - Technical aspects and complications of echocardiography
> - Echocardiography heart anatomy: chambers, valves, great vessels, pericardium, basic TEE views
> - TEE for perioperative diagnosis and treatment of ischemia
> - TEE for diagnosis of cardiac tamponade and constrictive pericarditis
> - TEE for diagnosis of pulmonary embolism
>
> ---
>
> *Data from* The American Board of Anesthesiology. Available at http://www.asahq.org/publicationsandservices/contentoutlineREV2003.pdf.

Table 2
Web sites with information relevant to TEE

Organization	Web address
American Board of Anesthesiology	www.theaba.org
American Society of Anesthesiologists	www.asahq.org
Society of Cardiovascular Anesthesiologists	www.scahq.org
American Society of Echocardiography	www.asecho.org
American College of Cardiology	www.acc.org
National Board of Echocardiography	www.echoboards.org
American Heart Association	www.americanheart.org

criteria are met, as defined by the National Board of Echocardiography, board certification in perioperative TEE is available to the anesthesiologist. The title of diplomate is designated to a physician who is board certified by the National Board of Echocardiography. Once board certified in perioperative TEE, an anesthesiologist may apply to become a fellow in the ASE.

Summary

There are benefits and risks to the use of TEE. The benefits are derived from the physiologic information that TEE provides, which may not be as readily obtained by any other technique. The risks of TEE are those related to mechanical trauma from the probe, as well as those of an incorrect TEE interpretation by the echocardiographer. Intraoperative TEE is a powerful monitoring and diagnostic tool. Performance of TEE requires special skills. As has been discussed, training guidelines exist.

As more clinical studies are published, the indications for intraoperative TEE are likely to expand. Class-I recommendations for intraoperative echocardiography have been listed. The authors have discussed some of the issues involved with each class-I indication.

Performance of the TEE is not an end in itself and should not distract the anesthesiologist from the primary goal of patient care. With proper training and experience, the anesthesiologist may learn how to use TEE to improve patient care.

References

[1] Thys DM, Abel M, Bollen BA, et al. Practice guidelines for perioperative transesophageal echocardiography: A report by the American Society of Anesthesiologists and the Society of Cardiovascular Anesthesiologists Task Force on Transesophageal Echocardiography. Anesthesiology 1996;84:986–1006.

[2] Cheitlin MD, Armstrong WF, Aurigemma GP, et al. ACC/AHA/ASE 2003 guideline update for the clinical application of echocardiography-summary article: a report of the American College of Cardiology/American Heart Association Task Force on Practice Guidelines (ACC/AHA/ASE Committee to Update the 1997 Guidelines for the Clinical Application of Echocardiography). J Am Coll Cardiol 2003;42:954–70.

[3] Cahalan MK, Abel M, Goldman M, et al. America Society of Echocardiography and Society of Cardiovascular Anesthesiologists task force guidelines for training in perioperative echocardiography. Anesth Analg 2002;94:1384–8.
[4] Shanewise JS, Cheung AT, Aronson S, et al. ASE/SCA guidelines for performing a comprehensive intraoperative multiplane transesophageal echocardiography examination: recommendations of the American Society of Echocardiography Council for Intraoperative Echocardiography and the Society of Cardiovascular Anesthesiologists Task Force for Certification in Perioperative Transesophageal Echocardiography. Anesth Analg 1999;89: 870–84.
[5] American Society of Anesthesiologists. Statement on transesophageal echocardiography. (Approved by House of Delegates on October 17, 2001, and last amended on October 25, 2005). Available at: http://www.asahq.org/publicationsAndServices/standards/TEE.pdf. Accessed August 26, 2006.
[6] Savage RM, Lytle BW, Aronson S, et al. Intraoperative echocardiography is indicated in high-risk coronary artery bypass grafting. Ann Thorac Surg 1997;64:368–73.
[7] Click RL, Abel MD, Schaff HV, et al. Intraoperative transesophageal echocardiography; 5 year prospective review of impact on surgical management. Mayo Clin Proc 2000;75:241–7.
[8] Mishra M, Chauhan R, Sharma KK, et al. Real-time intraoperative transesophageal echocardiography—how useful? Experience of 5,016 cases. J Cardiothorac Vasc Anesth 1998; 12:625–32.
[9] Couture P, Denault AY, McKenty S, et al. Impact on routine use of intraoperative transesophageal echocardiography during cardiac surgery. Can J Anaesth 2000;47:20–6.
[10] Michel-Cherqui M, Ceddaha A, Liu N, et al. Assessment of systematic use of intraoperative transesophageal echocardiography during cardiac surgery in adults: a prospective study of 203 patients. J Cardiothorac Vasc Anesth 2000;14:45–50.
[11] Sutton DC, Kluger R. Intraoperative transesophageal echocardiography: impact on adult cardiac surgery. Anaesth Intensive Care 1998;26:287–93.
[12] Bergquist BD, Bellows WH, Leung JM. Transesophageal echocardiography in myocardial revascularization: II. Influence on intraoperative decision making. Anesth Analg 1996;82: 1139–45.
[13] Cahalan MK. Assessment of global and regional left ventricular systolic function. Surgical Anatomy Wet Laboratory and Basic Transesophageal Echo 2002;February 18–20:146–9.
[14] Clements FM, Harpole DH, Quill T, et al. Estimation of left ventricular volume and ejection fraction by two-dimensional transesophageal echocardiography; comparison of short axis imaging and simultaneous radionuclide angiography. Br J Anaesth 1990;64:331–6.
[15] Cheung AT, Savino JS, Weiss SJ, et al. Echocardiographic and hemodynamic indexes of left ventricular preload in patients with normal and abnormal ventricular function. Anesthesiology 1994;81:376–87.
[16] Smith JS, Cahalan MK, Benefiel DJ, et al. Intraoperative detection of myocardial ischemia in high-risk patients: electrocardiography versus two-dimensional transesophageal echocardiography. Circulation 1985;72(5):1015–21.
[17] Hauser AM, Vellappillil G, Ramos RG, et al. Sequence of mechanical, electrocardiographic and clinical effects of repeated coronary artery occlusion in human beings: echocardiographic observations during coronary angiography. J Am Coll Cardiol 1985;5(2):193–7.
[18] Reichert CLA, Cees AV, Koolen JJ, et al. Transesophageal echocardiography in hypotensive patients after cardiac operations. J Thorac Cardiovasc Surg 1992;104:321–6.
[19] Van der Wouw PA, Koster RW, Delemarre BJ, et al. Diagnostic accuracy of transesophageal echocardiography during cardiopulmonary resuscitation. J Am Coll Cardiol 1997;30:780–3.
[20] Grewal KS, Malkowski MJ, Piracha AR, et al. Effect of general anesthesia on the severity of mitral regurgitation by transesophageal echocardiography. Am J Cardiol 2000;85:199–203.
[21] Gisbert A, Souliere V, Denault AY, et al. Dynamic quantitative echocardiographic evaluation of mitral regurgitation in the operative department. J Am Soc Echocardiogr 2006;19:140–6.

[22] Simon P, Owen AN, Havel M, et al. Transesophageal echocardiography in the emergency surgical management of patients with aortic dissection. J Thorac Cardiovasc Surg 1992; 103:1113–8.
[23] Stewart WJ, Secknus MA, Thomas JD, et al. Intraoperative echocardiography in the Ross procedure. J Am Coll Cardiol 1996;27:190A.
[24] Elkins RC. Pulmonary autograft—the optimal substitute for the aortic valve? N Engl J Med 1994;330:59–60.
[25] Gomez CB, Stutzbach PG, Guevara E, et al. Does intraoperative transesophageal echocardiography predict pulmonary valve dysfunction during the Ross Procedure. J Cardiothor Vasc Anesth 2002;16:437–40.
[26] Fyfe DA, Ritter SB, Snider AR, et al. Guidelines for transesophageal echocardiography in children. J Am Soc Echocardiogr 1992;5:640–4.
[27] Stevenson JG. Adherence to physician training guidelines for pediatric transesophageal echocardiography affects the outcome of patients undergoing repair of congenital cardiac defects. J Am Soc Echocardiogr 1999;12:165–72.
[28] Fyfe D. Transesophageal echocardiography guidelines: return to bypass or to bypass the guidelines? J Am Soc Echocardiogr 1999;12:343–4.
[29] Aronson S. Letter. J Am Soc Echocardiogr 1999;12:1008.
[30] Ramamoorthy C, Williams GD, Lynn AM. [Letter] J Am Soc Echocardiogr 1999;12:1008–9
[31] Russell IM, Silverman NH, Miller-Hance W, et al. Intraoperative transesophageal echocardiography for infants and children undergoing congenital heart surgery: the role of the anesthesiologist. J Am Soc Echocardiogr 1999;12:1009–10.
[32] Stevenson JG. Performance of intraoperative pediatric transesophageal echocardiography by anesthesiologists and echocardiographers: training and availability are more important than hats. J Am Soc Echocardiogr 1999;12:1013–4.
[33] Fyfe DA. Intraoperative transesophageal echocardiography in children with congenital heart disease: how, not who!. J Am Soc Echocardiogr 1999;12:1011–3.
[34] Ayres NA, Miler-Hance W, Fyfe DA, et al. Indications and guidelines for performance of transesophageal echocardiography in the patient with pediatric acquired of congenital heart disease. J Am Soc Echocardiogr 2005;18:91–8.
[35] Daniel WG, Mugge A, Martin RP, et al. Improvement in the diagnosis of abscesses associated with endocarditis by transesophageal echocardiography. N Engl J Med 1991;324:795–800.
[36] Applebaum RM, Cutler WM, Bhardwaj N, et al. Utility of transesophageal echocardiography during port-access minimally invasive cardiac surgery. Am J Cardiol 1988;82:183–8.
[37] Kallmeyer I, Collard C, Fox J, et al. The safety of intraoperative transesophageal echocardiography: a case series of 7200 cardiac surgical patients. Anesth Analg 2001;92:1126–30.
[38] Hogue CW, Lappas GD, Creswell LL, et al. Swallowing dysfunction after cardiac operations. Associated adverse outcomes and risk factors including intraoperative transesophageal echocardiography. J Thorac Cardiovasc Surg 1995;110:517–22.
[39] Daniel WG, Erbel R, Kasper W, et al. Safety of transesophageal echocardiography. A multicenter survey of 10,419 examinations. Circulation 1991;83:817–21.
[40] Lennon MJ, Gibbs NM, Weigtman WM, et al. Transesophageal echocardiography-related gastrointestinal complications in cardiac surgical patients. J Cardiothorac Vasc Anesth 2005; 19:141–5.
[41] Spence BC, Hartman GS, Gosselin BJ. Intraoperative esophageal dilation for TEE probe placement in a patient with an undiagnosed esophageal stricture. J Cardiothorac Vasc Anesth 2005;19:209–11.
[42] Shernan SK. When is intraoperative transesophageal echocardiography indicated? J Cardiothorac Vasc Anesth 2005;19:139–40.
[43] Joint Council on In-Training Examinations. American Board of Anesthesiology and American Society of Anesthesiologists. Content outline. Revised November 2003. Available at: http://www.asahq.org/publicationsandservices/contentoutlineREV2003.pdf.

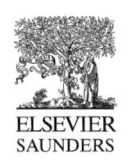

Assessment of Left Ventricular Global and Segmental Systolic Function with Transesophageal Echocardiography

David H. Odell, MD[a,b,c,]*, Michael K. Cahalan, MD[a]

[a]*Department of Anesthesiology, Room 3C-444, University of Utah School of Medicine, 30 North 1900 East, Salt Lake City, UT 84132-2304, USA*
[b]*Department of Internal Medicine, Division of Cardiology, Room 3C-444, University of Utah School of Medicine, 30 N, 1900 E, Suite 4A100, Salt Lake City, UT 84132-2304, USA*
[c]*Perioperative Echocardiography Service, Room 3C-444, University of Utah School of Medicine, 30 North 1900 East, Salt Lake City, UT 84132-2304, USA*

Anesthesiologists use transesophageal echocardiography (TEE) in the operating room, emergency room, and critical care settings. The individual indications differ widely, but evaluation of global and segmental left ventricular (LV) function is a universal requirement. In this article, the authors review a systematic approach to this evaluation.

Left-ventricle–focused TEE examination

The comprehensive TEE examination consists of 20 cross sections of the heart and great vessels [1]. However, in most patients, assessment of global and segmental LV systolic function requires only four of these cross sections: mid-esophageal (ME) four-chamber, ME two-chamber, ME long axis (LAX), and the transgastric (TG) mid-ventricular short axis (SAX) (Fig. 1). These four cross sections provide a comprehensive view of global LV systolic function as well as one or two views of each of the 16 standard segments used for assessment of segmental wall-motion abnormalities (SWMAs). This article briefly reviews the probe and transducer manipulations required for these cross sections.

To obtain the ME four-chamber cross section, advance the TEE probe to the ME level (usually about 30–32 cm of probe insertion as measured from

---

* Corresponding author.
E-mail address: David.Odell@hsc.utah.edu (D.H. Odell).

0889-8537/06/$ - see front matter © 2006 Elsevier Inc. All rights reserved.
doi:10.1016/j.atc.2006.08.004   *anesthesiology.theclinics.com*

ME 4 Chamber   ME 2 Chamber

ME Long Axis   Transgastric
                Mid Ventricular

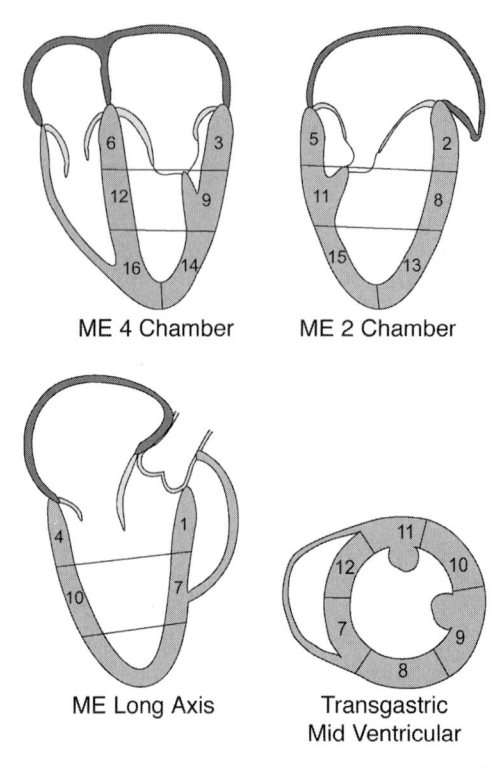

Fig. 1. The four TEE cross sections used in the global and segmental evaluation of LV systolic function are shown. The numbers correspond to the 16-segment model used most commonly in the identification of LV segments. 1, basal anteroseptal; 2, basal anterior; 3, basal lateral; 4, basal posterior; 5, basal inferior; 6, basal septal; 7, mid-anteroseptal; 8, mid-anterior; 9, mid-lateral; 10, mid-posterior; 11, mid-inferior; 12, mid-septal; 13, apical anterior; 14, apical lateral; 15, apical inferior; 16, apical septal. (*Adapted from* Shanewise JS, Cheung AT, Aronson S, et al. ASE/SCA guidelines for performing a comprehensive intraoperative multiplane transesophageal echocardiography examination: recommendations of the American Society of Echocardiography Council for Intraoperative Echocardiography and the Society of Cardiovascular Anesthesiologists Task Force for Certification in Perioperative Transesophageal Echocardiography. Anesth Analg 1999:89:875; with permission.)

the front incisors) and gently retroflex it to direct the ultrasound beam through the base of the heart and toward the apex. Both atria and ventricles are seen. The depth of scanning should be set to reveal the entire left ventricle, including the apex. While the multiplane angle is usually set at 0°, the angle may be advanced slightly (5–10°) to better visualize the tricuspid valve. In this cross section, the LV lateral wall is on the right side of the image, opposite the septal wall. To obtain the ME two-chamber cross section from the ME four-chamber image, center the image of the left ventricle on the video screen and then advance the multiplane transducer to approximately 90°. In the two-chamber cross section, the LV inferior wall is on the left and the anterior wall is on the right. Further advancement of the transducer to approximately 130° reveals the ME LAX cross section in which the LV posterior wall is seen on the left and the anteroseptal wall on the right immediately adjacent to the right ventricle. To obtain the TG mid-ventricular SAX image, advance the probe about 4 to 6 cm into the stomach and gently flex it. This cross section reveals all six of the LV mid-ventricular segments for a second time (see Fig. 1). Usually, this is the most valuable cross section of the four because it reveals myocardium supplied by all three of the major coronaries and because changes in global ventricular filling and ejection are appreciated easier in SAX than in LAX views. Should any of the above four cross sections be diagnostically inadequate, obtain other cross sections from the comprehensive examination as needed. In addition, whenever advancing or withdrawing the probe, it should be in the neutral position (neither flexed not retroflexed) and all probe manipulations should be done with the minimum possible force.

Assessment of global left ventricular systolic function

Multiple modalities may be used to measure LV function. The authors review only the three most common and clinically useful: fractional area change, fractional shortening, and myocardial velocity assessment. In urgent clinical situations, experienced practitioners estimate LV systolic function qualitatively, recognizing that only very marked abnormalities produce life-threatening consequences.

Fractional area change

The fractional area change of the left ventricle may be obtained with any of the four cross sections described above, but the TG mid-ventricular SAX view is usually the best choice because foreshortening of the left ventricle is a common problem with the LAX cross sections. The simple formula for this calculation is:

$$(EDA - ESA)/EDA, \text{ where EDA is end-diastolic area and ESA is end-systolic area}$$

Software packages available on ultrasound machines provide an easy way to make these measurements by using a track-ball device to trace the endocardial borders in both systole and diastole. By convention, the papillary muscles are included within the area measurements (Table 1). Although this measurement is obtained easily, its interpretation has inherent limitations. For example, when fractional area change is measured using the TG mid-ventricular cross section, an SWMA in the ventricular base or apex leads to over-estimation of global LV function. Also, fractional area change is dependent on ventricular preload and afterload. Thus, changes

Table 1
Normal LV systolic function values

Measurement	Men	Women
Fractional shortening	34% ± 9%	37% ± 7%
Fractional area change	59% ± 8%	62% ± 6%
Wall thickening	30% ± 7%	28% ± 8%

Reference values for LV function in subjects without clinical evidence of heart disease undergoing general anesthesia and controlled ventilation. Measurements obtained with two-dimensional TEE at the mid-ventricular transgastric SAX cross section. All values expressed as a percent change during systole.

Data from Skarvan K, Lambert A, Filipovic M, et al. Eur J Anaesthesiol 2001;18:713–22.

in fractional area change may not reflect changes in LV global function unless loading conditions remain constant.

Fractional shortening

Fractional shortening is a second method of evaluating LV function. It is analogous to fractional area change in that it measures the change in dimension (instead of cross-sectional area as used in fractional area change) occurring during systole. The equation for this measurement is:

(LVED − LVES)/LVED, where LVED is the LV
end-diastole diameter and LVES is LV end-systole diameter

Fractional shortening has greater historical than practical value. It was the principal measure of LV function in the early days of echocardiography when only M-mode technology was available. However, it is a commonly sited measurement in reports and studies. The authors include it in this review for those reasons. Again, the TG mid-ventricular cross section is the most useful for this measurement with the M-mode cursor placed across the myocardium of interest. Software on the ultrasound machine provides an easy method to make these measurements. Fractional shortening has the same limitations as fractional area change when used for the assessment of global LV function. In fact, given the one-dimensional nature of M-mode, fractional shortening may not reflect overall ventricular function in the presence of any SWMA.

Tissue Doppler

Tissue Doppler imaging is a relatively new use of pulsed-wave Doppler technology adapted to measure myocardial velocities instead of blood-flow velocities [2]. During normal LV contraction, the mitral annulus descends toward the apex of the heart. Tissue Doppler imaging measures the velocity of this descent (S_m) and S_m correlates with traditional measures of LV function, including ejection fraction and the rate of rise of LV systolic pressure (dP/dt) [3,4]. In addition, S_m decreases in the presence of myocardial ischemia and responds as expected with changes in inotropy [5,6]. The four-chamber cross section is best for measuring S_m. The sampling volume is placed at the lateral insertion point of the mitral valve into the left ventricle and the cross section is aligned so that the sampling cursor is directly parallel with the motion of the annulus (Fig. 2). S_m is an easy and reproducible measurement. However, like fractional area change and fractional shortening, it should be interpreted with caution when preload changes. Ama and colleagues tested its load dependence in 42 hemodynamically stable patients with normal segmental LV function after coronary surgery. S_m did not change significantly in response to a 20% increase or decrease in mean arterial pressure induced by phenylephrine or nitroglycerine. However, it increased significantly when preload was augmented by rapid infusion of colloid [7]. In summary, S_m is less dependent on afterload than fractional area change and fractional shortening, but like these other two measures remains critically dependent on preload. The few measures of LV function that appear to be both preload- and afterload-independent are not practical for clinical use.

Assessment of segmental left ventricular systolic function

Within seconds after the onset of myocardial ischemia, affected segments of the heart cease normal contraction. This fact is the basis for the use of TEE for the detection of myocardial ischemia. For example, in 50 patients undergoing cardiovascular surgery, new severe SWMAs occurred in 24 patients and ischemic ST-segment changes occurred in only 6 [8]. Three patients who sustained

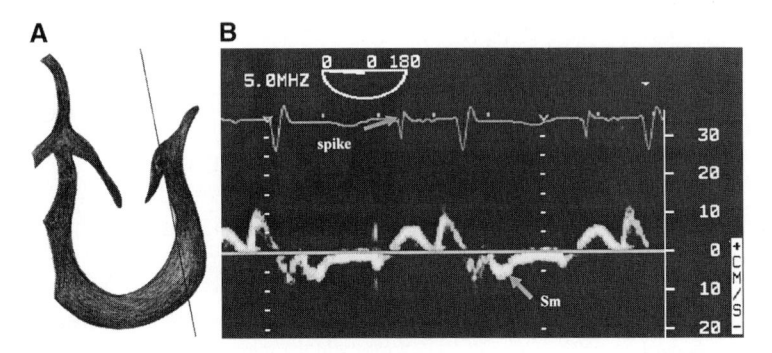

Fig. 2. (*A*) Placement of the tissue Doppler sampling volume in the lateral mitral annulus using the ME four-chamber cross section. (*B*) Resulting trace demonstrating the characteristic waveforms. Sm and arrow indicate downward deflection caused by the descent of the mitral annulus during systole. The following upward deflections are due to the return of the annulus toward the base of the heart in diastole. (*From* Ama R, Segers P, Roosens C, et al. The effects of load on systolic mitral annular velocity by tissue Doppler imaging. Anesth Analg 2004;99:334; with permission.)

intraoperative myocardial infarctions developed severe SWMAs in the corresponding area of myocardium, which persisted until the end of surgery, but only 1 of these 3 had ischemic ST-segment changes intraoperatively. Subsequent studies in comparable patients confirmed these advantages of TEE over ECG monitoring [9–11]. Moreover, when multiple TEE cross sections are monitored (not just the one cross section as was done in the above studies), the detection rate of SWMAs more than doubles [12,13]. The same four cross sections listed above (ME four-chamber, two-chamber, LAX and the TG mid-ventricular SAX) are optimal for evaluating myocardial segments using the standard 16-segment model [1].

Limitations of TEE in the detection of ischemia should be recognized. When an area of myocardium is clearly in view, segmental contraction can be difficult to evaluate if the heart rotates or translates markedly during systole or if discoordinated contraction occurs due to bundle branch block or ventricular pacing. Interpretation of septal motion is the most problematic because it often is confounded by discoordinated contraction patterns. However, a simple rule applies: When the septum is viable and nonischemic, it thickens appreciably during systole, although its inward motion may begin slightly before or after the inward motion of the other ventricular segments. Consequently, a valid system for SWMA assessment first must compensate for global motion of the heart and then evaluate both regional endocardial motion and myocardial thickening. A marked worsening of segmental wall motion and wall thickening (in the absence of similar global changes) is required to make the diagnosis of ischemia; less-pronounced changes are not consistently interpreted, even by experts (Table 2). Because not all hearts contract normally and not all parts of the normal heart contract to the same degree, not all SWMAs are indicative of myocardial

Table 2
Classes of segmental LV systolic function

Functional classes	Radial shortening[a]	Myocardial thickening[b]
Normal	≥30%	+++
Mild hypokinesis	10%–30%	++
Severe hypokinesis	>0% and <10%	+
Akinesis	0	0
Dyskinesis	Systolic lengthening	Systolic thinning

[a] Radial shortening is defined as the decrease in length during systole of an imaginary radius from the endocardium to the center of the LV cavity in the mid-ventricular SAX cross section. A floating reference system is used to compensate for any rotational or translational motion of the heart.

[b] Myocardial thickening is defined as the increase in distance between the endocardial and epicardial borders during systole.

Data from Smith JS, Cahalan MK, Benefiel DJ, et al. Intraoperative detection of myocardial ischemia in high-risk patients: electrocardiography versus two-dimensional transesophageal echocardiography. Circulation 1985;72:1015–21.

ischemia. For example, myocardial infarction, myocardial stunning, and myocarditis can cause SWMAs. Echocardiographic contrast agents can delineate myocardial blood flow, but to date have not been proven to be practical for differentiating an infarcted from an acutely stunned myocardium [14]. Fortunately, dobutamine may facilitate this differential diagnosis because it can improve segmental function in stunned but not infarcted myocardium [15]. For clinical purposes, when stunned myocardium is suspected following cardiopulmonary bypass, graft status should be reevaluated and segmental myocardial function closely monitored for signs of improvement. A trial of low-to-moderate–dose dobutamine may improve the function of stunned myocardium. If worsening occurs, if graft status is questionable, or if hemodynamics are tenuous, additional revascularization should be considered. Intraoperative stress-testing has been evaluated and appears safe in the setting of cardiac surgery, but it is not used outside of research settings currently to the authors' knowledge [16,17].

The limitations noted above should not obscure the physiologic fact that a sudden, severe decrease or cessation of LV segmental contraction is almost always due to myocardial ischemia.

Summary

The evaluation of LV global and segmental systolic function is a primary application for perioperative TEE. Although the practical techniques customarily used for these applications have limitations, they afford direct measures of function not otherwise available to the clinician in the operating room or intensive care setting.

References

[1] Shanewise JS, Cheung AT, Aronson S, et al. ASE/SCA guidelines for performing a comprehensive intraoperative multiplane transesophageal echocardiography examination: recommendations of the American Society of Echocardiography Council for Intraoperative Echocardiography and the Society of Cardiovascular Anesthesiologists Task Force for Certification in Perioperative Transesophageal Echocardiography. Anesth Analg 1999;89: 870–84.
[2] Pai RG, Bodenheimer MM, Pai SM, et al. Usefulness of systolic excursion of the mitral annulus as an index of left ventricular systolic function. Am J Cardiol 1991;67:222–4.
[3] Mishiro Y, Oki T, Yamada H, et al. Evaluation of left ventricular contraction abnormalities in patients with dilated cardiomyopathy with the use of pulsed tissue Doppler imaging. J Am Soc Echocardiogr 1999;12:913–20.
[4] Yamada H, Oki T, Mishiro Y, et al. Effect of aging on diastolic left ventricular velocities measured by pulsed tissue Doppler imaging in healthy subjects. J Am Soc Echocardiogr 1999;12:574–81.
[5] Gorcsan J III, Strum DP, Mandarino WA, et al. Quantitative assessment of alterations in regional left ventricular myocardial contractility with color-coded tissue Doppler echocardiography. Comparison with sonomicrometry and pressure–volume relations. Circulation 1997;20(95):2423–33.

[6] Alam M, Wardell J, Andersson E, et al. Effects of first myocardial infarction on left ventricular systolic and diastolic function with the use of mitral annular velocity determined by pulsed wave doppler tissue imaging. J Am Soc Echocardiogr 2000;13:343–52.
[7] Ama R, Segers P, Roosens C, et al. The effects of load on systolic mitral annular velocity by tissue Doppler imaging. Anesth Analg 2004;99:332–8.
[8] Smith JS, Cahalan MK, Benefiel DJ, et al. Intraoperative detection of myocardial ischemia in high-risk patients: electrocardiography versus two-dimensional transesophageal echocardiography. Circulation 1985;72:1015–21.
[9] Leung JM, O'Kelly B, Browner WS, et al. Prognostic importance of postbypass regional wall-motion abnormalities in patients undergoing coronary artery bypass graft surgery. Anesthesiology 1989;71:16–25.
[10] van Daele ME, Sutherland GR, Mitchell MM, et al. Do changes in pulmonary capillary wedge pressure adequately reflect myocardial ischemia during anesthesia? A correlative preoperative hemodynamic, electrocardiographic, and transesophageal echocardiographic study. Circulation 1990;81:865–71.
[11] Comunale ME, Body SC, Ley C, et al. The concordance of intraoperative left ventricular wall-motion abnormalities and electrocardiographic S-T changes: association with outcome after coronary revascularization. Anesthesiology 1998;88:945–54.
[12] Shah PM, Kyo S, Matsumura M, et al. Utility of biplane transesophageal echocardiography in left ventricular wall motion analysis. J Cardiothorac Vasc Anesth 1991;5:316–9.
[13] Rouine-Rapp K, Ionescu P, Balea M, et al. Detection of intraoperative segmental wall-motion abnormalities by transesophageal echocardiography: the incremental value of additional cross sections in the transverse and longitudinal planes. Anesth Analg 1996;83:1141–8.
[14] Aronson S, Lee BK, Wiencek JG, et al. Assessment of myocardial perfusion during CABG surgery with two-dimensional transesophageal contrast echocardiography. Anesthesiology 1991;75:433–40.
[15] Voci P, Bilotta F, Caretta Q, et al. Low-dose dobutamine echocardiography predicts the early response of dysfunctioning myocardial segments to coronary artery bypass grafting. Am Heart J 1995;129:521–6.
[16] Seeberger MD, Cahalan MK, Chu E, et al. Rapid atrial pacing for detecting provokable demand ischemia in anesthetized patients. Anesth Analg 1997;84:1180–5.
[17] Seeberger MD, Skarvan K, Buser P, et al. Dobutamine stress echocardiography to detect inducible demand ischemia in anesthetized patients with coronary artery disease. Anesthesiology 1998;88:1233–9.

Noninvasive Technologies for Tissue Perfusion

James Ramsay, MD, FRCP(C)

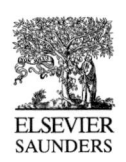

Anesthesiology Critical Care Medicine, Emory University School of Medicine, Emory University Hospital, 1364 Clifton Road, Atlanta GA 30322, USA

The adequacy of vital organ perfusion ideally should be monitored or determined with a device that measures tissue oxygenation, an impractical task for vital organs remote from the body surface. Tissue perfusion or oxygenation should not be confused with arterial oxygenation, as the oxygenation in the arterial blood may be perfectly normal while vital organs are being underperfused. Transcutaneous oxygen electrodes can measure oxygenation beneath the skin; these devices are used to assess wound healing, determine the appropriate level for amputation, and measure effectiveness of hyperbaric oxygen therapy in wound healing. They have not found widespread clinical utility in the operating room or ICU. Transcranial cerebral oximetry may be used to measure the oxygen saturation of underlying brain tissue, with potential utility in procedures or conditions where brain blood flow may be altered or threatened. In states of reduced perfusion tissue carbon dioxide content (CO_2) increases; more specifically, the gradient between tissue and arterial CO_2 widens [1]. Gastric tonometry, or measurement of the pCO_2 in the gastric mucosa by means of a specially designed nasogastric tube, uses this principle to determine the perfusion status of the intestinal tract. Although this technique has shown in several studies to be a valuable indicator of the adequacy of intestinal and whole body perfusion, factors such as user dependence, the need for a nasogastric tube, and the need for histamine receptor blockade and withholding of enteric feeding have contributed to a failure to adopt [2]. Other noninvasive techniques to measure tissue oxygenation or CO_2 status, such as sublingual tissue capnometry, have received significant experimental attention in the resuscitation literature, but have not been studied in the perioperative setting and remain

E-mail address: james.ramsay@emoryhealthcare.org

largely experimental [2]. Techniques for measuring whole-body oxygenation are invasive, such as central venous or mixed venous oximetry.

In the clinical setting, the perfusion of vital organs usually is assessed by measuring the cardiac output (CO), and usually by thermodilution using a pulmonary artery catheter (PAC). This article describes four techniques of measuring CO without the need for a PAC: indirect partial-rebreathing Fick, blood flow velocity measurement by Doppler, arterial pressure waveform analysis, and thoracic bioimpedance. Most clinical assessments have compared less invasive or noninvasive techniques with thermodilution to achieve clinical relevance and acceptability. In the absence of another readily available standard this is probably appropriate; however there is some variability inherent with thermodilution itself [3–5].

Cardiac output using the Fick principle

The Fick principle is named for Adolph Fick, who stated in 1890 that oxygen consumption is equal to the rate of oxygen pickup by the red blood cells in the lung, times the cardiac output [6]. The rate of oxygen pickup is defined as the arterio–venous difference in oxygen content. Rearranging this equation, the cardiac output is equal to the oxygen consumption divided by the arterio–venous difference in oxygen content:

Original Fick : $\dot{V}O_2 = (CaO_2 - C\bar{v}O_2) \times CO$

Rearranged : $CO = \dot{V}O_2/(CaO_2 - C\bar{v}O_2)$

where VO_2 = total body oxygen consumption
CO = cardiac output
CaO_2 = arterial blood content of oxygen
CvO_2 = mixed venous blood content of oxygen

Oxygen consumption can be measured with respiratory gas analysis, but this is cumbersome. Measuring oxygen content of blood is invasive; arterial blood and mixed venous blood samples (ie, from the pulmonary artery) are required.

In 1988, Capek and colleagues described a novel application of the Fick principle to determine cardiac output by measurement of CO_2 production [7]. The Fick equation for CO_2 is as follows:

$\dot{V}CO_2 = (C\bar{v}CO_2 - CaCO_2) \times CO$

Rearranged : $CO = \dot{V}CO_2/(C\bar{v}CO_2 - CaCO_2)$

where $\dot{V}CO_2$ = total body carbon dioxide production

CO = cardiac output
$C\bar{v}CO_2$ = mixed venous blood content of CO_2
$CaCO_2$ = arterial blood content of CO_2

If these parameters had to be measured, this still would be a cumbersome and invasive procedure; however the novel application is to use both indirect determination of CO_2 elimination, and a differential form of the CO_2 Fick equation, where respiratory gas measurements are made in two conditions: baseline and after a brief period of rebreathing. End tidal CO_2 concentration is used instead of arterial CO_2 measurement, and it is assumed that during rebreathing there will be a change in arterial CO_2 and CO_2 elimination, but little change in mixed venous CO_2. When measurements are made in the two conditions of nonrebreathing and rebreathing, then the equations are subtracted to create the differential Fick equation, mixed venous CO_2 drops out:

$$\text{Nonrebreathing}: CO = \dot{V}CO_{2nrb}/(C\bar{v}CO_{2nrb} - CaCO_{2nrb})$$

$$\text{Rebreathing}: CO = \dot{V}CO_{2rb}/(C\bar{v}CO_{2rb} - CaCO_{2rb})$$

$$\text{Differential}: CO = \text{change in } \dot{V}CO_2/\text{change in } CaCO_2$$

The change in $CaCO_2$ is derived by multiplying the change in end tidal CO_2 by the slope of the CO_2 dissociation curve, and the change in VCO_2 is measured using the CO_2 sensor (ie, capnometer) and a flow meter. The reader is referred to the original paper by Capek [7] for a full description and the various assumptions made in the mathematical model. Use of end tidal CO_2 means only blood flow passing through ventilated alveoli is being measured by this technique. Therefore, there needs to be a correction made for intrapulmonary shunt.

This concept has been commercialized and marketed as the NICO monitor (Novametrix Medical Systems Incorporated, Wallingford Connecticut) (Fig. 1). A small partial rebreathing circuit adjusted in length for patient size, which can be included or excluded by activating a valve, is placed in the breathing circuit of an intubated patient. The device automatically measures cardiac output every 3 minutes by making baseline measurements after 60 seconds without rebreathing; introducing the rebreathing circuit for 50 seconds, then performing repeat measurements; then calculating the differential Fick as described previously. After 70 seconds the cycle is repeated. This monitor is truly noninvasive, requiring only analysis of respiratory gas (CO_2) and flow. It requires simultaneous measurement of oxygen saturation to estimate intrapulmonary shunt (from standard equations) and can be used only in intubated patients.

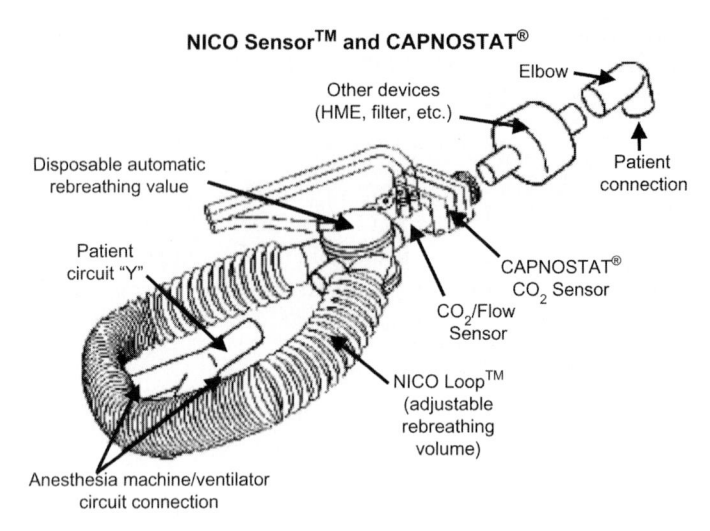

Fig. 1. The NICO airway sensor—a combination of a flow sensor, mainstream CO_2 sensor, an adjustable dead space tubing, and a pneumatic valve—is connected between the tracheal tube of the patient and the Y piece of the breathing circuit. *Abbreviation:* HME, heat and moisture exchanger. (*Reproduced from* Botero M, Lobato E. Advances in noninvasive cardiac output monitoring: an update. J Cardiothorac Vasc Anesth 2001;15:631–40; with permission.)

Clinical results have varied with setting and patient population. As with all noninvasive CO monitors, comparisons must be made with the clinical gold standard of thermodilution, bearing in mind the limitations and inherent variability with the latter technique. In a study comparing four different methods of CO measurement after cardiac surgery, Botero and colleagues found the indirect Fick technique using the NICO monitor to correlate as well as or better than thermodilution to ultrasound transit-time flowmetry [3]. In two studies in the critical care setting, de Abreu and colleagues [8,9] found it to be a reasonable monitor of nonshunted pulmonary blood flow. As might be expected, where there is severe or changing lung disease, or where spontaneous ventilation with varying tidal volume is occurring, the correlation with thermodilution is less acceptable [10,11]. In a pediatric study, the correlation was best for children with more than 0.6 m^2 body surface area and a tidal volume of greater than 300 mL [12]. In a recent comparative study using a porcine model, the NICO monitor responded to changes in cardiac output relatively slowly and correlated less well with aortic transit time ultrasound at the extremes of cardiac output than other less invasive techniques [13]. Although the limitations with regard to the need for intubation, mechanical ventilation, and relatively stable shunt are real, this monitor requires no technical expertise or ongoing manipulation/correction. Additionally, it is completely noninvasive and can be set up to provide values within minutes.

Measurement of blood velocity: cardiac ultrasound and esophageal Doppler devices

The principle of blood flow velocity measurement with ultrasound is well known to echocardiographers. When a sound signal of a given frequency is directed at a moving object, the signal reflected back to the source is altered in frequency proportional to the velocity of the object. This is called the Doppler effect, named after the Austrian physicist Christian Doppler who first described it. The Doppler equation quantifies this effect:

$$\Delta f = v \times \cos(\theta) \times 2f_t/c$$

where: Δf is the difference between transmitted and received frequencies
f_t is the transmitted frequency
v is blood velocity
c is the speed of sound in blood
(θ) is the angle of incidence between the sound source and the motion
This equation can be rearranged to determine velocity of blood flow:

$$V = \Delta f / \cos(\theta) \times c/2f_t$$

The second part of the equation is essentially a constant, and $\cos(\theta)$ is assumed to be 1 (the ultrasound is parallel to the blood flow), leaving only the frequency of reflected ultrasound to be measured. The frequency is measured continuously, permitting a continuous velocity signal; the velocity–time integral (or mean velocity times duration of ejection) is multiplied by the cross-sectional area of the vessel to determine the stroke volume [14] (Fig. 2). The two most important limitations are the ability to obtain a good view or signal with which to measure velocity and the ability to obtain a view parallel to the blood flow. The latter is very important, as $\cos(\theta)$ is assumed to be one. As the angle increases above 20°, a large error is introduced.

Cardiac output can be measured using the Doppler principle and technique with an echocardiography probe and machine, using views that permit directing the ultrasound signal parallel or nearly parallel to the blood flow. With transthoracic echocardiography, the window to the heart is the suprasternal notch such that flow in the descending aorta may be measured. With transesophageal echocardiography, the midesophageal views of the pulmonary artery or the transgastric long axis view of the ascending aorta may be used. Using the latter view, Perrino and colleagues described the use of transesophageal echocardiography (TEE) to measure cardiac output during cardiac surgery, finding a good correlation with thermodilution [15,16]. Perrino also presented a very lucid description of the use of Doppler techniques in his recent coauthored textbook [17]. An advantage to the echocardiography approach is the ability to measure the cross-sectional area of the vessel

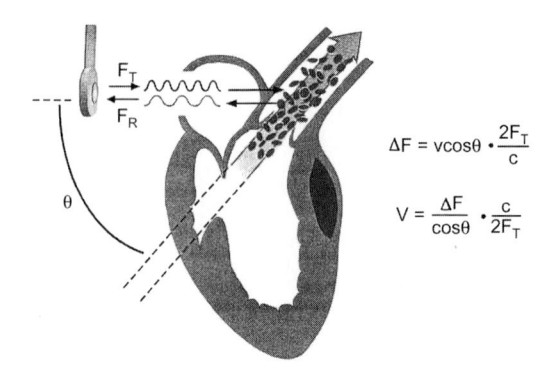

Fig. 2. Physiologic and mathematical basis of the Doppler equation. The Doppler equation calculates blood flow velocity based on two variables: the Doppler frequency shift (*delta* F) and the cosine of the angle of incidence between the ultrasound beam and the blood flow. The Doppler frequency shift is measured by the echocardigraphic system (either proprietary esophageal monitor or echocardiography machine) but cosine *theta* is unknown, and in proprietary devices, it is assumed to be 1. V = blood flow velocity; F_T = transmitted signal frequency; F_R = reflected signal frequency; delta F = difference between F_R and F_T; c = speed of sound in tissue; *theta* = angle of incidence between the orientation of the ultrasound beam and that of the blood flow. To calculate stroke volume, the velocity–time integral (continuous velocity signal) is multiplied by the cross-sectional area of the blood vessel, either measured or assumed from a nomogram. (*Reproduced and text modified from* Perrino AC. Doppler technology and technique. In: Perrino AC Jr, Reeves ST, editors. A practical approach to transesophageal echocardiography. Philadelphia: Lippincott Williams and Wilkins; 2003. p. 77–93; with permission.)

being studied at the same time, rather than using a nomogram. The main disadvantages are the need for echocardiography skill (and a machine) and the inability to obtain adequate images in some patients, regardless of view.

Two manufacturers have produced esophageal Doppler devices that measure the velocity signal in the descending aorta. In both cases, flow in the great vessels above the site of measurement is accounted for using a correction factor based on patient size, age, and sex. With one of the devices where the Doppler probe is disposable probe (Deltex Cardio Q monitor, Deltex Medical, Chichester United Kingdom), a nomogram is used to determine aortic cross-sectional area. With the other (Arrow Hemosonic monitor, Arrow International, Reading, Pennsylvania), a reusable probe with a sterile sleeve permits measurement of the diameter of the aorta using ultrasound. Numerous studies have been published over the last 10 years with these monitors, and recent reviews have compared noninvasive techniques [18,19] and compared the esophageal Doppler with thermodilution [20]. The overview of these studies appears to be that values obtained with these dedicated esophageal monitors correlate better with changes in cardiac output measured by other techniques, especially thermodilution, than with absolute values. In the recent comparative study by Bajorat and colleagues [13], the speed and accuracy of the Hemosonic monitor was good, provided a good signal could be obtained. Although placement of a probe in the esophagus is noninvasive compared with placing a catheter in a blood vessel, it is somewhat invasive. A significant drawback is the need to have a stable velocity signal. Small changes in probe position, which can occur spontaneously or with any patient movement, can result in a change or loss of signal, making it less useful in awake patients.

Pulse contour analysis technique

The pulse contour technique of measuring cardiac output relies on the principle that the arterial pressure waveform is related to the stroke volume. This originally was described by Frank and colleagues in 1930 [21] and has been studied with varied success ever since. A recent publication describing a novel time-averaged approach to this technique reviews the traditional Windkessel model of the circulation, which is the underlying principle of arterial waveform analysis [22] (Fig. 3).

Although it is possible to obtain an arterial waveform with noninvasive monitors, pulse contour cardiac output devices currently available require an invasive arterial waveform. In addition, two of the three require an external calibration with a known cardiac output. One relies on lithium indicator dilution (PulseCO, LiDCO Limited, Cambridge, United Kingdom), where the radial artery lithium concentration is measured after a venous injection of lithium. The other is calibrated with a transpulmonary thermodilution

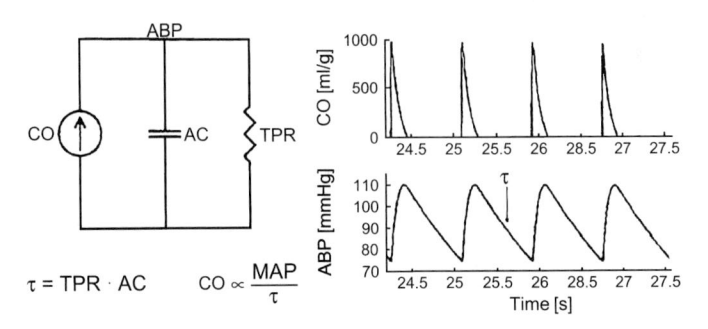

Fig. 3. A mathematical model for deriving cardiac output from an arterial pressure waveform. According to the "Windkessel" model, which assumes Ohm's law (described for electrical circuits) applies to the circulation (*left*), ABP should decay like a pure exponential during each diastolic interval with a time constant (T) equal to the product of the TPR and the nearly constant AC. Thus, an exponential is fitted to the diastolic interval of each ABP pulse to determine T (*right*) and the time-averaged ABP (MAP) is divided by T to estimate proportional CO. Newer arterial waveform analysis techniques may use significant modifications of this equation or different equations altogether. *Abbreviations:* ABP, arterial blood pressure; AC, arterial system compliance; MAP, mean arterial pressure; TPR, total peripheral resistance. (*Reproduced and text modified from* Mukkamala R, Reisner H, Hojman M, et al. Continuous cardiac output monitoring by peripheral blood pressure waveform analysis. IEEE Trans Biomed Eng 2006: 53:459–67; with permission. © Copyright 2006 IEEE.)

technique (PiCCO, Pulsion Medical Systems, Munich, Germany), where a central venous injection of cold or room temperature injectate is sensed by a thermistor-tipped catheter placed in the femoral artery. Both the lithium indicator dilution and transpulmonary thermodilution techniques (ie, the calibration techniques for the noninvasive pulse contour) have been shown to correlate well with standard thermodilution. Neither of these pulse contour techniques is truly noninvasive; however, they do not require a pulmonary artery catheter. The third and most recently introduced technique (Flotrac, Edwards Lifesciences LLC, Irvine, California) does not require external calibration, but it has not been compared adequately with other techniques to warrant conclusions regarding reliability or clinical utility.

Although all techniques of pulse contour analysis use the arterial waveform, just how the waveform is analyzed differs significantly. In the case of PulseCO, a proprietary algorithm uses beat duration, ejection duration, mean arterial pressure, and the modulus and phase of the first waveform harmonic in order compute beat-to-beat stroke volume [23]. Both this latter publication and a more recent independent evaluation of this system in 22 postoperative patients showed the pulse contour analysis to compare well with lithium indicator dilution [24]. Certain patient populations cannot be analyzed adequately with this technique, including those on lithium therapy and patients with significant cardiac dysrhythmias, severe aortic incompetence, or a poor arterial waveform. Calibrations with lithium indicator dilution are recommended every 8 hours; if done more frequently, serum lithium levels may interfere with the calibration. A major advantage of the PulseCO system is that the calibration with lithium can be done with a peripheral venous catheter; it therefore only requires the peripheral venous catheter and radial arterial catheter.

The PiCCO system uses a more traditional Windkessel model for waveform analysis [25]. The proprietary algorithm was revised recently to take into account the shape of the systolic portion of the arterial waveform [26]. Earlier studies with this system showed a fair correlation with thermodilution [27,28]; in patients after cardiac surgery, the new algorithm correlated well with thermodilution during changes in preload [26]. Both long radial artery catheters [29] and brachial artery catheters [30] appear to be acceptable alternatives to femoral artery catheters for the transpulmonary thermodilution calibrations. In addition to providing stroke volume and CO, this system can be used to calculate extravascular lung volume.

The most recent entry into the field of pulse contour cardiac output analysis is the Flotrac sensor, with a general description available in one review publication [31]. The product information available from the manufacturer states the proprietary algorithm takes into account the pulse pressure, known determinants of arterial system compliance (such as age, sex, and body surface area), and other undefined aspects of the arterial waveform to calculate stroke volume without the need for external calibration. There are no clinical comparison or validation studies other than abstracts. A different, novel time-averaged technique for analysis of the arterial pressure waveform briefly referred to previously [22] appears to have the potential to not require external calibration, but there are no commercial devices.

Bioimpedance

Cardiac output measurement by thoracic bioimpedance analysis was described in 1966 by Kubicek and colleagues, with a potential application to study cardiovascular effects of flight [32]. When a small alternating current is applied to the thorax by means of electrodes on the neck and lower thoracic area, there is a change in impedance of the thoracic cavity,

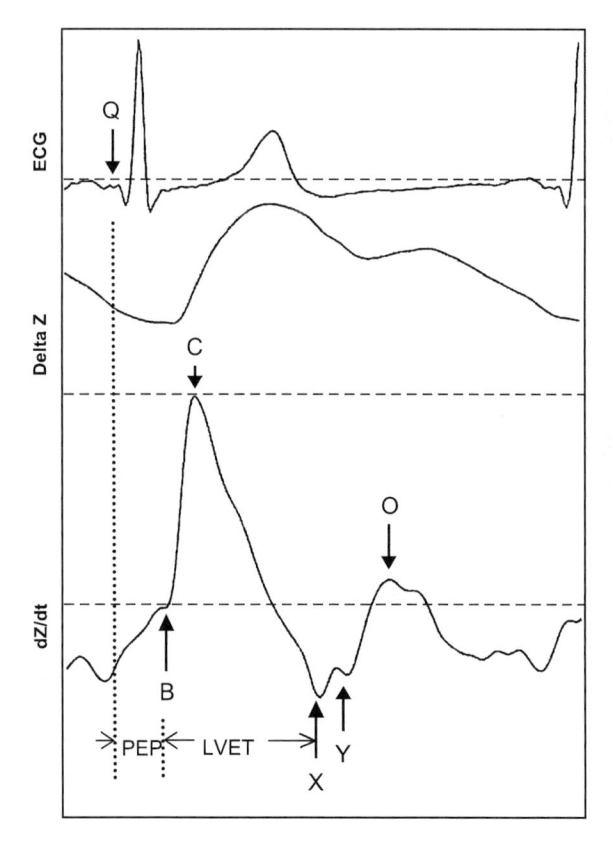

Fig. 4. Thoracic impedance (*Delta* Z) and the first derivative of impedance (dZ/dt) from a bioimpedance monitor. The velocity index describes the maximum deflection of the first derivative of the impedance (C point); the pre-ejection period (PEP) is measured from ventricular depolarization (Q point) to aortic valve opening (B point) to aortic valve closure (X point). The equation used to derive stroke volume is given in the text. (*Reproduced from and text modified from* Packer M, Abraham WT, Mehra MR, et al. Utility of impedance cardiography for the identification of short-term risk of clinical decompensation in stable patients with chronic heart failure. J Am Coll Cardiol 2006:47:2245–52; with permission. © Copyright 2006 American College of Cardiology Foundation.)

as fluid is ejected by the heart as shown in Fig. 4. The thoracic impedance value is processed to obtain the first derivative of impedance, and with these values, the stroke volume is calculated as follows:

$$\text{Stroke Volume} = p(L^2/Z_o^2) \times (DZ)_{max}(RVET)$$

where: $p(L^2/Z_o^2)$ is the conversion from ohm-seconds to milliliters
P = blood conductivity
L = length of conducting material
Z_o = steady state impedance
DZ_{max} is the maximum change in impedance with time
RVET is right ventricular ejection time

Over the last 40 years, numerous mathematical techniques have been used to modify this basic equation, and to derive cardiac-related parameters, including ventricular ejection time and stroke volume. There are at least two devices available for clinical use (BioZ ICG monitor, Cardiodynamics, San Diego, California, and Aesculon Electrical Velocimetry, Ospyka Medical GmbH, Berlin, Germany). Although there has been some enthusiasm expressed for this technique, a recent meta-analysis concluded that correlation with thermodilution, especially in patients with cardiac pathology, was not acceptable in the publications before 1999 [33]. Revisions to the analysis techniques continue to be described. In two studies in cardiac surgical patients, the correlation with thermodilution appears to be more acceptable, using the most recent analysis techniques of impedance obtained from the

Table 1
Less invasive cardiac output measurement techniques

Technique	Invasiveness	Limitations
Partial rebreathing indirect Fick	Requires intubated patient	Measures nonshunted pulmonary blood flow; requires stable respiratory pattern
Doppler flow	Esophageal probe required	Patient needs to be immobile; user experience provides best results; probe may need repositioning; nomogram used for aortic diameter (1 of 2 devices)
Arterial waveform analysis	Requires arterial catheter; one technique requires central line	Two of three available devices require calibration with other CO technique; one of three devices very new (no calibration needed)
Bioimpedance	Truly noninvasive (surface electrodes)	Pre-1999 studies suggest only modest correlation with thermodilution; new algorithms may be better

current monitors [34–36]. Novel approaches to bioimpedance continue to appear, such as incorporating electrodes into an endotracheal tube rather than on the thoracic chest wall [37].

Although the limitations of bioimpedance in critically ill patients and those who have severe cardiopulmonary pathology have been described, there has been significant interest from the cardiology community in using this technique to follow outpatients who have cardiac disease. A recent report by Packer and colleagues [38] found that use of impedance-derived parameters (they used parameters other than cardiac output) in heart failure patients was helpful in identifying those at risk for decompensation.

Summary

As outlined in Table 1, the nonthermodilution techniques available to measure cardiac output are noninvasive and clinically applicable to a variable degree. The truly noninvasive monitors are bioimpedance and CO_2 rebreathing. The latter, however, requires the patient to be intubated, and the former continues to be evaluated with regard to correlation with the thermodilution standard. Esophageal Doppler devices are relatively noninvasive in that they do not require vascular cannulation, but they do require an immobile patient and some user expertise. Pulse contour analysis requires an arterial catheter, and two of the three available monitors require external calibration, while the third has not been validated adequately. The reader can see that all four approaches continue to be refined, with new analysis algorithms and monitors continuing to appear on the market. In the absence of true tissue oxygenation monitors, it seems likely that some or all of these alternatives to thermodilution will play a greater role in the care of patients where measurement of cardiac output is desired.

References

[1] Lima A, Bakker J. Noninvasive monitoring of peripheral perfusion. Intensive Care Med 2005;31:1316–26.
[2] Maciel AT, Creteur J, Vincent JL. Tissue capnometry: does the answer lie under the tongue? Intensive Care Med 2004;30:2157–65.
[3] Botero M, Kirby D, Lobato EB, et al. Measurement of cardiac output before and after cardiopulmonary bypass: comparison among aortic transit-time ultrasound, thermodilution, and noninvasive partial CO_2 rebreathing. J Cardiothorac Vasc Anesth 2004;18: 563–72.
[4] Jansen JR. The thermodilution method for the clinical assessment of cardiac output. Intensive Care Med 1995;21:691–7.
[5] Thrush DN, Varolotta D. Thermodilution cardiac output: comparison between automated and manual injection of indicator. J Cardiothorac Vasc Anesth 1992;6:17–9.
[6] Guyton AC, Jones CE, Coleman TG. Circulatory physiology: cardiac output and its regulation. 2nd edition. Philadelphia: WB Saunders; 1973. p. 21–5.
[7] Capek JM, Roy RJ. Noninvasive measurement of cardiac output using partial CO_2 rebreathing. IEEE Trans Biomed Eng 1988;35:653–61.

[8] de Abreu MG, Quintel M, Ragaller M, et al. Partial carbon dioxide rebreathing: a reliable technique for noninvasive measurement of nonshunted pulmonary capillary blood flow. Crit Care Med 1997;25:675–83.
[9] de Abreu MG, Geiger S, Winkler T, et al. Evaluation of a new device for noninvasive measurement of nonshunted pulmonary capillary blood flow in patients with acute lung injury. Intensive Care Med 2002;28:318–23.
[10] Tachibana K, Imanaka H, Takuechi M, et al. Noninvasive cardiac output measurement using partial carbon dioxide rebreathing is less accurate at settings of reduced minute ventilation and when spontaneous breathing is present. Anesthesiology 2003;98:830–7.
[11] Valiatti JL, Amaral JL. Comparison between cardiac output values measured by thermodilution and partial carbon dioxide rebreathing in patients with acute lung injury. Sao Paulo Med J 2004;122:233–8.
[12] Levy RJ, Chiavacci RM, Nicolson SC, et al. An evaluation of a noninvasive cardiac output measurement using partial carbon dioxide rebreathing in children. Anesth Analg 2004;99:1642–7.
[13] Bajorat J, Hofmockel R, Vagts DA, et al. Comparison of invasive and less-invasive techniques of cardiac output measurement under different haemodynamic conditions in a pig model. Eur J Anaesthesiol 2006;23:23–30.
[14] Singer M, Clarke J, Bennett ED. Continuous hemodynamic monitoring by esophageal Doppler. Crit Care Med 1989;17:447–52.
[15] Perrino AC, Harris SN, Luther MA. Intraoperative determination of cardiac output using multi-plane transoesphageal echocardiography: a comparison to thermodilution. Anesthesiology 1998;89:350–7.
[16] Gray PE, Perrino AC. Hemodynamic-induced changes in aortic valve area: implications for Doppler cardiac output determinations. Anesth Analg 2001;92:584–9.
[17] Perrino AC. Doppler technology and technique. In: Perrino ACJR, Reeves ST, editors. A practical approach to transesophageal echocardiography. Philadelphia: Lippincott Williams and Wilkins; 2003. p. 77–93.
[18] Chaney JC, Derdak S. Minimally invasive hemodynamic monitoring for the intensivist: current and emerging technology. Crit Care Med 2002;30:2338–45.
[19] Laupland KB, Bands CJ. Utility of esophageal Doppler as a minimally invasive hemodynamic monitor: a review. Can J Anaesthesiol 2002;49:393–401.
[20] Dark PM, Singer M. The validity of transesophageal Doppler ultrasonography as a measure of cardiac output in critically ill adults. Intensive Care Med 2004;30:2060–6.
[21] Frank O. Wellen-und Windkesselthrorie (Estimation of the stroke volume of the human heart using the Windkessel theory). Zeitschrift Fur Biologie 1930;90:405–9.
[22] Mukkamala R, Reisner H, Hojman HM, et al. Continuous cardiac output monitoring by peripheral blood pressure waveform analysis. IEEE Trans Biomed Eng 2006;53:459–67.
[23] Linton NW, Linton RA. Estimation of changes in cardiac output from the arterial blood pressure waveform in the upper limb. Br J Anaesth 2001;86:486–96.
[24] Pittman J, Gar-Yosef S, SumPing J, et al. Continuous cardiac output monitoring with pulse contour analysis: a comparison with lithium indicator dilution cardiac output measurement. Crit Care Med 2005;33:2015–21.
[25] Wesseling KH, Jansen JR, Settels JJ, et al. Computation of aortic flow from pressure in humans using a non-linear, three-element model. J Appl Physiol 1993;74:2566–73.
[26] Felbinger TW, Reuter DA, Eltzschig HK, et al. Comparison of pulmonary arterial thermodilution and arterial pulse contour analysis: evaluation of a new algorithm. J Clin Anesth 2002;14:296–301.
[27] Della Rocca G, Costa MG, Pompei L, et al. Continuous and intermittent cardiac output measurement: pulmonary artery catheter versus aortic transpulmonary technique. Br J Anaesth 2002;88:350–6.
[28] Della Rocca G, Costa MG, Coccia C, et al. Cardiac output monitoring: aortic transpulmonary thermodilution and pulse contour analysis agree with standard thermodilution methods in patients undergoing lung transplantation. Can J Anaesthesiol 2003;50:707–11.

[29] Orme RM, Pigott DW, Mihm FG. Measurement of cardiac output by transpulmonary arterial thermodilution using a long radial artery catheter. A comparison with intermittent pulmonary artery thermodilution. Anaesthesia 2004;59:590–4.
[30] Wouters PF, Quaghebeur B, Sergeant P, et al. Cardiac output monitoring using a brachial arterial catheter during off-pump coronary artery bypass grafting. J Cardiothorac Vasc Anesth 2005;19:160–4.
[31] Manecke GR. Edwards FloTrac sensor and Vigileo monitor: easy, accurate, reliable cardiac output assessment using the arterial pulse wave. Expert Rev Med Devices 2005;2:523–7.
[32] Kubicek WG, Karnegis JN, Patterson RP, et al. Development and evaluation of an impedance cardiac output system. Aerosp Med 1966;37:1208–12.
[33] Raaijmakers E, Faes TJ, Scholten RJ, et al. A meta-analysis of three decades of validating thoracic impedance cardiography. Crit Care Med 1999;27:1203–13.
[34] Schmidt C, Theilmeier G, VanAken H, et al. Comparison of electrical velocimetry and transoesophageal Doppler echocardiography for measuring stroke volume and cardiac output. Br J Anaesth 2005;95:603–10.
[35] Bernstein DP, Lemmens HJ. Stroke volume equation for impedance cardiography. Med Biol Eng Comput 2005;43:443–50.
[36] Van de Water JM, Miller TW, Vogel RL, et al. Impedance cardiography; the next vital sign technology. Chest 2003;123:2028–33.
[37] Wallace AW, Salahieh A, Lawrence A, et al. Endotracheal cardiac output monitor. Anesthesiology 2000;92:178–89.
[38] Packer M, Abraham WT, Mehra MR, et al. Utility of impedance cardiography for the identification of short-term risk of clinical decompensation in stable patients with chronic heart failure. J Am Coll Cardiol 2006;47:2245–52.

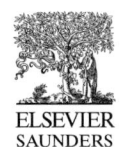

Monitoring of the Brain and Spinal Cord

Leslie C. Jameson, MD*, Tod B. Sloan, MD, MBA, PhD

University of Colorado at Denver and Health Sciences Center, Campus Box B113, 4200 East 9th Avenue, Denver, CO 80262, USA

Over the last 30 years, intraoperative neurophysiologic monitoring (IOM) of the brain and spinal cord has become an established technique to provide functional neurologic assessment during axial skeletal, head and neck, spinal cord, and some intracranial procedures. IOM techniques have been developed to assess neuronal electrophysiology (eg, electroencephalogram, evoked potentials, and electromyography), blood flow (eg, cerebral blood flow and transcranial Doppler ultrasonography), oxygenation (eg, cerebral oximetry), and even neural tissue pH values (eg, intraparenchymal electrodes). Changing surgical techniques and the necessity to prevent new injuries or prevent exacerbation of existing neurologic injury have driven refinement and innovation. This article focuses on the commonly used intraoperative monitoring modalities: somatosensory evoked potentials (SSEP); motor evoked potential (MEP), electromyography (EMG), and brain stem auditory evoked responses (BAER). An anesthesiologist with an in-depth understanding of these techniques effectively assists the surgeon and monitoring physician in assuring the patient who has neural risk that he/she will have the best possible outcome.

In many centers, IOM has become common, as surgeons have recognized that these techniques enhance their intraoperative decision making. Studies have shown improved outcome in specific surgical procedures making IOM a key component of the surgical technique. For example, facial nerve monitoring during acoustic neuroma resection unequivocally reduces long-term postoperative facial nerve injury, leading to an improved quality of life and reduction in subsequent medical costs [1]. Longitudinal studies comparing outcomes of patients having IOM with retrospective non-IOM controls have been used to meet evidence-based principles [2]. As such, IOM has

---

* Corresponding author.
E-mail address: leslie.jameson@uchsc.edu (L.C. Jameson).

become a standard of care in axial skeletal [2–4], head and neck [5], base of skull, and posterior fossa surgeries [6,7]. It also is being explored for use during intracranial aneurysm clipping, tumor resection [8–10], and hip arthroplasty [11].

Somatosensory evoked potential

The most commonly used electrophysiologic technique to monitor functional continuity of nerve, spinal cord, and brain is SSEP. In this technique, a mixed motor/sensory nerve is stimulated, thus initiating sensory and motor transmissions that are recorded as muscle contractions (twitch) or an averaged electroencephalogram (EEG) response recorded from the scalp over sensory cortex. Although any mixed motor sensory nerve can be used, in practical terms the nerves stimulated tend to be large and superficial, such as median (C_6-T_1), ulnar (C_8-T_1), common peroneal (L_4-S_1), and posterior tibial (L_4-S_2) [3,12,13].

The length of the neural tract involved makes the SSEP potentially one of the most widely applicable monitoring techniques; peripheral nerves, brachial or lumbosacral plexus, spinal cord tracts, brainstem structures, and sensory cortex can be assessed independently. It is thought that the incoming volley of neural activity from the upper extremity represents primarily the activity in the pathway of proprioception and vibration (Fig. 1). Stimulation of the peripheral nerve causes a response that ascends the ipsilateral dorsal column, has synapses near the nucleatus cuneatus, decussates near the cervico–medullary junction, ascends by means of the contralateral medial lemniscus, has synapses in the ventroposterolateral nucleus of the thalamus, and finally projects to the contralateral parietal sensory cortex [3]. The neural pathway from the lower extremity is similar to the upper extremity except that a portion of the lower extremity response appears to travel by means of antero–lateral spinocerebellar pathways.

Intraoperative use of the SSEP primarily includes surgical procedures where spinal cord injury is recognized, and unfortunately, can be a frequent devastating complication. Axial skeletal surgery for scoliosis in teenagers and degenerative spine disease in older adults are by far the most commonly monitored surgical procedures. Other examples of procedures in which SSEP monitoring has been used are shown in Table 1. As will be discussed later, the SSEP often is combined with other forms of monitoring (especially electromyography and MEPs).

The use of the SSEP in spine surgery is supported by several basic studies in animals, which indicate that changes in the cortical amplitude of the somatosensory evoked response from hind limb stimulation correlates with loss of sensory and motor function during spine distraction [14,15]. Changes in axial skeletal and therefore spinal cord configuration during surgical manipulation can cause simultaneous changes in sensory and motor pathways.

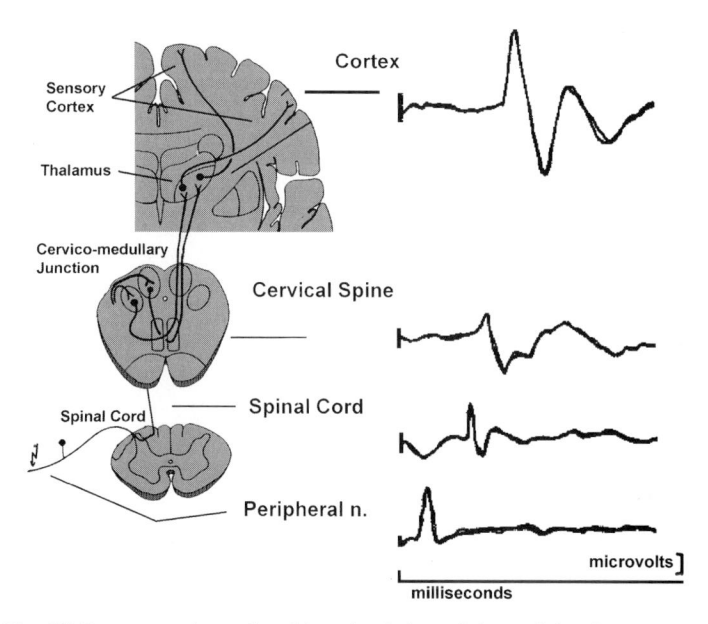

Fig. 1. The SSEP response is produced by stimulation of the peripheral nerve (*arrow*). The response in the nerve can be recorded (shown is a response recorded at the popliteal fossa from posterior tibial nerve stimulation). The response that ascends through the dorsal spinal columns and can be recorded epidurally over the cervical spine and over the sensory cortex.

The value of the SSEP in human surgery has been documented by the Scoliosis Research Society (SRS) and the European Spinal Deformities Society. These organizations reviewed over 51,000 surgical cases and noted that the overall injury rate was 0.55% (1 in 182 cases), well below the rate of 0.7% to 4% reported in spine surgery with instrumentation when SSEP monitoring was not used. These organizations concluded that "these results confirm the clinical efficacy of SSEP spinal cord monitoring" by an experienced IOM team to reduce neurologic injury [16]. The SRS issued a position statement that concluded "neurophysiological monitoring can assist in the early detection of (potential) complications and possibly prevent postoperative morbidity in patients undergoing operations on the spine" [13]. Such statements made SSEP monitoring during scoliosis correction a virtual standard of care. IOM has become common in many different types of axial skeletal and spinal cord surgery. A 1995 survey of US surgeons confirmed that 88% of surgeons used SSEP in over 50% of their spinal surgery cases [13].The changes seen during spine distraction are related to change in spinal cord perfusion, either from direct cord compression, or disruption of the arterial blood supply [3].

The SSEP has been used for many other types of surgery where neural function is placed at risk. For example, it has been used during dorsal root entry zone lesioning (DREZ) [17]. During these procedures, the

Table 1
Surgical procedure and recommended IOM and anesthetic regimen

Surgery	Somatosensory evoked potential	Motor evoked potential	Electromyography Free run	Electromyography Stimulated	Brain stem auditory evoked responses	Volatile	Intravenous anesthesia	Neuromuscular blockade
Spine skeletal								
Cervical	●	●					●	No
Thoracic	●	●					●	No
Lumbar instrumentation			●	●		●		No
Lumbar disc			●	●		●		No
Head and neck								
Parotid			●	●		●		No
Radical neck			●	●		●		No
Thyroid			●	●		●		No
Cochlear implant			●	●		●		No
Mastoid			●	●		●		No
Neurosurgery								
Spine								
Vascular	●	●					●	No
Tumor	●	●					●	No
Posterior fossa								
Acoustic neuroma	●	⊞	●	●	●	●		No
Cerebellopontine	●	●	●	●	⊞		●	No
Vascular					⊞		●	No
Supratentorial								
MCA aneurysm	●	●					●	No
Tumor motor cortex	●	●					●	No
Orthopedic joint								
Hip, knee, shoulder	●		●			●		No

SSEP can be used to identify the optimal location of the desired lesioning, thereby helping to avoid unwanted spinal cord injury. Resection of a spinal cord tumor can be directed by SSEP response to surgical action.

The value of the SSEP is not isolated to the spinal column. For example, the SSEP technique has been considered indispensable for intraoperative evaluation and monitoring during surgical procedures on peripheral nerves and plexus regions. In addition to detecting surgical misadventure caused by change in the axial skeleton, SSEP monitoring can detect potential nerve injury related to positioning, usually a stretch or pressure injury. Ulnar nerve injury, thought to be as high as 4.8% in the prone position, can be detected by recording the response to ulnar nerve stimulation in the wrist or forearm. Direct stimulation of nerves allows identification of residual function through damaged nerves (neuroma in continuity) and identification of a preganglionic or postganglionic injury in plexus lesions; this allows selective and focused repair. The SSEP technique has the capacity to detect neural continuity in some situations in which the clinical examination is not possible, or in which function may be insufficient to allow an accurate clinical examination [18].

SSEP monitoring is used frequently during surgery on the posterior fossa to assess the integrity of the brainstem. When combined with other techniques (notably auditory and cranial nerve monitoring) the safety of these procedures can be increased. The SSEP also has been used during supratentorial neurosurgery. In general, monitoring is most effective when used for localization of the sensory strip by recording the cortical component (N_{20}) of the median nerve SSEP. Bipolar recording strips placed on the cortex identify the gyrus separating the motor and sensory strip (rolandic fissure) through the location of a phase reversal of the response [19,20].

The SSEP also has been effective for assessing the viability of specific neural pathways (particularly identification of ischemia). Like EEG, SSEP remains normal until cortical blood flow is reduced to about 20 cc/min/100 g and is altered and then lost at blood flows between 15 and 18 cc/min/100 g, levels above those associated with irreversible cell death. Thus during axial surgery, SSEP monitoring can identify hypoperfusion caused by deliberate hypotension or anemia from hemodilution before permanent injury. Levels of hypotension or anemia not usually associated with injury may in a specific individual cause neuron damage and permanent injury if not corrected [21].

Similarly, SSEP is useful during carotid endarterectomy and neurovascular surgery (eg, intracranial arteriovenous malformation, intracranial aneurysm surgery, and interventional neuroradiological procedures) to detect hypoperfusion. Studies have shown that the SSEP abnormality correlates with clinical outcome and serum S-100B protein indicative of cell damage [22,23]. Combinations of surgical actions (eg, retractor pressure, hypotension, temporary clipping, and hyperventilation) can combine to produce neuron ischemia. For example, evoked potentials have been used to minimize cortical injury from retractor pressure. Such injuries are estimated to occur in 5% of intracranial aneurysm procedures and 10% of cranial base procedures. In the postoperative period, monitoring also can be used to identify ischemia from vasospasm after subarachnoid hemorrhage from aneurysm rupture or hemorrhagic stroke [6].

With respect to anesthesia, the cortical SSEP is depressed; amplitude is decreased, and there is increased latency in a dose-dependent manner by inhalational agents. It can be obtained, however, in most patients with 0.5 minimum alveolar concentration (MAC) of a volatile anesthetic supplemented by intravenous medications, usually narcotics or intravenous hypnotics. Intravenous agents also can be used; etomidate and ketamine have been shown to increase rather than decrease cortical amplitude. Complete muscle relaxation may improve the responses recorded near muscles (such as over the cervical spine); however, relaxation may not be acceptable if EMG or motor evoked potentials also are being performed. Total intravenous anesthesia (TIVA), most commonly a propofol/narcotic infusion, maintains or minimally decreases cortical responses. Thus in patients with significant preoperative neurologic findings or requiring additional IOM studies, TIVA may be required to allow effective monitoring [24,25].

Although the SSEP has an excellent track record of detecting reversible injury during spine and intracranial surgery, it often is combined with other monitoring techniques to focus the attention on structures not monitored by the SSEP (eg, the motor pathways and nerve pathways not included in the SSEP pathways). Finally, it is important to note that in the view of some surgeons, anesthesiologists, and IOM physicians, intraoperative wake-up test remains the gold standard and is recommended by some for confirming possible injury when the monitoring techniques become persistently abnormal during a surgical procedure [26].

Motor evoked potentials

Despite reports of improved outcomes obtained with SSEP monitoring, case reports of isolated motor injury with normal sensory function appeared, making it clear that a means to separately monitor motor function was needed. This is a consequence of the topographic locations of the sensory (posterior) and motor tracts (anterior) in the spinal cord and the difference in blood supply to these pathways.

The blood supply to the motor tracts consists of a single anterior spinal artery that continues from the foramen magnum to the filum terminate and is supplied by 5 to 10 radicular arteries. The anterior spinal artery supplies 75% of the cord including the descending motor tracts. The paucity of arterial supply in the anterior cord produces watershed areas, particularly in the thoracic spine. The anterior circulation supplies neurons and synapses that are more sensitive to hypoperfusion injury (eg, anemia, hypotension, blood vessel compression) than the posterior cord. The posterior spinal arteries provide relatively luxuriant flow to the posterior cord. Each vertebral body supplies the posterior vessels [27]. In the intracranial circulation, blood flow through the lenticulostriate vessels from the middle cerebral artery into the internal capsule again creates a watershed area making motor function more vulnerable to hypoperfusion than the ascending sensory tracts. MEP provides unique information about the functional status of the anterior spinal cord and internal capsule [9,10,28].

MEP requires direct stimulation of the motor cortex [29]. Transcranial stimulation can be achieved by either focused magnetic or electrical energy. This produces EMG responses through the motor pathway (Fig. 2). Cortical pyramidal cells are activated directly (producing descending D waves) or indirectly (producing descending I waves). Waves can travel down the spinal axonal motor pathways and be monitored with epidural electrodes. These responses temporally summate at the anterior horn cells and produce a peripheral nerve response that activates a compound muscle action potential, the more commonly used EMG response using needle pairs near the muscles [30].

Current techniques in IOM nearly exclusively use electrical stimulation (tceMEP). Between four and six (interstimulus interval 2.0 m seconds) transcranial electrical stimuli of 150 to 400 V each are administered through

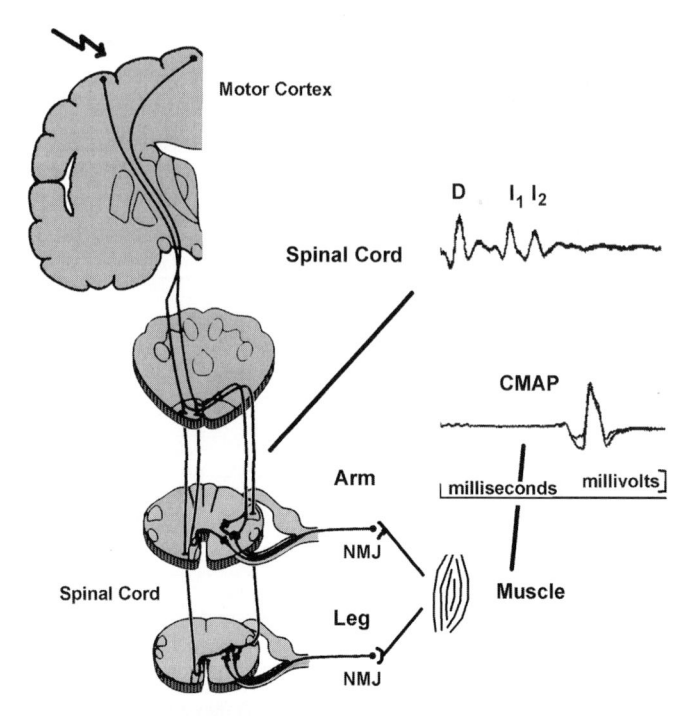

Fig. 2. Motor evoked potentials are produced by stimulation of the motor cortex (*arrow*). The response can be recorded epidurally over the spinal column as a D wave followed by a series of I waves. The pathway synapses in the anterior horn of the spinal cord and the response travel to the muscle by means of the neuromuscular junction (NMJ). The response typically is recorded near the muscle as a compound muscle action potential (CMAP).

corkscrew electrodes over the motor cortex. A compound muscle action potential (CMAP) is recorded in the upper (eg, abductor pollicis brevis) and lower (eg, tibialis anterior and lateral gastronomies) extremity muscles with either surface or needle electrodes [31]. The surgeon is notified before tceMEP stimulation. In the past, stimulation of the spinal cord with either epidural electrodes or percutaneous needles has been used. Other recording techniques that allow complete neuromuscular blockade have included spinal stimulation with epidural recording electrodes or compound nerve action potentials (CNAP). Both techniques primarily monitor antidromic sensory responses and are not specific for motor pathway monitoring. They should not be confused with a true MEP [29].

Developing standardized criteria for significant tceMEP change has proven difficult because of the large variability in response even in normal awake subjects, a situation that is magnified during general anesthesia. TIVA using propofol or propofol/ketamine mixture plus narcotic usually is used to obtain stable reproducible tceMEP. Exposure to volatile anesthetics significantly reduces amplitude or eliminates tceMEP (Fig. 3) [24,32,33]. Benzodiazepines, etomidate, barbiturates, and even high-dose propofol decrease the probability of generating a tceMEP. Only ketamine decreases the threshold for the MEP response [24,34]. Neuromuscular-blocking drugs must be avoided or their

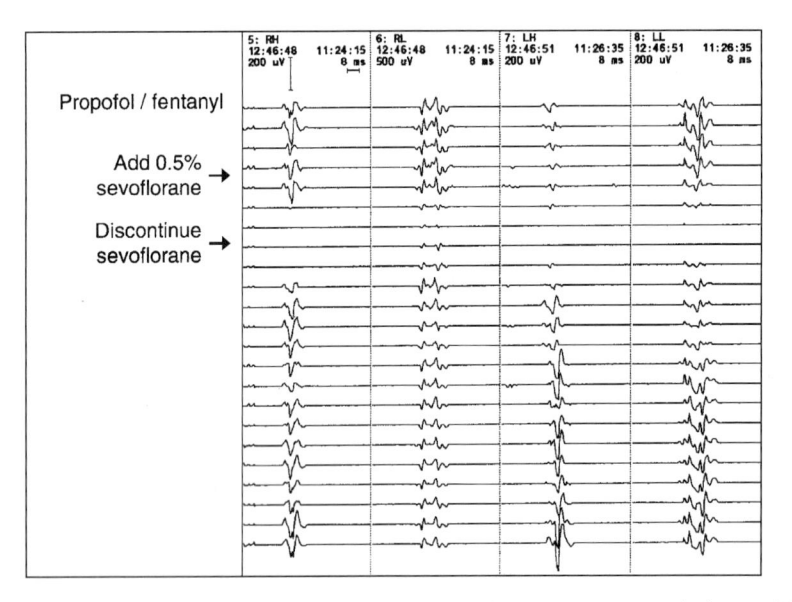

Fig. 3. The effect of the administration of 0.5% of sevoflurane on motor evoked potentials. Traces are generated by three pulse transcranial electrical stimulation with response recorded in tibialis anterior and thenar muscles. (*Adapted from* MacDonald DB, Al Zayed Z, Khoudeir I, et al. Monitoring scoliosis surgery with combined multiple pulse transcranial electric motor and cortical somatosensory-evoked potentials from the lower and upper extremities. Spine 2003;28:194–203; with permission.)

effects very carefully monitored to guarantee EMG change is not caused by neuromuscular blockade. TIVA anesthesia, multiple stimuli, and a stimulus voltage limited to 400V have been reported to produce a tceMEP in 92% of patients. Failures were related to pre-existing neurologic disorders (1.9%) or equipment difficulties [31].

In addition to the difficulties with anesthetic management, concerns about safety may have contributed to the reluctance to use tceMEP. In a 2002 survey of the literature, published complications included: tongue laceration (n = 29), cardiac arrhythmia (n = 5), scalp burn at the site of stimulating electrodes (n = 2), jaw fracture (n = 1), and awareness (n = 1). Concerns about neuropsychiatric effects, headaches, and endocrine abnormalities have not been reported. Common relative tceMEP contraindications include epilepsy, cortex lesion, skull defects, high intracranial pressure, intracranial apparatus (electrodes, vascular clips, and shunts), and cardiac pacemakers or other implanted pumps. The effect of these relative contraindications on outcome is unknown. The absolute number and the incidence of even minor complications are low [35].

The most frequent use of tceMEP is in corrective axial skeletal surgery. Two recent studies [33,36] examined tceMEP effect on spine surgery outcome and reported a high correlation with outcome. In the largest study, 11.3% had tceMEP change; in the five patients with permanent tceMEP change, all had partial permanent neurologic injury [36]. In cervical spine surgery, tceMEP, used as a standard of care, is believed to decrease morbidity [37], in part because it may allow differentiation between cervical cord myelopathy from peripheral neuropathy [38].

Use of tceMEP in intracranial surgery can be divided into two categories, vascular lesions and parenchymal lesions. Direct motor cortex stimulation [9] has been used successfully to define the edge of motor cortex tumors. Reversible change usually was associated with transient postoperative motor weakness. Irreversible tceMEP change was associated with permanent disabling paresis. These results correlated with earlier studies that found the degree of tceMEP change correlated with degree of postoperative paresis [39]. Similar correlation of tceMEP with outcome has been seen with aneurysm clipping in the basilar, carotid, and middle cerebral circulations.

Electromyography

EMG provides useful information in a large array of surgical situations (see Table 1), posterior fossa, head and neck, spine, and major joint replacement surgery. EMG is monitored by placing two electrodes near or in a muscle, then displaying the electrical activity generated by muscle contraction. The response also may be converted to sound. Monitoring is conducted as passive, free-running EMG, where continuous activity is observed and recorded, or stimulated EMG, where an electrical stimulus is applied to a nerve and the response recorded. EMG has proven particularly effective in identifying nerves such as those encased in tumor (eg, acoustic neuroma) or scar (eg, repeat spine surgery). EMG electrodes may record activity of only 1% to 2% of the muscle fibers in a given muscle. For example, the monitored response in the tibialis anterior with 270,000 muscle fibers is generated by only 18 to 34 muscle fibers [40]. The most commonly monitored nerves are cervical (C2-7), lumbosacral (L2-S2), facial (posterior fossa), and recurrent laryngeal (vocal cords) (Table 2).

Patterns of EMG activity represent mechanisms of reversible injury (Fig. 4). A normal EMG during light general anesthesia has low-amplitude, high-frequency activity. As the depth of anesthesia increases, the amplitude approaches zero. Deep general anesthesia, however, can increase the difficulty in generating a spontaneous or stimulated response [40], thus reducing test sensitivity. Fortunately, this is rarely a problem, and the anesthesiologist only must avoid the use of nondepolarizing muscle relaxants during the procedure.

Abnormal EMG activity is described as burst or neurotonic activity. A burst is short asynchronous polyphasic wave caused by abrupt direct nerve trauma, tugging, stretch, or fluid irrigation. Modifying the surgical activity allows burst activity to immediately resolve with little chance for permanent injury. Neurotonic activity is a prolonged repetitive series of synchronous discharges that can last many minutes to hours. Neurotonic activity is associated with significant stretch or compression by retractors or surgical position (eg, spine distraction, or dural tear with nerve rootlet

Table 2
Nerve roots and muscles most commonly monitored

Nerve		Muscle
Spinal cord		
Cervical	C 2-4	Trapezoids, sternocleidomastoid
	C 5, 6	Biceps, deltoid
	C 6, 7	Flexor carpi radialis
Thoracic	C 8-T 1	Adductor pollicis
	T 2-6	Specific intercostals
	T 5-12	Specific area rectus abdominus
Lumbar	L 2	Adductor longus
	L 2-4	Vastus medialis
Sacral	L 4-S 1	Tibialis anterior
	L 5-S 1	Peroneus longus
	S 1-2	Gastrocnemius
	S 2-4	Anal sphincter
Cranial nerves		
	III, IV, VI	Ocular muscles
	V	Masseter
	VII	Obicularis oculi, oris; mentalis temporalis
	IX	Pharyngeal muscles
	X	Vocal cords
	XI	Trapezius, sternocleidomastoid
	XII	Tongue

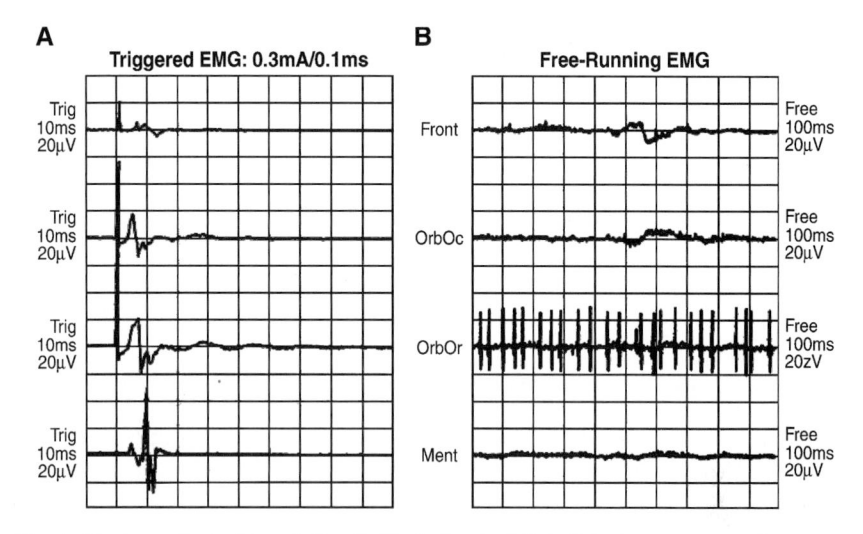

Fig. 4. Electromyelographic activity of obicularis oris. (*A*) Activity in response to direct nerve stimulation. (*B*) Spontaneous activity, including neurotonic discharges associated with nerve injury. (*Adapted from* Edwards BM, Kileny PR. Intraoperative neurophysiologic monitoring: indications and techniques for common procedures in otolaryngology–head and neck surgery. Otolaryngol Clin North Am 2005;38:631–42; with permission.)

herniation). Here prompt action is necessary, or postoperative damage likely will lead to motor dysfunction (motor fibers) or chronic postoperative pain syndromes (sensory fibers) [5,41].

Otolaryngologists and neurosurgeons were early adopters of cranial nerve EMG as a standard of care for facial nerve during resection of acoustic neuromas (vestibular schwannoma) and cerebellopontine angle tumors. Free-running EMG and stimulated EMG of the obicularis oculi, obicularis oris, mentalis, and temporalis muscles are used to warn of injury, identify the facial nerve, and predict long-term function. Facial nerve monitoring (FNM) is considered the standard of care by the National Institutes of Health, American Association of Neurological Surgeons, and the American Academy of Otolaryngology [5].

Other procedures where EMG monitoring has become local standard of care include radical neck (c.n. VII, X, XI), thyroid (c.n. X), parotid (c.n. VII), auditory implant procedures (c.n. VII), and base of skull procedures (c.n. III, IV, VI, IX, X, XI, XII). In microvascular decompression for hemifacial spasm and trigeminal neuralgia, intraoperative stimulation of c.n. VII and V both before and after moving the offending vessel has led to more accurate identification of the offending vessel with better postoperative results [5,7]. Similarly, free-running EMG monitoring has been used to guide lower extremity limb lengthening and avoid sciatic nerve injury during hip arthroplasty [11].

EMG also has been used extensively to identify when a pedicle screw breaches or fractures the pedicle during spine instrumentation. This can help prevent chronic irritation of the dorsal root ganglion; this can lead to postoperative radicular pain and unstable fixation. In large studies, the frequency of incorrect pedicle screw placement is about 5% to 6%. EMG activity following stimulation of the pedicle screw (PSS) is more effective (94%) than fluoroscopy 63% and palpation alone 11% [40]. Generally, PSS with EMG response greater than 16 mA suggests the screw is within the pedicle, and a response less than 10 mA suggests fracture of the pedicle. Response less than 6 mA suggests direct contact with the dorsal nerve root, and a response less than 5mA suggests an unstable screw [42].

Brainstem auditory evoked potentials

BAER is produced by stimulating the cochlea with clicks and recording the brainstem response. BAER monitoring is used to assess c.n. VIII function during acoustic neuroma and cerebellopontine tumor resection, microvascular decompression of cranial nerves VII and V, and vertebral and basilar artery aneurysm clipping. It also helps assess brainstem function in comatose patients. Five distinct BAER waves are described, with waves I, III and V usually being used for monitoring (Table 3) [43]. Several studies have shown improved hearing outcome in patients with good hearing before surgery [44]. Small case series have reported that BAER can detect hypoperfusion of the brainstem or cochlea during aneurysm clipping or retraction of the cerebellum [43]. Fortunately, the impact of general anesthetic drugs on BAER response is small.

Impact of monitoring on the anesthesiologist

Providing adequate IOM monitoring conditions relies on the knowledge and adaptability of the anesthesiologist. Physiological factors within the anesthesiologist's control help define the health of the neural tracts (ie, maintaining stable perfusion, eg, adequate blood pressure and O_2 delivery). During pediatric spine procedures, extremes of hypotension and reductions in hemoglobin/hematocrit have been reported as safe. Most management protocols in children call for moderate reductions in BP and oxygen

Table 3
Anatomic generators of brainstem auditory evoked potentials

Wave	Generator	Functional indication
I	Auditory nerve	Cochlea and VIII nerve intact
II	Cochlear nucleus	Stimulus received; relayed to contralateral nucleus
III	Pons	Signal received from ipsi- and contralateral nucleus
V	Mesencephalon	Signal received from ipsi- and contralateral pons
I-III latency		Cochlea and nerve function
III-V latency		Brainstem function

carrying capacity (hemodilution). Adults may be less tolerant of these ranges. When changes in IOM occur, increasing BP, confirming normal laboratory values and reviewing anesthetic management can prove critical in improving patient outcome by correcting a critical abnormality and providing critical information in the decision to change surgical technique [24,25].

The appropriate choice of the type and depth of anesthesia allow the IOM provider to associate waveforms' change with surgical activity. Developing an effective anesthesia plan requires knowledge of which specific IOM modalities are being performed during a surgical procedure. Volatile anesthetics depress evoked responses in a dose-dependent manner, with BAER being very resistant to change and MEP being often unobtainable with their use. TIVA, propofol, with or without ketamine, and narcotics provide stable general anesthetic and optimize all IOM studies. EMG is resistant to all hypnotic and analgesic agents. Muscle relaxants should be avoided, or their effect very carefully monitored to maintain two or more twitches during train-of-four neuromuscular stimulation (see Table 1) [24,32] .

Summary

IOM has become commonly used by many surgeons to enhance their intraoperative decision making and reduce the morbidity and mortality of selected procedures. The ability to perform these tests rests on the anesthesiologist's ability to provide the patient with an anesthetic plan that provides comfort and monitoring. When events occur, the anesthesiologist's knowledge and ability to manipulate the patient's physiologic condition become integral to the decision making. A good understanding of the neural anatomy, impact of physiology, and anesthetic medications can allow effective IOM and good team decision making when changes in IOM occur.

References

[1] Wilson L, Lin E, Lalwani A. Cost-effectiveness of intraoperative facial nerve monitoring in middle ear or mastoid surgery. Laryngoscope 2003;113:1736–45.
[2] Forbes HJ, Allen PW, Waller CS, et al. Spinal cord monitoring in scoliosis surgery. Experience with 1168 cases. J Bone Joint Surg Br 1991;45:759–63.
[3] Toleikis JR. Intraoperative monitoring using somatosensory evoked potentials. A position statement by the American Society of Neurophysiological Monitoring. J Clin Monit Comput 2005;19:241–58.
[4] Padberg AM, Wilson-Holden TJ, Lenke LG, et al. Somatosensory and motor-evoked potential monitoring without a wake-up test during iddiopathic scoliosis surgery: An accepted standard of care. Spine 1998;23:1392–400.
[5] Edwards BM, Kileny PR. Intraoperative neurophysiologic monitoring: indications and techniques for common procedures in otolaryngology-head and neck surgery. Otolaryngol Clin North Am 2005;38:631–42.
[6] Freye E. Cerebral monitoring in the operating room and the intensive care unit - an introductory for the clinician and a guide for the novice wanting to open a window to the brain. Part II: sensory-evoked potentials (SSEP, AEP, VEP). J Clin Monit Comput 2005;19:77–168.

[7] Mooij JJ, Mustafa MK, van Weerden TW. Hemifacial spasm: intraoperative electromyographic monitoring as a guide for microvascular decompression. Neurosurgery 2001;49:1365–70 [discussion 1370–1].
[8] Quinones-Hinojosa A, Alam M, Lyon R. Transcranial motor evoked potentials during basilar artery aneurysm surgery: technique application for 30 consecutive patients. Neurosurgery 2004;54:916–24.
[9] Neuloh G, Schramm J. Motor evoked potential monitoring for the surgery of brain tumors and vascular malformations. Adv Tech Stand Neurosurg 2004;29:171–228.
[10] Neuloh G, Schramm J. Monitoring of motor evoked potentials compared with somatosensory evoked potentials and microvascular Doppler ultrasonography in cerebral aneurysm surgery. J Neurosurg 2004;100:389–99.
[11] Brown DM, McGinnis WC, Mesghali H. Neurophysiologic intraoperative monitoring during revision total hip arthroplasty. J Bone Joint Surg Am 2002;84-A(Suppl 2):56–61.
[12] Nuwer MR, Dawson EG. Intraoperative evoked potential monitoring of the spinal cord: enhanced stability of cortical recordings. Electroencephalogr Clin Neurophysiol 1984;59:318–27.
[13] Nuwer MR, Dawson EG, Carlson LG, et al. Somatosensory evoked potential spinal cord monitoring reduces neurologic deficits after scoliosis surgery: results of a large multi-center survey. Electroencephalogr Clin Neurophysiol 1995;96:6–11.
[14] Jones SJ, Edgar MA, Ransford AO, et al. A system for the electrophysiological monitoring of the spinal cord during operations for scoliosis. J Bone Joint Surg Br 1983;65:134–9.
[15] Nordwall A, Axelgaard J, Harada Y, et al. Spinal cord monitoring using evoked potentials recorded from feline vertebral bone. Spine 1979;4:486–94.
[16] Dawson EG, Sherman JE, Kanim LE, et al. Spinal cord monitoring. Results of the Scoliosis Research Society and the European Spinal Deformity Society survey. Spine 1991;16(Suppl 8):S361–4.
[17] Friedman WA. Somatosensory evoked potentials in neurosurgery. Clin Neurosurg 1988;34:187–238.
[18] Labrom RD, Hoskins M, Reilly CW, et al. Clinical usefulness of somatosensory evoked potentials for detection of brachial plexopathy secondary to malpositioning in scoliosis surgery. Spine 2005;30(18):2089–93.
[19] Hacke W, Zeumer H, Berg-Dammer E. Monitoring of hemispheric or brainstem functions with neurophysiologic methods during interventional neuroradiology. AJNR Am J Neuroradiol 1983;4:382–4.
[20] Emerson RG, Turner CA. Monitoring during supratentorial surgery. J Clin Neurophysiol 1993;10:404–11.
[21] Horiuchi K, Suzuki K, Sasaki T, et al. Intraoperative monitoring of blood flow insufficiency during surgery of middle cerebral artery aneurysms. J Neurosurg 2005;103:275–83.
[22] Schick U, Dohnert J, Meyer JJ, et al. Prognostic significance of SSEP, BAEP and serum S-100B monitoring after aneurysm surgery. Acta Neurol Scand 2003;108:161–9.
[23] Manninen P, Sarjeant R, Joshi M. Posterior tibial nerve and median nerve somatosensory evoked potential monitoring during carotid endarterectomy. Can J Anaesth 2004;51:937–41.
[24] Banoub M, Tetzlaff JE, Schubert A. Pharmacologic and physiologic influences affecting sensory evoked potentials. Anesthesiology 2003;99:716–37.
[25] Sloan TB, Heyer EJ. Anesthesia for intraoperative neurophysiologic monitoring of the spinal cord. J Clin Neurophysiol 2002;19:430–43.
[26] Papastefanou SL, Henderson LM, Smith NJ, et al. Surface electrode somatosensory-evoked potentials in spinal surgery: implications for indications and practice. Spine 2000;25:2467–72.
[27] Gillilan L. The arterial blood supply of the human spinal cord. J Comp Neurol 2004;110:75–103.

[28] Sakuma J, Suzuki K, Sasaki T, et al. Monitoring and preventing blood flow insufficiency due to clip rotation after the treatment of internal carotid artery aneurysms. J Neurosurg 2004; 100:960–2.
[29] Toleikis J, Skelly JP, Carlvin AO, et al. Spinally elicited peripheral nerve responses are sensory rather than motor. Clin Neurophysiol 2000;111:736–42.
[30] Deletis V. Intraoperative monitoring of the functional integrity of the motor pathways. Adv Neurol 1993;63:201–14.
[31] Legatt AD. Current practice of motor evoked potential monitoring: Results of a survey. J Clin Neurophysiol 2002;19:454–60.
[32] Sloan T. Evoked potentials. Anesthesia and motor evoked potentials monitoring. In: D V, S J, editors. Neurophysiology in neurosurgery. San Diego (CA): Academic Press; 2002. p. 451–74.
[33] MacDonald DB, Al Zayed Z, Khoudeir I, et al. Monitoring scoliosis surgery with combined multiple pulse transcranial electric motor and cortical somatosensory-evoked potentials from the lower and upper extremities. Spine 2003;28:194–203.
[34] Inoue S, Kawaguchi M, Kakimoto M, et al. Amplitude and intrapatient variability of myogenic motor evoked potentials to transcranial electrical stimulation during ketamine/N_2O- and propofol/N_2O-based anesthesia. J Neurosurg Anesthesiol 2002;14:213–7.
[35] MacDonald DB. Safety of intraoperative transcranial electrical stimulation motor evoked potential monitoring. J Clin Neurophysiol 2002;19:416–29.
[36] Langeloo DD, Lelivelt A, Louis Journee H, et al. Transcranial electrical motor evoked potential monitoring during surgery for spinal deformity: a study of 145 patients. Spine 2003;28(10):1043–50.
[37] Freedman B, Potter B, Kuklo T. Managing neurologic complications in cervical spine surgery. Current Opinion in Orthopedics, 2005. 16(3): p. 169–177.
[38] Chistyakov AV, Soustiel JF, Hafner H, et al. The value of motor and somatosensory evoked potentials in evaluation of cervical myelopathy in the presence of peripheral neuropathy. Spine 2004;29:e239–47.
[39] Zhou HH, Kelly PJ. Transcranial electrical motor evoked potential monitoring for brain tumor resection. Neurosurgery 2001;48:1075–81.
[40] Leppanen R. Intraoperative monitoring of segmental spinal nerve root function with free-run and electrically triggered electromyography and spinal cord function with reflexes and f-responses. A position statement by the American Society of Neurophysiological Monitoring. J Clin Monit Comput 2005;19:437–61.
[41] Holland NR. Intraoperative electromyography. J Clin Neurophysiol 2002;19(5):444–53.
[42] Danesh-Clough T, Taylor P, Hodgson B, et al. The use of evoked EMG in detecting misplaced thoracolumbar pedicle screws. Spine 2001;26:1313–6.
[43] Legatt AD. Mechanisms of intraoperative brainstem auditory evoked potential changes. J Clin Neurophysiol 2002;19:396–408.
[44] Tonn JC, Schlake HP, Goldbrunner R, et al. Acoustic neuroma surgery as an interdisciplinary approach: a neurosurgical series of 508 patients [see comment]. J Neurol Neurosurg Psychiatry 2000;69:161–6.

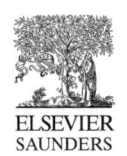

Depth of Anesthesia Monitoring

T. Andrew Bowdle, MD, PhD

Division of Cardiothoracic Anesthesiology, Department of Anesthesiology, Mail Stop 356540, Room AA-117C, University of Washington, Seattle, WA 98195, USA

Anesthetic drug effects have traditionally been measured by the observation of heart rate, blood pressure, breathing pattern, and the presence or absence of movement. While these are useful measures, the cardiopulmonary effects of anesthetics are side effects, rather than direct indicators of the sedative and hypnotic effects, which are the main reason that anesthetics are given in the first place. Clearly, patients can experience intraoperative awareness in the absence of clinical signs of light anesthesia, such as changes in heart rate or blood pressure, or even movement. Therefore, a more direct and reliable method of measuring anesthetic drug effects on the brain is highly desirable and has been the object of research for many years. Electroencephalography (EEG) is an obvious brain monitoring modality because it is noninvasive and continuous. Many anesthetic drugs produce characteristic effects on the EEG, and these have been extensively studied. However, efforts to use EEG monitoring as a real-time clinical tool were not successful until relatively recently. The development of relatively inexpensive, fast microcomputers was a critical prerequisite [1].

The first product available for routine intraoperative EEG monitoring of anesthetic depth was produced by Aspect Medical Systems (Newton, Massachusetts) and given the name BIS from bispectral analysis, which is part of the algorithm used to interpret the EEG. The US Food and Drug Administration in 1996 approved the BIS sensor. By 2001, 4 million patients had been monitored. BIS is by far the most extensively used and studied depth-of-anesthesia monitor, and necessarily much of the material in this article concerns the BIS product (A search of PubMed for the term "bispectral index" yielded 852 citations at the time this article was created). The Aspect Medical Systems website (www.aspectmedical.com) provides access to bibliographies, educational material and technical information. There are several

E-mail address: bowdle@u.washington.edu

other depth-of-anesthesia monitors now available and these will also be described to the extent that information is available.

The BIS algorithm

The cortical EEG of a normal, awake subject is characterized by fast, low-amplitude activity. The administration of most, but not all, anesthetic drugs initially results in increased amplitude, followed at larger doses by decreased frequency and increased regularity, and finally, at very deep levels, periods of isoelectric (flat) EEG interspersed with bursts of undulating EEG activity (burst suppression). There are some individual differences in the EEG effects of various anesthetic drugs that will be discussed elsewhere in this article. The BIS algorithm (or similar algorithms for other EEG-based depth-of-anesthesia monitors) uses a statistical process to analyze the EEG and compute an index on a linear scale from 0 to 100, where 0 is an isoelectric EEG. The algorithm is empirical and is not based upon a physical law or a simple equation. The main variables incorporated in the algorithm are the frequency and power spectrum of the EEG, the amount of burst suppression, and the degree of synchronization of the EEG.

Synchronization is another effect of anesthetics on the EEG. The complex raw EEG waveform is made up of several underlying sine-wave components. When the sine waves are consistently in phase with each other, the EEG may be described as synchronized. Anesthetics tend to increase the degree of synchronization. Quantifying synchronization requires the analysis of the phase relationships of the component sine waves, in addition to measurements of the amplitude and frequency of the waveforms. Bispectral analysis is a mathematical technique used by the BIS monitor to analyze the degree of synchronization of the EEG. The details of the BIS algorithm have been partially described in the literature [2].

Clinical validation

The BIS index is a number from 0 to 100. A variety of clinical studies were performed to validate the index and define the relationship to clinical end-points [3–9]. The probability of explicit recall decreases dramatically below a BIS index of 70, and below 60 the probability of explicit recall becomes extremely small. At BIS index values below 40, the index is determined primarily by the degree of "suppression" or isoelectricity of the EEG. The BIS index values correlate to the reduction in cerebral metabolic rate measured from positron emission tomographic scanning during administration of hypnotic drugs [10].

Numerous studies have shown that the use of the BIS index to guide the administration of anesthetic drug results in administration, on average, of less anesthetic drug [11]. While few patients experience intraoperative awareness because of inadequate anesthesia, the vast majority of patients tend to receive more than enough anesthetic when anesthesia is administered without the guidance of depth-of-anesthesia monitoring. When average anesthetic doses are adjusted downward with the guidance of depth-of-anesthesia monitoring, the result tends to be faster wake-up and recovery from anesthesia. Liu and colleagues [11] recently performed a meta-analysis of 11 randomized controlled trials of BIS monitoring for ambulatory surgery, comprising 1380 patients. They found that the use of BIS monitoring reduced anesthetic consumption by 19%, reduced the incidence of nausea and vomiting to 32% from 38%, and reduced recovery room stay by 4 minutes.

Movement

Surgeons generally do not want their patients to move during surgery and every anesthesiologist has heard the refrain "the patient is waking up" from the surgical team when the patient has moved. Interestingly, movement during surgery is only rarely associated with truly "waking up" since movement is common and intraoperative awareness is relatively rare. Case reports of intraoperative awareness also show that intraoperative awareness is not necessarily associated with movement, even in patients who have not received neuromuscular blocking drugs [12]. Clearly, movement and hypnosis are not closely linked, and there is a physiological basis for considering these properties of a general anesthetic as being somewhat distinct. Considerable evidence suggests that immobility during anesthesia is related primarily to anesthetic effects in the spinal cord, while hypnosis occurs in the brain [13,14]. Rampil measured isoflurane minimum alveolar concentration (MAC) (effective dose 50% for movement) in rats before and after surgical decerebration and found that MAC was unchanged by removal of cortical and forebrain structures [15]. Antognini [16,17] devised a goat model in which isoflurane could be delivered selectively to the brain or to the entire body. Isoflurane MAC was twice as large when only the brain received isoflurane, as when isoflurane was administered to the entire body [17]. Halothane MAC was over three times larger when administered only to the brain [16]. Some goats moved despite EEG isoelectricity.

Not surprisingly, EEG analysis is not a particularly good way to measure the effects of anesthetic drugs on the spinal cord, and is not a particularly reliable method for predicting whether patients will move during surgery. Sebel and colleagues [6] investigated the relationship between BIS index values and movement in response to skin incision in a multicenter study in which each of seven centers used a different anesthetic technique. For the center that used isoflurane as the only anesthetic agent, there was a sigmoid-shaped relationship between the probability of movement and the BIS index, with a 50% probability of movement corresponding to a BIS of 40

(Fig. 1). This is consistent with the notion that the spinal cord, rather than the brain, is primarily responsible for movement during anesthesia, since a BIS index of 40 corresponds to a relatively deep level of hypnosis. For the other six centers in which varying amounts of opioid were combined with isoflurane, propofol, or nitrous oxide, the probability of movement at a BIS of 40 was reduced to around 10% or less, with one center having no movement at all, and the relationship between the BIS index and probability of movement was relatively weak. Clearly, opioids strongly inhibit movement during anesthesia, probably at sites in the spinal cord. Valjus and colleagues [18] found a similar result when they compared the effects of remifentanil or esmolol during a propofol and nitrous-oxide anesthetic in which the state entropy (a method of EEG interpretation; see below) was held constant at 50 ± 5 (similar to a BIS of 50). All of the patients in the esmolol group moved in response to surgical stimulation, while none of the patients in the remifentanil group moved.

The drugs behind the number

Opioids have an interesting and complex effect on the interpretation of the EEG. Opioids given by themselves have relatively weak hypnotic effects, although large doses of opioids will produce unconsciousness [19]. Likewise, smaller doses of opioids have relatively weak effects on the EEG, but larger

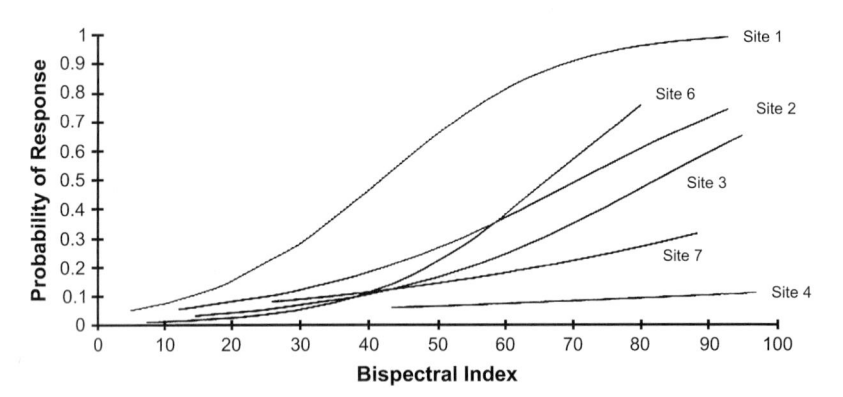

Fig. 1. The probability of movement in response to a surgical stimulus versus BIS index (bispectral index) for seven centers in a multicenter study. Each center employed a different anesthetic technique, and variable amounts of opioid were used. When isoflurane was the sole anesthetic agent, there was a sigmoid-shaped relationship with a probability of movement of about 50% at a BIS index of 40 (*Site 1*). For the other six centers in which varying amounts of opioid were combined with isoflurane, propofol, or nitrous oxide, the probability of movement at a BIS index of 40 was reduced to around 10% or less. Site 5 had no movement in response to a surgical stimulus, thus, a relationship to BIS could not be determined. (*From* Sebel PS, Lang E, Rampil IJ, et al. A multicenter study of bispectral electroencephalogram analysis for monitoring anesthetic effect. Anesth Analg 1997;84:896; with permission.)

doses produce dramatic EEG slowing [19]. When opioids are combined with typical hypnotic drugs, such as propofol, there is a synergistic effect that dramatically strengthens the anesthetic effect of the combination of drugs [20]. In addition, opioids are particularly effective at preventing movement in response to a stimulus. This effectiveness is not necessarily reflected in the EEG since the effects are mostly subcortical. Bouillon and colleagues [20] studied the effects of the combination of remifentanil and propofol on the BIS index, entropy, responsiveness to laryngoscopy, and hypnosis. They found that small amounts of remifentanil dramatically reduced the amount of propofol needed to prevent responsiveness. Pharmacodynamic modeling suggested that for various proportions of propofol and remifentanil, all of which achieve 95% effectiveness for preventing responsiveness, BIS or entropy index values would be lower for combinations containing a relatively larger proportion of propofol (Fig. 2) [20]. This is the expected result, since the doses of remifentanil used have relatively small effects on the EEG. This is an important finding with clinical implications. A depth-of-anesthesia monitoring index value has to be interpreted in the context of the drugs that have been given to produce it. Anesthetic regimens containing opioids are likely to produce less-responsive patients at any given monitoring index value, compared with anesthetic regimens containing no opioids or lesser amounts of opioids. The study of Valjus and colleagues [18], described previously, provides a dramatic example of this principal. At a constant entropy index value of 50, patients receiving remifentanil did not move during surgery, while all patients receiving esmolol instead of remifentanil moved in response to surgical stimulus.

Another way of looking at the relationship between depth-of-anesthesia index values and anesthetic drugs is to realize that no EEG patterns are pathognomonic for a particular drug-induced state. Natural sleep is an extreme example of the need to interpret index values in the context of which drugs have been given. The EEG during natural sleep may resemble the EEG during anesthesia and depth-of-anesthesia index values will decline during natural sleep [21]. The response of a sleeping person to a surgical stimulus is entirely different from the response of a person under general anesthesia, yet the depth-of-anesthesia index values before the surgical stimulus may be identical. A "box and a number" are not enough. The anesthesiologist must know what drugs have been used to produce a particular index value and how those drugs may affect the responses of the patient to surgical stimulation.

Muscle action potentials and other high-frequency artifacts

EEG signals are quite small and require substantial amplification. Muscle action potentials (recorded as the electromyogram [EMG]), 60-Hz noise from electrical equipment, noise from external pacemaker generators and

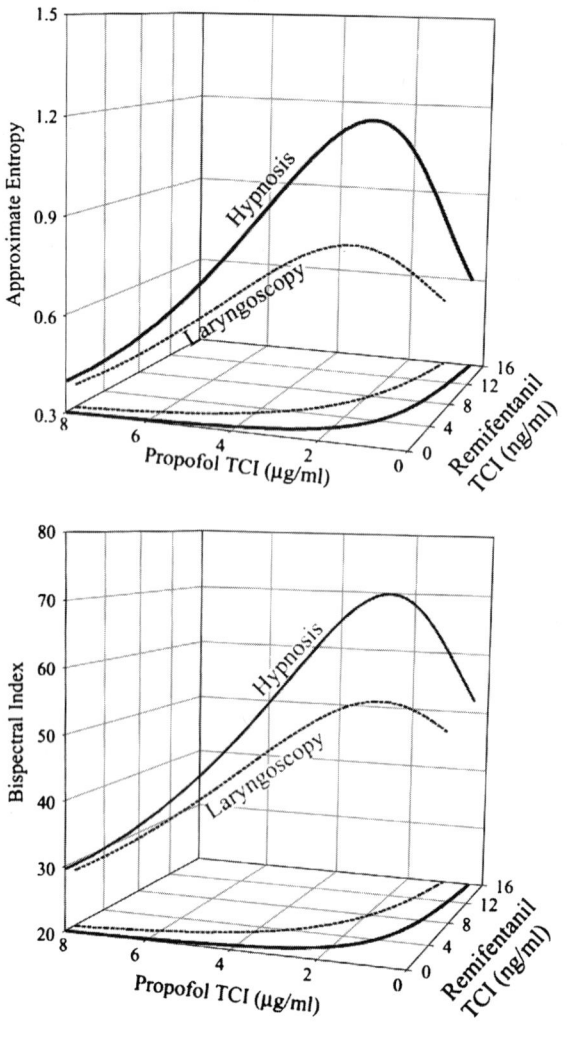

Fig. 2. Simulation of approximate entropy (*top*) and BIS index (*bottom*) values for equipotent combinations of propofol and remifentanil for 95% probability of no response to shouting and shaking (*solid lines*) and 95% probability of no response to laryngoscopy (*dashed lines*). Combinations containing relatively greater amounts of propofol and relatively lesser amounts of remifentanil result in a 95% probability of no response at lower values of entropy or BIS. TCI, target-controlled infusion. (*From* Bouillon TW, Bruhn J, Radulescu L, et al. Pharmacodynamic interaction between propofol and remifentanil regarding hypnosis, tolerance of laryngoscopy, bispectral index, and electroencephalographic approximate entropy. Anesthesiology 2004;100:1369; with permission.)

electrocautery can significantly contaminate the EEG signal. The EEG frequency spectrum ranges from about 0 to 30 Hz. EMG and other sources of high-frequency noise generally exceed 30 Hz but overlap significantly with the EEG spectrum and will cause spurious elevation of the depth-of-anesthesia index (Fig. 3). This could be prevented by aggressively filtering higher frequencies to eliminate EMG and other noise. However, such filtering may also filter important high-frequency EEG activity. Since the higher-frequency EEG activity is associated with wakefulness and lighter levels of anesthesia, filtering this activity could conceivably make a monitor less useful for avoiding intraoperative awareness.

The BIS monitor evaluates the presence of EMG or other high-frequency noise and lights up an EMG signal-strength indicator on the monitor screen to alert the user that the BIS index is likely to be spuriously elevated by high-frequency artifact. The onset of a BIS index value above the recommended range (eg, >60) and increased EMG activity may either represent truly light anesthesia with a BIS index value that is truly high, or it may represent increased EMG activity with a BIS index value that is not truly high but is spuriously elevated by the EMG activity. In this circumstance, if clinical judgment suggests the possibility of light anesthesia, it is prudent to administer additional anesthetic. Administration of a muscle relaxant (Usually only a small dose is required.) will usually eliminate the EMG activity and restore conditions for reliable EEG signal acquisition. The true BIS index value can then be ascertained. The BIS index value typically falls following administration of a muscle relaxant when an EMG artifact is present, since the EMG activity usually elevates the BIS index value.

While the main effect of muscle relaxants on BIS is to eliminate the EMG activity that may result in a spurious BIS value, there is also evidence that

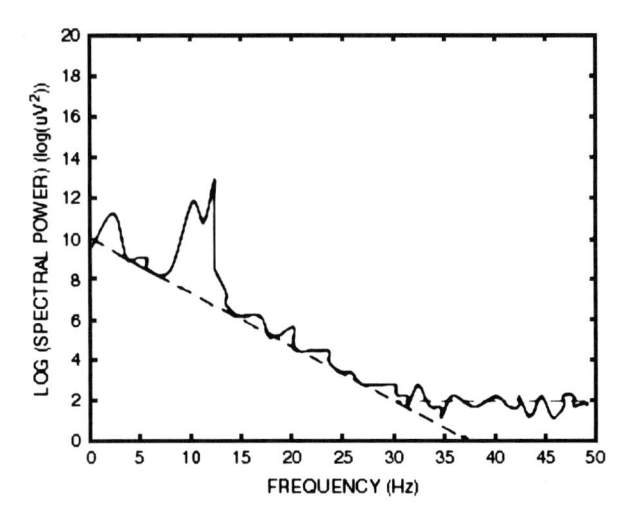

Fig. 3. The power spectrum (on a logarithmic scale) of a signal recorded from the forehead plotted against the frequency. EEG dominates the spectrum at frequencies <30 Hz (*sloping line*) while EMG dominates the spectrum at frequencies >30 Hz (*horizontal line*). (*From* Viertio-Oja H, Maja V, Sarkela M, et al. Description of the entropy algorithm as applied in the Datex–Ohmeda S/5 entropy module. Acta Anaesthesiol Scand 2004;48(2):157; with permission.)

some muscle relaxants may increase anesthetic depth, either by a deafferentation effect associated with muscle relaxation, or by direct action of the muscle relaxant or its metabolites in the brain. For example, pancuronium has been shown to reduce halothane dose requirement in humans [22] and to prolong the duration of EEG burst suppression in dogs anesthetized with isoflurane [23].

EMG artifacts in the EEG are by far the most common problem in interpreting the index values from depth-of-anesthesia monitors. Clinicians using these monitors have to be aware of the presence or absence of EMG activity at all times. EMG activity is particularly problematic when depth-of-anesthesia monitoring is used to evaluate the depth of sedation during procedural sedation or intensive care unit sedation [24,25]. Under those circumstances, EMG activity frequently prevents the computation of valid index values.

External cardiac-pacemaker generators (but not permanently implanted cardiac pacemakers), such as those used during cardiac surgery, frequently produce high-frequency artifacts that interfere with EEG interpretation, as has been noted in the literature [26]. In the author's experience, external cardiac pacing virtually always lights up the EMG signal-strength bar on the BIS monitor and elevates the BIS index. This can be easily confirmed by noting the change in EMG signal strength and BIS index when the pacemaker is turned on and off.

Low-amplitude EEG

EEG signals should be interpreted carefully when the EEG amplitude is unusually low. A low-amplitude signal can be discerned from observing the raw EEG, and is one of the reasons that display of the raw EEG signal is important. Low-amplitude EEG can occur congenitally, though this is rare [27], or can be acquired due to brain pathology or to edema of the scalp. In the author's experience, edema of the scalp due to third-space fluid accumulation during long surgical procedures is a relatively common cause of an acquired low-amplitude EEG signal. In the presence of a low-amplitude EEG signal, a low signal-to-noise ratio pertains, making the EEG interpretation more vulnerable to influence by high-frequency artifacts. The extreme example of this situation is a flat EEG, which should produce an index value of 0, but may produce a high index value because the monitor confuses high-frequency artifacts for EEG [28]. This can occur in brain-dead subjects and may create confusion during organ donation.

Anesthetic drugs that don't produce typical EEG effects

Depth-of-anesthesia monitoring using EEG interpretation depends upon incorporating the EEG effects of commonly used anesthetic drugs in a computer algorithm for analyzing the raw EEG and computing a depth-of-anesthesia index number. The algorithms have been devised using such drugs as propofol, midazolam, and isoflurane. However, not all anesthetic drugs are accounted for by the available algorithms. Nitrous oxide produces EEG effects that are distinct from the potent inhalational agents, and in most studies nitrous oxide has produced little or no change in BIS or entropy index values [29–32]. Since nitrous oxide is a relatively weak hypnotic, but a good analgesic, it can probably be thought of as having a role similar to opioids, which also have relatively little effect on the EEG (when given in smaller doses). Ketamine is an unusual intravenous anesthetic because it produces EEG activation, an increase in high-frequency activity in the EEG, which may elevate the BIS index or other EEG-derived indexes, depending upon the dose used [33–41]. Smaller doses of ketamine may not have a noticeable effect on the BIS index. The EEG effects of etomidate and dexmedetomidine have not been extensively studied, but the BIS index does appear to track the effects of these drugs [42–45]. Halothane produces greater amounts of high-frequency EEG activity, compared with the newer volatile anesthetic agents, and appears to produce a relatively higher BIS index value, compared with an equivalent dose (based on MAC) of sevoflurane, in adults and children, but not in infants [46,47].

Paradoxical delta activity

Occasionally during general anesthesia there will be a sudden onset of dramatic slowing in the EEG, with the appearance of high-amplitude slow (delta) waves, which is unexplained by the administration of anesthetic drugs or obvious changes in the condition of the patient. This has been termed "paradoxical slowing" or "paradoxical delta" [48,49]. The physiological explanation for this EEG phenomenon is not known. Depth-of-anesthesia monitor index values will decline under these circumstances because slow activity can also be produced by deep anesthesia. In the author's experience, these events are characterized by a sudden fall in the index with no obvious cause, accompanied by high-amplitude slow activity in the raw EEG, followed by a gradual (eg, 5–10 min) return to a higher index value that is more consistent with the clinical circumstances. Paradoxical slowing can be disconcerting when it takes place in a setting where cerebral ischemia is also a possible cause of EEG slowing, such as during cardiac surgery or cerebral vascular surgery, and can only be distinguished from cerebral ischemia with certainty in retrospect.

Anesthetic depth: the consequences of too much or too little

Definitions: implicit recall, explicit recall, and responsiveness

The word "unconsciousness" has frequently been used to describe general anesthesia, but there is currently no mechanistic, physiologic explanation of consciousness or unconsciousness. Sleep is often considered to be a form of unconsciousness, yet general anesthesia is clearly different from natural sleep. One practical means of testing for consciousness is to determine responsiveness, defined as the ability to follow commands. However, even responsiveness is ambiguous because when anesthetic drugs have been given, subjects may respond to command but have no recollection of doing so. Are these subjects conscious or unconsciousness? Only they know for sure and they aren't able to tell us. Interestingly, most anesthesiologists rarely test for responsiveness during an anesthetic. If we routinely test for responsiveness, we might be surprised to find that many of our patients were responsive, since responsiveness persists at much deeper levels of anesthesia than does explicit recall. While explicit recall becomes very uncommon at the BIS index range of 60 to 70, responsiveness may persist to a BIS index as low as 40 (Fig 4) [4]. Thus, from a practical standpoint, the success of a general anesthetic has to be determined afterwards by the absence of explicit recall. If the patient has no recollections, the anesthetic is considered adequate.

Evidence indicates that subjects having no explicit recall may nevertheless process information, particularly auditory information, during general anesthesia [50]. For example, subjects given test words during general anesthesia have been able to pick these words out from a list with greater than random accuracy, a process that has been called implicit recall [51]. Explicit recall is "things you know," while implicit recall is "things your brain knows that you don't." The clinical significance of implicit recall, if any, is unknown. Implicit recall may occur at depth-of-anesthesia index values well below

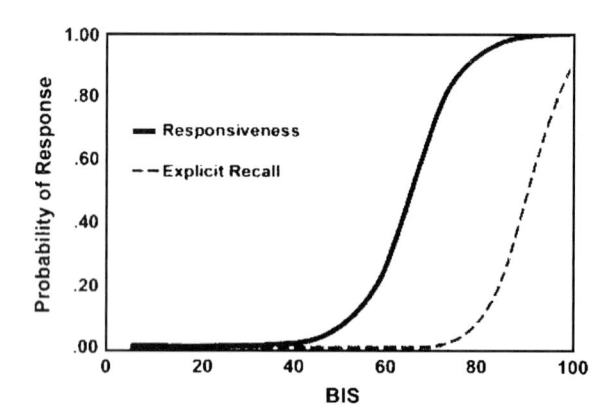

Fig. 4. Probability of responsiveness (to command) and explicit recall at various BIS index values. These are pooled data from volunteers who received either isoflurane, midazolam, or propofol. Note that responsiveness can occur at levels of the BIS index not associated with recall. (*Adapted from* Glass PS, Bloom M, Kearse L, et al. Bispectral analysis measures sedation and memory effects of propofol, midazolam, isoflurane, and alfentanil in healthy volunteers. Anesthesiology 1997;86:843; with permission.)

the levels associated with explicit recall (eg, implicit recall may occur at a BIS index value of 40, while explicit recall is likely only at BIS >70) [52]. Not all investigators have been able to replicate this phenomenon [53].

The consequences of too little: intraoperative awareness

For the purposes of this article, intraoperative awareness is defined as explicit recall that occurs during general anesthesia. The ability to recall the events afterwards is an essential feature of this definition. Intraoperative "consciousness" without recall and intraoperative responsiveness (following commands) without recall are not included in this definition. Intraoperative awareness may vary in duration and intensity and is necessarily based upon the subjective experience of the patient. Because intraoperative awareness is subjective, observers may disagree about whether a particular patient's experience is true intraoperative awareness or some other experience, such as dreaming or recollection of events occurring before or after the anesthetic. Some have suggested that a report of intraoperative awareness must contain information that can be objectively confirmed, such as verbatim reporting of a conversation that took place in the operating room during the anesthetic that can also be recalled by the operating room staff [54]. However, such a standard for diagnosing intraoperative awareness would almost certainly exclude cases of true intraoperative awareness that simply cannot be objectively confirmed [55]. Studies of intraoperative awareness should report the actual experiences related by patients purporting to experience intraoperative awareness so that peer reviewers and others can assess for themselves whether the experiences reported reasonably represent intraoperative awareness or not. Some cases of purported intraoperative awareness must ultimately be classified as "possible awareness" when the patient's history is not universally convincing. However, in anesthetic practice (in contrast to the research setting) the anesthesia provider should be very cautious in denying a report of intraoperative awareness by an individual patient, since case studies have suggested that intraoperative awareness can result in lasting psychiatric disability. For such patients to have their claims met with skepticism is probably counterproductive [56–58]. There is a chilling report of intraoperative awareness written by a physician who experienced intraoperative awareness due to the failure of a propofol infusion pump [59].

There have been three large prospective studies of the incidence of intraoperative awareness and several smaller studies. Myles and colleagues [60] interviewed 10,811 patients within 24 hours of surgery at an Australian tertiary-care hospital (without obstetric or pediatric surgical services) and found an incidence of intraoperative awareness of 0.1%. They also measured patient satisfaction. Not surprisingly, intraoperative awareness was powerfully associated with patient dissatisfaction. Sandin and colleagues [61] prospectively studied 11,785 patients from two hospitals in Sweden and found an incidence of intraoperative awareness ranging from 0.10%, for patients not receiving neuromuscular blocking drugs during anesthetic maintenance, to 0.18%, for patients receiving a neuromuscular blocking drug. Sebel and colleagues [62] performed a multicenter, prospective study in the United States of 19,576 patients and found an overall incidence of intraoperative awareness of 0.13%. Davidson and colleagues [63] recently reported an incidence of intraoperative awareness of 0.8% in a prospective study of 864 children. In only one of the seven cases of awareness was neuromuscular blockers used during anesthetic maintenance. The incidence of intraoperative awareness varies depending upon the type of surgical procedure. Numerous studies have suggested that the rate of intraoperative awareness is particularly high during cardiac surgery, ranging from about 0.4% to 1% [60,62,64–68]. Trauma and obstetric surgery have also been associated with relatively high rates of awareness. There is no evidence that any particular anesthetic techniques or particular anesthetic drugs are more likely than others to prevent intraoperative awareness (aside from avoidance of obvious, deliberately light anesthesia). While there seems to be a popular notion that total intravenous anesthesia is more likely to result in awareness, the available evidence actually suggests that this is not the case [61,69–71].

Some anesthesiologists express doubt about the reported incidence of intraoperative awareness because their personal experience suggests that the incidence is substantially lower than is generally reported in the literature. However, these individual impressions may be misleading. Moerman and colleagues [72] studied 26 patients referred to them because of intraoperative awareness and found that in 70% of cases, for a variety of reasons, the anesthesiologist was never informed about the intraoperative awareness. Unless anesthesiologists specifically and deliberately seek a history of intraoperative awareness from their patients, many cases are apparently missed in routine clinical practice. Interestingly, while some anesthesiologists doubt the importance of intraoperative awareness as a clinical problem, many patients seem to be quite concerned. McCleane and Cooper [73] surveyed 247 patients before surgery and found that 50% were concerned about the prospect of intraoperative awareness. Following apparently uneventful surgery, 25% were still concerned about the prospect of intraoperative awareness during some future anesthetic encounter. This study was reported in 1990, before there was public attention focused on intraoperative awareness because of publicity about the BIS monitor.

According to one hypothesis, depth-of-anesthesia monitoring possibly reduces the incidence of intraoperative awareness. However, the opposite hypothesis is also entertained—that depth-of-anesthesia monitoring has led to a reduction in the average amount of anesthetic administered, as studies have shown, and this reduced use of anesthesia increases the risk of intraoperative awareness [74]. Two prospective studies have suggested that intraoperative monitoring with BIS can significantly reduce the incidence of intraoperative awareness. In a retrospective case-comparison study, 5057 consecutive BIS-monitored cases from two hospitals in Sweden were compared with 7826 non–BIS-monitored cases from the same institutions [75]. There were 2 cases of intraoperative awareness (during intubation; both had BIS values >60) in the BIS-monitored series compared with 14 in the non–BIS-monitored series ($P < .039$). In a prospective, randomized, international multicenter trial, 2503 "high risk" (eg, cardiac anesthesia, trauma, obstetrics) patients were assigned to BIS or non-BIS monitoring [60]. There were 2 cases of intraoperative awareness in the BIS-monitored group (during laryngoscopy with BIS index 79–82 and during cardiac surgery with BIS index 55–59), compared with 11 in the non–BIS-monitoring group ($P = .022$).

While intraoperative awareness is more likely at depth-of-anesthesia monitoring index values above the recommended range (eg, >60 for BIS), clearly it is possible for index values to exceed the recommended range without the occurrence of intraoperative awareness, and the sufficient conditions to produce intraoperative awareness are not known. Ekman and colleagues [75] reported the distribution of BIS index values >60 found in their study of 5057 consecutive BIS-monitored patients. They found an average time with BIS index >60 of 1.9 minutes during induction of anesthesia (range 0–10 min) and 2.0 minutes during maintenance (range 0–178 min). Only 2 patients had intraoperative awareness, which occurred during intubation with BIS index values >60.

Additional studies of the effect of depth-of-anesthesia monitoring on intraoperative awareness are clearly needed. There are no published studies on this topic with monitors other than the BIS monitor. However, in comparison to other monitoring devices used in anesthesiology, the availability of two studies showing benefit of depth-of-anesthesia monitoring is remarkable. Proving that monitoring devices of any kind improve outcome has been quite difficult. Pulse oximetry has not been shown to affect outcome [76–78], yet most anesthesiologists would consider pulse oximetry to be indispensable. Pulmonary artery catheters have frequently been alleged to worsen outcome [79,80], although recent randomized prospective studies have suggested that perhaps pulmonary artery catheters do not worsen outcome, but do not improve it either [81].

The Joint Commission on Accreditation of Hospitals Organization has published a "sentinel event alert" concerning intraoperative awareness (available at http://www.jointcommission.org/SentinelEvents/SentinelEventAlert/sea_32.htm;). The American Society of Anesthesiologists has published a practice advisory on intraoperative awareness and "brain function monitoring" (available at http://www.asahq.org/publicationsAndServices/AwareAdvisoryFinalOct05.pdf).

Dreaming during anesthesia

When asked specifically about dreaming, approximately 6% of patients in large series reported that they were dreaming during anesthesia [62,82].

Although dreaming and intraoperative awareness may be difficult to distinguish in some cases, dream content frequently appears to be distinct from the content of intraoperative awareness, and generally patients appear to distinguish between dreaming and intraoperative awareness. The significance of intraoperative dreaming is unknown. Whether dreaming is a manifestation of excessively light anesthesia or a veiled form of intraoperative awareness is unknown, although Leslie and colleagues [82] reported that the incidence of dreaming was lower in BIS-monitored patients in comparison to a control group (2.7% versus 5.7%; $P = .004$).

Processing time

An important limitation with computerized EEG interpretation for depth-of-anesthesia monitoring is the time required to process the signal and compute the index value for display on the monitor screen. This processing time is substantial, requiring some seconds, although usually less than a minute, and can be easily observed clinically when administering a bolus of an intravenous induction agent to an awake patient. At a time when the patient is clearly unconscious, the index value displayed by the monitor will lag behind, continuing to be in the awake range for a number of seconds. Pilge and colleagues [83] attempted to further quantify the processing delays inherent in the BIS monitor, the Cerebral State Monitor (CSM) (Danmeter, Odense, Denmark), and the Narcotrend monitor (Monitor-Technik, Bad Bramstedt, Germany) by feeding the devices with artificially generated signals corresponding to the awake state and various depths of anesthesia along with various transitions between these states. They found time delays of 14 to 155 seconds for all of the devices. For a sudden transition from "general anesthesia" to "awake," the delays were 15, 30 and 65 seconds for CSM, BIS and Narcotrend, respectively. They also found that the processing delays varied depending upon the type of signal presented and the order of changes from one type of signal to another. Processing delays may be an inherent limitation on the effectiveness of using processed EEG data for avoidance of intraoperative awareness. Clearly, the anesthesiologist must use judgment in adjusting anesthetic depth in the face of various kinds of stimulation and not rely entirely on the depth-of-anesthesia monitoring, particularly when there will be sudden transitions of anesthetic depth or intensity of stimulus. This may be particularly important during induction of anesthesia and laryngoscopy, and may help to explain the three cases of awareness during laryngoscopy that occurred despite BIS monitoring in the two prospective studies of the use of BIS monitoring to prevent intraoperative awareness [60,75].

Processing time can also be critically important in understanding the results of certain studies of depth-of-anesthesia monitoring. For example, a study by Barr and colleagues [84] involved alternating periods of wakefulness and loss of responsiveness induced by turning a propofol infusion on and off. They concluded that BIS index values did not discriminate wakefulness from unconsciousness during propofol infusion. However, the lag time in BIS index values attributable to processing was not taken into account and probably contributed to the apparent discrepancy between the clinical state of the subjects and the BIS index values. Their study serves as a further reminder that the shift from consciousness to unconsciousness is not instantly reflected by the depth-of-anesthesia index values.

Intraoperative awareness despite the use of depth-of-anesthesia monitoring

No monitoring device is perfect, and there should be no surprise if depth-of-anesthesia monitoring fails to perform in some cases. Obviously failures have to be kept to a minimum for monitoring to be useful. The worst kind of failure for a depth-of-anesthesia monitor would be intraoperative awareness that occurs despite an index value in the recommended range for general anesthesia (eg, <60 for BIS). Index ranges are established based on the probability of finding a particular state (eg, awake versus asleep) within a particular range of index values. In other words, the probability of awareness will be very low if the patient has an index below a certain level, but the probability will not be zero, and awareness would be expected to occur occasionally with an index value within the recommended range. However, the actual failure rate for the recommended ranges in a large population is not known with certainty for any of the monitors. For the BIS monitor only, two prospective studies show that BIS monitoring is effective for reducing the incidence of intraoperative awareness compared with no depth-of-anesthesia monitoring, which suggests that the recommended index range for general anesthesia for BIS probably has a very low failure rate [60,75]. Case reports are important for providing additional, albeit anecdotal, information about monitoring failures. A cluster of reports of intraoperative awareness that occurs with index values within the recommended range would certainly suggest a problem with the recommended range. Interestingly, case reports of intraoperative awareness that occur with index values in the recommended range have been rare. Mychaskiw [85] reported a case of intraoperative awareness during sternotomy apparently at a BIS index value of 47, based on review of the BIS values recorded on the anesthesia record. However, subsequent to publication of the case report, analysis of the flash memory of the monitor (BIS monitors have a flash memory that stores around 30 days of cases under typical conditions of use.) revealed BIS index values >60 occurred at the approximate time of the awareness episode and were not recorded on the anesthesia record. This additional information was published in a subsequent report [86]. Rampersad and Mulroy [87] subsequently published another report of intraoperative awareness with BIS index values <60 recorded every 15 minutes on the anesthesia record. The flash memory was apparently not accessed for additional data. In addition to these reports, there is one case of intraoperative awareness with a BIS index value <60 during cardiac surgery contained in the multicenter prospective randomized trial of BIS monitoring for the prevention of intraoperative awareness [60]. There may be other case reports that have not come to the attention of this author. However, considering the large number of patients that have been monitored, the number of case reports remains remarkably small. Cases of intraoperative awareness that occur during depth-of-anesthesia monitoring with index values within the recommended range should be reported in the peer-reviewed literature. If possible, the memory of the monitor should be accessed to be sure that the index values recorded in the anesthetic record are indicative of the range of index values that actually occurred during the episode of intraoperative awareness.

The consequences of too much: increased perioperative mortality?

While the focus on depth-of-anesthesia monitoring has mainly concerned avoidance of intraoperative awareness, a growing body of evidence suggests that anesthetics, particularly volatile anesthetics, may produce long-lasting harmful effects. Furthermore, if these long-lasting harmful effects are dose-related, there would be a rationale for limiting anesthetic administration to the minimum effective dose.

Monk and colleagues [88] studied 1064 patients in a prospective observational study of 1-year postoperative mortality. They found that "deep hypnotic time" (BIS index <45) was an independent predictor of increased mortality. This study did not discover the mechanism by which "deep" anesthesia would promote mortality. The notion that anesthetics might produce dose-related, long-lasting toxicity challenges the dogma that the effects of anesthetic drugs are entirely reversible. Interestingly, a variety of studies in animals and in vitro suggest the possibility of irreversible effects of anesthetic drugs.

Eckenhoff and colleagues [89] found that inhaled anesthetics enhance oligomerization and cytotoxicity of Alzheimer-disease–associated peptides in vitro. Futterer and colleagues [90] examined the proteome of the rat brain 72 hours following desflurane anesthesia and found changes in cytosolic protein expression. Culley and colleagues [87,91–93] have performed a series of experiments studying the effects of anesthesia on memory and learning in rats. They found that a 2-hour 1.2% isoflurane anesthetic attenuated performance on a previously learned task in aged rats, but improved it in adult rats. However, acquisition of new spatial memory was impaired in both young and aged rats for 14 days following isoflurane anesthesia, persisting for up to 28 days in aged rats. Animal studies have suggested that anesthesia may be harmful to newborns by producing an unusual amount of apoptosis (programmed cell death). Ketamine, halothane, nitrous oxide, isoflurane, diazepam, midazolam, and other drugs have been shown to increase apoptotic neurodegeneration in developing rat or mouse brain [94,95]. Whether this occurs in humans is unknown, and the implications of these findings have been debated [96–98]. Sevoflurane produces dose-related epileptiform discharges, reminiscent of enflurane, that occur at deep levels of sevoflurane anesthesia [99]. Whether anesthetic-induced epileptiform activity is harmful is unknown, but some have recommended limiting the dose of sevoflurane by EEG depth-of-anesthesia monitoring [99].

These studies raise many questions and certainly not enough is understood about long-lasting anesthetic drug effects to make specific changes in clinical practice. However, if long-lasting anesthetic drug effects were confirmed in humans, there could be a compelling rationale for depth-of-anesthesia monitoring to help limit anesthetic exposure to the minimum effective dose.

Pediatric depth-of-anesthesia monitoring

The normal EEG in children differs significantly from the adult EEG and undergoes age-related changes during development. From infancy to adulthood the amplitude of the EEG decreases and the frequency spectrum shifts to higher frequencies. The BIS algorithm was developed entirely from samples of adult EEG. Thus, depth-of-anesthesia monitoring based on EEG in children might be expected to present some problems. Nevertheless, several studies suggest that BIS and other EEG algorithms may be useful in children, although data are limited for children under 1 year of age [99–101]. BIS monitoring has been shown to result in lower anesthetic drug doses and faster recovery from anesthesia for children over 3 years of age [102]. A recent study of intraoperative awareness in children found a higher incidence than is usually found in adults, providing a compelling rationale for monitoring children [63]. Child-sized electrodes are available for the BIS monitor.

Sevoflurane is frequently used for inhalation induction of anesthesia in children. BIS index values during sevoflurane induction show a biphasic response, with an abrupt drop following loss of consciousness, associated with very-low–frequency EEG activity followed by an increase in BIS index values as end-tidal sevoflurane concentrations rise, associated with a shift to faster EEG activity [103,104]. Very deep sevoflurane anesthesia has been associated with epileptiform activity in children and adults [99], reminiscent of enflurane, and this may be associated with high BIS index values (which is paradoxical, since the patient is deeply anesthetized) [105]. Epileptiform activity induced by inhalational agents has not been specifically demonstrated to be harmful, but as a general principle seizure activity may be harmful to the brain. Therefore, Constant and colleagues [99] have proposed that depth-of-anesthesia monitoring could be especially useful in children for avoiding overly deep sevoflurane anesthesia and thereby minimizing the possibility for epileptiform activity.

Additional studies of depth-of-anesthesia monitoring in children are needed. Given the potential confounding effects of age-related changes in the baseline EEG, practitioners should proceed cautiously. However, the potential benefits for depth-of-anesthesia monitoring in children appear to be at least as valuable as in adults, if not more so.

Alternatives to BIS

The appearance of alternative products and technologies to BIS for monitoring depth of anesthesia was inevitable and desirable. No useful and successful technology is likely to remain unchallenged in the marketplace for long, and the emergence of competitors to the BIS system was all but guaranteed. However, the availability of multiple devices for monitoring depth of anesthesia complicates the situation for anesthesiologists interested in applying depth-of-anesthesia monitoring in their practices. If BIS was the only technology available, the decision would be to use BIS or not to use BIS. The anesthesiologist must now determine whether or not to use depth-of-anesthesia monitoring and also determine which device to use. Unfortunately, there is no "gold standard" for anesthetic depth, making comparison of different devices extremely difficult. Even different software versions of the same device, or changes in the patient sensor, may give different results. To make things even more confusing, the some proprietary names for the devices and their associated software and sensors have changed as technology is exchanged between companies or when major changes are made in the products. Thus the anesthesiologist consumer must be quite wary and should expect that a significant process of "due diligence" will be required. BIS technology is by far the best documented in the peer-reviewed literature, making evaluation of the BIS system easier in comparison to the other products. However, alternatives to BIS are increasingly being described in the literature. A summary follows of the currently available products along with key citations from the peer-reviewed literature.

SEDLine

Formerly known as the Patient State Analyzer (PSA) 4000 from Physiometrix, the SEDLine monitor from Hospira, Inc. (www.hospira.com, Lake Forest, Illinois) is an EEG monitor that superficially resembles the BIS monitor. The PSA 4000 was originally provided with a somewhat complex EEG electrode array involving two anterior electrodes, a midline central electrode, and a midline posterior electrode held in place by a head strap. The PSA 4000 monitor produced a dimensionless scale from 0 to 100, called a patient state index (PSI), with 0 representing an isoelectric EEG. The PSA monitor thus used an index similar to that used by the BIS monitor. Using this electrode array, Drover and colleagues [106] compared standard practice to EEG-guided propofol titration of propofol–alfentanil–nitrous-oxide anesthesia in a multicenter, prospective, randomized study of 259 surgical patients. Propofol was adjusted to a PSI target level of 25 to 50. The group titrated with EEG guidance received less propofol and emerged more quickly from anesthesia, a result previously obtained in similar studies of the BIS monitor. The EEG electrode array used in the study by Drover and colleagues has since been replaced with a self-adhesive electrode strip placed on the forehead, resembling the BIS sensor. White and colleagues [107] compared the Physiometrix PSA 4000 with a self-adhesive electrode strip sensor to the BIS monitor with the XP-version sensor in 22 American Society of Anesthesiologists grade-I and -II patients receiving propofol, fentanyl, desflurane, and nitrous oxide general anesthesia for laparosopic surgery. Various endpoints were reported and, in general, the results were similar for the PSA 4000 and BIS monitors. However, the number of patients studied was very small, and the investigators noted the "relatively limited database for the PSI (Patient State Index)" that is available in the peer-reviewed literature, and recommended that "further studies with the PSA monitor are clearly needed in larger populations of surgical patients undergoing different types of surgical procedures...It would also be important to determine whether use of the PSI for titrating volatile anesthetics during surgical procedures facilitates the early recovery process while avoiding intraoperative recall, analogous to the recent studies with the BIS and auditory evoked potential monitors" [107]. Indeed, a Medline search (April 2006) in using the terms "PSA 4000" or "Patient State Analyzer" found only four citations at the time this manuscript was created.

A-Line AEP Monitor/2

The A-Line AEP Monitor/2 by Danmeter (www.danmeter.dk) combines features of EEG analysis and auditory evoked potentials to produce the A-Line Autoregressive Index (AAI), which is scaled from 0 to 100. As of April 2006, the Danmeter website contained a large amount of useful technical information, including a bibliography. A previous version of this monitor, the A-Line AEP, used only auditory evoked potentials, without EEG analysis, to monitor depth of anesthesia. Obviously these two versions are not comparable and should be considered separately.

The A-Line monitor uses the middle-latency auditory evoked response (mLAER). Auditory evoked potentials result from auditory stimuli and are made up of positive and negative waves. Each wave results from transmission of an auditory signal through specific anatomic sites in the pathway from the ear to the cerebral cortex. Middle latency potentials (20–80 ms after stimulation) correspond to transmission from the thalamus to the auditory cortex [108]. Increasing depth of anesthesia decreases the amplitude and increases the latency of the mLAER. Scalp electrodes may be used to record the mLAER, which has to be separated from the overlying EEG signal. The A-Line monitor uses a specialized technique to rapidly extract the mLAER signal from the EEG, referred to as "autoregressive" or ARX processing.

Prolongation of the negative wave of the mLAER beyond 47 ms distinguished between subjects with and without recall during anesthesia [109,110]. However, a significant limitation to the use of mLAER for the measurement of anesthetic depth is that it becomes severely attenuated and cannot be detected soon after loss of consciousness. This phenomenon can be seen in the study of Ekman and colleagues [111] in which sevoflurane was administered in gradually increasing concentrations. BIS decreased to 25 to 30 from 50 to 55 as sevoflurane increased from about 1.5% to 3%, while the AAI was relatively unchanged. Kreuer and colleagues [112] found no significant change in the AAI between 3% and 9% desflurane. Thus, the AAI may be useful for measuring depth of anesthesia at "lighter" levels of anesthesia, or for avoiding consciousness during anesthesia, but may not be useful for distinguishing gradations of "deeper" levels of anesthesia.

A logical next step would be to use the mLAER for measuring the lighter depths of anesthesia while using spontaneous EEG to measure the deeper levels, which is the approach taken by the next-generation monitor. At low amplitude of mLAER, the AAI is based entirely on the spontaneous EEG. Vereecke and colleagues [113] administered propofol to volunteers and showed that the AAI based on combined mLAER and EEG tracked the estimated plasma concentration of propofol administered by computer-assisted continuous infusion more effectively than mLAER alone. The investigators attributed the improved performance to the detection and quantification of EEG burst suppression when EEG interpretation is included in the algorithm (mLAER would be flat and the AAI based on mLAER would have reached a constant plateau value during EEG burst suppression). Weber and colleagues [114] reported on an interesting study in which they removed the earphones (used to administer the auditory stimulus) from awake and anesthetized subjects, producing instantaneous loss of the mLAER and transition to the mode of spontaneous EEG analysis. The AAI values were significantly lower as a result of discontinuing the auditory stimulus, suggesting a discontinuity in the algorithm. However, the AAI values were still in an appropriate range for subjects who were awake and for subjects who were anesthetized. As of April 2006, no peer-reviewed clinical study has confirmed the validity of the A-Line AEP Monitor/2 with combined mLAER and EEG analysis.

Those accustomed to the BIS index scale of 0 to 100 should note that while the AAI has the same 0-to-100 scale, the values have different meaning. While a BIS index range of 45 to 60 is suggested for surgical anesthesia, AAI value of >50 corresponds to the awake state, while surgical anesthesia is suggested to be in the range of 15 to 25.

Entropy

Entropy was originally defined as a physical concept related to the amount of disorder in a system. In thermodynamics, entropy is proportional to the logarithm of the number of available microstates. Entropy was defined for information theory by Shannon [115] in terms of the irregularity, complexity, or unpredictability characteristics of a signal. Generally speaking, the EEG signal is most complex in the awake state and becomes more regular as anesthetic depth increases. Burst suppression and isoelectric (flat) EEG are examples of highly regular patterns that occur during deep anesthesia. On a scale where maximum entropy is 1, and minimal entropy is 0, an isoelectric EEG would have an entropy of 0. The entropy concept has been adapted to the interpretation of EEG for the purpose of gauging anesthetic depth for the Datex–Ohmeda S/5 Entropy Module. The Datex–Ohmeda algorithm has been described in an article by Vierto-Oja and colleagues [116]. Several studies suggest that entropy is a useful measure of anesthetic drug effects for propofol, sevoflurane, and the combination of propofol and remifentanil, giving results roughly similar to BIS [20,34,117–123].

Interestingly, the Datex–Ohmeda algorithm computes two different entropy numbers, designated "state entropy" and "response entropy" [116]. These two different methods of calculation revolve around distinguishing EEG from EMG artifacts. State entropy is computed for the frequency range from 0.8 to 32 Hz. Most of the power in the EEG spectrum for this frequency range will consist of EEG activity. The response entropy is computed for the frequency range of 0.8 to 47 Hz. Between 32 and 47 Hz, most of the power will consist of EMG (muscle) activity, so the response entropy should be more sensitive to EMG activity than the state entropy. The reasoning behind this approach is that an increase in EMG activity may indicate that the patient is responding to some stimulus by increasing tone in the facial muscle near the sensor electrodes, possibly serving as an early warning of impending arousal. Essentially, this approach attempts to use EMG activity as useful information rather than as a nuisance artifact contaminating the EEG signal. However, clinical experience shows that EMG activity can also occur in the absence of any other signs of arousal. Does this approach actually yield useful information? Valjus and colleagues [18] performed an interesting experiment in which they randomly assigned 51 patients to receive remifentanil or esmolol during a propofol–nitrous-oxide general anesthetic given for gynecologic laparoscopy. State entropy and response entropy were recorded. State entropy was held constant at 50 ± 5 (similar to a BIS of 50) by adjustment of the propofol infusion. The hypothesis was that response entropy would be higher in the esmolol group. Presumably analgesia associated with remifentanil administration would reduce EMG activity, movement, and responsiveness, and this would be reflected in lower response entropy in the remifentanil group. However, the results showed no difference in response entropy between the two groups, despite the finding that all of the patients in the esmolol group moved at some time during surgery, while no patients in the remifentanil group moved. These results call into question the utility of the response entropy as computed by the Datex–Ohmeda algorithm.

Other monitors

Snap

The Snap monitor (Everest Biomedical Instruments, Chesterfield, Missouri, www.snaphandheld.com) is an EEG monitor. Its most noteworthy feature appears to be compact size. The original Snap monitor consisted of a module inserted into a Handspring Visor personal-digital-assistant–style handheld computer. This was superseded by the Snap II monitor, which is somewhat larger, albeit still relatively small. Peer-reviewed reports concerning this monitor are very limited [124].

Cerebral State Monitor

The CSM is an EEG monitor from Danmeter (www.danmeter.dk). Unlike Danmeter's A-Line AEP Monitor/2, there is no evoked potential feature with the CSM. Like the Snap, this monitor is especially compact. It is also capable of wireless communication with a patient monitor or computer. Peer-reviewed reports concerning this monitor are very limited [125].

Narcotrend

The Narcotrend EEG monitor (www.narcotrend.de) is an EEG monitor that was not available in the United States as of April 2006. Several studies have suggested that this monitor produces reasonable results, roughly similar to BIS [126–145].

Summary

Depth-of-anesthesia monitoring with EEG or EEG combined with mLAER is becoming widely used in anesthesia practice. Evidence shows that this monitoring improves outcome by reducing the incidence of intraoperative awareness while reducing the average amount of anesthesia that is administered, resulting in faster wake-up and recovery, and perhaps reduced nausea and vomiting. As with any monitoring device, there are limitations in the use of the monitors and the anesthesiologist must be able to interpret the data accordingly. The limitations include the following.

- The currently available monitoring algorithms do not account for all anesthetic drugs, including ketamine, nitrous oxide and halothane.
- EMG and other high-frequency electrical artifacts are common and interfere with EEG interpretation.
- Data processing time produces a lag in the computation of the depth-of-anesthesia monitoring index.
- Frequently the EEG effects of anesthetic drugs are not good predictors of movement in response to a surgical stimulus because the main site of action for anesthetic drugs to prevent movement is the spinal cord.
- The use of depth-of-anesthesia monitoring in children is not as well understood as in adults.

Several monitoring devices are commercially available. The BIS monitor is the most thoroughly studied and most widely used, but the amount of information about other monitors is growing. In the future, depth-of-anesthesia monitoring will probably help in further refining and better understanding the process of administering anesthesia.

References

[1] Rampil IJ. A primer for EEG signal processing in anesthesia. Anesthesiology 1998;89(4): 980–1002.
[2] Sigl JC, Chamoun NG. An introduction to bispectral analysis for the electroencephalogram. J Clin Monit 1994;10(6):392–404.
[3] Gan TJ, Glass PS, Windsor A, et al. Bispectral index monitoring allows faster emergence and improved recovery from propofol, alfentanil and nitrous oxide anesthesia. Anesthesiology 1997;87:808–15.
[4] Glass PS, Bloom M, Kearse L, et al. Bispectral analysis measures sedation and memory effects of propofol, midazolam, isoflurane, and alfentanil in healthy volunteers. Anesthesiology 1997;86(4):836–47.
[5] Sebel PS, Bowles SM, Saini V, et al. EEG bispectrum predicts movement during thiopental/ isoflurane anesthesia. J Clin Monit 1995;11(2):83–91.
[6] Sebel PS, Lang E, Rampil IJ, et al. A multicenter study of bispectral electroencephalogram analysis for monitoring anesthetic effect. Anesth Analg 1997;84:891–9.
[7] Flaishon R, Windsor A, Sigl J, et al. Recovery of consciousness after thiopental or propofol. Bispectral index and isolated forearm technique. Anesthesiology 1997;86(3):613–9.
[8] Iselin-Chaves IA, Flaishon R, Sebel PS, et al. The effect of the interaction of propofol and alfentanil on recall, loss of consciousness, and the bispectral index. Anesth Analg 1998; 87(4):949–55.
[9] Kearse LA Jr, Rosow C, Zaslavsky A, et al. Bispectral analysis of the electroencephalogram predicts conscious processing of information during propofol sedation and hypnosis. Anesthesiology 1998;88(1):25–34.
[10] Alkire MT. Quantitative EEG correlations with brain glucose metabolic rate during anesthesia in volunteers. Anesthesiology 1998;89(2):323–33.
[11] Liu SS. Effects of bispectral index monitoring on ambulatory anesthesia. A meta-analysis of randomized controlled trials and a cost analysis. Anesthesiology 2004;101:311–5.
[12] Saucier N, Walts LF, Moreland JR. Patient awareness during nitrous oxide, oxygen, and halothane anesthesia. Anesth Analg 1983;62(2):239–40.
[13] Sonner JM, Antognini JF, Dutton RC, et al. Inhaled anesthetics and immobility: mechanisms, mysteries, and minimum alveolar anesthetic concentration. Anesth Analg 2003; 97(3):718–40.
[14] Eger EI 2nd, Koblin DD, Harris RA, et al. Hypothesis: inhaled anesthetics produce immobility and amnesia by different mechanisms at different sites. Anesth Analg 1997;84(4): 915–8.
[15] Rampil IJ, Mason P, Singh H. Anesthetic potency (MAC) is independent of forebrain structures in the rat. Anesthesiology 1993;78(4):707–12.
[16] Antognini JF, Carstens E, Atherley R. Does the immobilizing effect of thiopental in brain exceed that of halothane? Anesthesiology 2002;96(4):980–6.
[17] Antognini JF, Schwartz K. Exaggerated anesthetic requirements in the preferentially anesthetized brain. Anesthesiology 1993;79(6):1244–9.
[18] Valjus M, Ahonen J, Jokela R, et al. Response entropy is not more sensitive than state entropy in distinguishing the use of esmolol instead of remifentanil in patients undergoing gynaecological laparoscopy. Acta Anaesthesiol Scand 2006;50(1):32–9.

[19] Bowdle TA, Ward RJ. Induction of anesthesia with small doses of sufentanil or fentanyl: dose versus EEG response, speed of onset and thiopental requirement. Anesthesiology 1989;70:26–30.

[20] Bouillon TW, Bruhn J, Radulescu L, et al. Pharmacodynamic interaction between propofol and remifentanil regarding hypnosis, tolerance of laryngoscopy, bispectral index, and electroencephalographic approximate entropy. Anesthesiology 2004;100: 1353–72.

[21] Nieuwenhuijs D, Coleman EL, Douglas NJ, et al. Bispectral index values and spectral edge frequency at different stages of physiologic sleep. Anesth Analg 2002;94:125–9.

[22] Forbes AR, Cohen NH, Eger EI 2nd. Pancuronium reduces halothane requirement in man. Anesth Analg 1979;58(6):497–9.

[23] Schwartz AE, Navedo AT, Berman MF. Pancuronium increases the duration of electroencephalogram burst suppression in dogs anesthetized with isoflurane. Anesthesiology 1992; 77(4):686–90.

[24] Fraser GL, Riker RR. Bispectral index monitoring in the intensive care unit provides more signal than noise. Pharmacotherapy 2005;25(5 Pt 2):19S–27S.

[25] LeBlanc JM, Dasta JF, Kane-Gill SL. Role of the bispectral index in sedation monitoring in the ICU. Ann Pharmacother 2006;40(3):490–500.

[26] Vretzakis G, Dragoumanis C, Ferdi H, et al. Influence of an external pacemaker on bispectral index. Eur J Anaesthesiol 2005;22(1):70–2.

[27] Schnider TW, Luginbuhl M, Petersen-Felix S, et al. Unreasonably low bispectral index values in a volunteer with genetically determined low-voltage electroencephalographic signal. Anesthesiology 1998;89(6):1607–8.

[28] Myles PS, Cairo S. Artifact in the bispectral index in a patient with severe ischemic brain injury. Anesth Analg 2004;98(3):706–7.

[29] Anderson RE, Jakobsson JG. Entropy of EEG during anaesthetic induction: a comparative study with propofol or nitrous oxide as sole agent. Br J Anaesth 2004;92(2):167–70.

[30] Rampil IJ, Kim JS, Lenhardt R, et al. Bispectral EEG index during nitrous oxide administration. Anesthesiology 1998;89:671–7.

[31] Barr G, Jakobsson JG, Owall A, et al. Nitrous oxide does not alter bispectral index: study with nitrous oxide as sole agent and as an adjunct to i.v. anaesthesia. Br J Anaesth 1999; 82(6):827–30.

[32] Coste C, Guignard B, Menigaux C, et al. Nitrous oxide prevents movement during orotracheal intubation without affecting BIS value. Anesth Anal 2000;91(1):130–5.

[33] Hirota K, Kubota T, Ishihara H, et al. The effects of nitrous oxide and ketamine on the bispectral index and 95% spectral edge frequency during propofol-fentanyl anaesthesia. Eur J Anaesthesiol 1999;16(11):779–83.

[34] Hans P, Dewandre PY, Brichant JF, et al. Comparative effects of ketamine on bispectral index and spectral entropy of the electroencephalogram under sevoflurane anaesthesia. Br J Anaesth 2005;94(3):336–40.

[35] Friedberg BL. The effect of a dissociative dose of ketamine on the bispectral index (BIS) during propofol hypnosis. J Clin Anesth 1999;11(1):4–7.

[36] Friedberg BL, Sigl JC. Clonidine premedication decreases propofol consumption during bispectral index (BIS) monitored propofol-ketamine technique for office-based surgery. Dermatol Surg 2000;26(9):848–52.

[37] Roffey P, Mikhail M, Thangathurai D. Ketamine interferes with bispectral index monitoring in cardiac patients undergoing cardiopulmonary bypass. J Cardiothorac Vasc Anesth 2000;14(4):494–5.

[38] Sakai T, Singh H, Mi WD, et al. The effect of ketamine on clinical endpoints of hypnosis and EEG variables during propofol infusion. Acta Anaesthesiol Scand 1999;43(2): 212–6.

[39] Suzuki M, Edmonds HL Jr, Tsueda K, et al. Effect of ketamine on bispectral index and levels of sedation. J Clin Monit Comput 1998;14(5):373.

[40] Vereecke HE, Struys MM, Mortier EP. A comparison of bispectral index and ARX-derived auditory evoked potential index in measuring the clinical interaction between ketamine and propofol anaesthesia. Anaesthesia 2003;58(10):957–61.
[41] Wu CC, Mok MS, Lin CS, et al. EEG-bispectral index changes with ketamine versus thiamylal induction of anesthesia. Acta Anaesthesiol Sin 2001;39(1):11–5.
[42] Lallemand MA, Lentschener C, Mazoit JX, et al. Bispectral index changes following etomidate induction of general anaesthesia and orotracheal intubation. Br J Anaesth 2003; 91(3):341–6.
[43] El-Kerdawy HM, Zalingen EE, Bovill JG. The influence of the alpha2-adrenoceptor agonist, clonidine, on the EEG and on the MAC of isoflurane. Eur J Anaesthesiol 2000;17(2): 105–10.
[44] Triltsch AE, Welte M, von Homeyer P, et al. Bispectral index-guided sedation with dexmedetomidine in intensive care: a prospective, randomized, double blind, placebo-controlled phase II study. Crit Care Med 2002;30(5):1007–14.
[45] Turkmen A, Altan A, Turgut N, et al. The correlation between the Richmond agitation-sedation scale and bispectral index during dexmedetomidine sedation. Eur J Anaesthesiol 2006;23(4):300–4.
[46] Edwards JJ, Soto RG, Bedford RF. Bispectral index values are higher during halothane vs. sevoflurane anesthesia in children, but not in infants. Acta Anaesthesiol Scand 2005;49(8): 1084–7.
[47] Edwards JJ, Soto RG, Thrush DM, et al. Bispectral index scale is higher for halothane than sevoflurane during intraoperative anesthesia. Anesthesiology 2003;99(6):1453–5.
[48] Bischoff P, Kochs E, Haferkorn D, et al. Intraoperative EEG changes in relation to the surgical procedure during isoflurane-nitrous oxide anesthesia: hysterectomy versus mastectomy. J Clin Anesth 1996;8(1):36–43.
[49] Kochs E, Bischoff P, Pichlmeier U, et al. Surgical stimulation induces changes in brain electrical activity during isoflurane/nitrous oxide anesthesia. A topographic electroencephalographic analysis. Anesthesiology 1994;80(5):1026–34.
[50] Ghoneim MM, Block RI. Learning and memory during general anesthesia: an update. Anesthesiology 1997;87(2):387–410.
[51] Deeprose C, Andrade J, Harrison D, et al. Unconscious auditory priming during surgery with propofol and nitrous oxide anaesthesia: a replication. Br J Anaesth 2005;94(1): 57–62.
[52] Iselin-Chaves IA, Willems SJ, Jermann FC, et al. Investigation of implicit memory during isoflurane anesthesia for elective surgery using the process dissociation procedure. Anesthesiology 2005;103(5):925–33.
[53] Kerssens C, Ouchi T, Sebel PS. No evidence of memory function during anesthesia with propofol or isoflurane with close control of hypnotic state. Anesthesiology 2005;102(1): 57–62.
[54] Eger EI 2nd, Sonner JM. How likely is awareness during anesthesia? Anesth Analg 2005; 100(5):1544.
[55] Bowdle TA, Sebel PS, Ghoneim MM, et al. How likely is awareness during anesthesia? Anesth Analg 2005;100:1545.
[56] Osterman JE, Hopper J, Heran WJ, et al. Awareness under anesthesia and the development of posttraumatic stress disorder. Gen Hosp Psychiatry 2001;23(4):198–204.
[57] Osterman JE, van der Kolk BA. Awareness during anesthesia and posttraumatic stress disorder. Gen Hosp Psychiatry 1998;20(5):274–81.
[58] Lennmarken C, Bildfors K, Enlund G, et al. Victims of awareness. Acta Anaesthesiol Scand 2002;46(3):229–31.
[59] Rowan KJ. Awareness under TIVA: a doctor's personal experience. Anaesth Intensive Care 2002;30(4):505–6.
[60] Myles PS, Leslie K, McNeil J, et al. Bispectral index monitoring to prevent awareness during anaesthesia: the B-Aware randomized controlled trial. Lancet 2004;363:1757–63.

[61] Sandin RH, Enlund G, Samuelsson P, et al. Awareness during anaesthesia: a prospective case study. Lancet 2000;355:707–11.
[62] Sebel PS, Bowdle TA, Ghoneim MM, et al. The incidence of awareness during anesthesia: a multicenter United States study. Anesth Analg 2004;99:833–9.
[63] Davidson AJ, Huang GH, Czarnecki C, et al. Awareness during anesthesia in children: a prospective cohort study. Anesth Analg 2005;100(3):653–61.
[64] Dowd NP, Cheng DCH, Karski JM, et al. Intraoperative awareness in fast-track cardiac anesthesia. Anesthesiology 1998;89:1068–73.
[65] Domino KB, Posner KL, Caplan RA, et al. Awareness during anesthesia: a closed claims analysis. Anesthesiology 1999;90:1053–61.
[66] Phillips AA, McLean RF, Devitt JH, et al. Recall of intraoperative events after general anaesthesia and cardiopulmonary bypass. Can J Anaesth 1993;40:922–66.
[67] Ranta S, Jussila J, Hynynen M. Recall of awareness during cardiac anaesthesia: influence of feedback information to the anesthesiologist. Acta Anaesthesiol Scand 1996;40: 554–60.
[68] Ranta SO-V, Hernanen P, Hynynen M. Patient's conscious recollections from cardiac anesthesia. J Cardiothorac Vasc Anesth 2002;16:426–30.
[69] Enlund M. TIVA, awareness, and the Brice interview. Anesth Analg 2006;102(3):967.
[70] Enlund M, Hassan HG. Intraoperative awareness: detected by the structured Brice interview? Acta Anaesthesiol Scand 2002;46(4):345–9.
[71] Nordstrom O, Engstrom AM, Persson S, et al. Incidence of awareness in total i.v. anaesthesia based on propofol, alfentanil and neuromuscular blockade. Acta Anaesthesiol Scand 1997;41(8):978–84.
[72] Moerman N, Bonke B, Oosting J. Awareness and recall during general anesthesia. Facts and feelings. Anesthesiology 1993;79:454–64.
[73] McCleane GJ, Cooper R. The nature of pre-operative anxiety. Anaesthesia 1990;45(2): 153–5.
[74] Kalkman CJ, Drummond J. Monitors of depth of anesthesia, quo vadis? Anesthesiology 2002;96:784–7.
[75] Ekman A, Lindholm M-L, Lennmarken C, et al. Reduction in the incidence of awareness using BIS monitoring. Acta Anaesthesiol Scand 2004;48:20–6.
[76] Moller JT, Johannessen NW, Espersen K, et al. Randomized evaluation of pulse oximetry in 20,802 patients: II. Perioperative events and postoperative complications. Anesthesiology 1993;78(3):445–53.
[77] Moller JT, Pedersen T, Rasmussen LS, et al. Randomized evaluation of pulse oximetry in 20,802 patients: I. Design, demography, pulse oximetry failure rate, and overall complication rate. Anesthesiology 1993;78(3):436–44.
[78] Pedersen T, Moller AM, Pedersen BD. Pulse oximetry for perioperative monitoring: systematic review of randomized, controlled trials. Anesth Analg 2003;96(2):426–31.
[79] Dalen JE, Bone RC. Is it time to pull the pulmonary artery catheter? JAMA 1996;276(11): 916–8.
[80] Connors AF Jr, Speroff T, Dawson NV, et al. The effectiveness of right heart catheterization in the initial care of critically ill patients. SUPPORT investigators. JAMA 1996; 276(11):889–97.
[81] Shah MR, Hasselblad V, Stevenson LW, et al. Impact of the pulmonary artery catheter in critically ill patients: meta-analysis of randomized clinical trials. JAMA 2005;294(13):1664–70.
[82] Leslie K, Myles PS, Forbes A, et al. Dreaming during anaesthesia in patients at high risk of awareness. Anaesthesia 2005;60(3):239–44.
[83] Pilge S, Zanner R, Schneider G, et al. Time delay of index calculation: analysis of cerebral state, bispectral, and narcotrend indices. Anesthesiology 2006;104(3):488–94.
[84] Barr G, Anderson RE, Owall A, et al. Being awake intermittently during propofol-induced hypnosis: a study of BIS, explicit and implicit memory. Acta Anaesthesiol Scand 2001; 45(7):834–8.

[85] Mychaskiw G 2nd, Horowitz M, Sachdev V, et al. Explicit intraoperative recall at a bispectral index of 47. Anesth Analg 2001;92(4):808–9.
[86] Rampil I. False negative BIS? Maybe, maybe not! Anesth Analg 2001;93(3):798–9.
[87] Rampersad SE, Mulroy MF. A case of awareness despite an "adequate depth of anesthesia" as indicated by a bispectral index monitor. Anesth Analg 2005;100(5):1363–4.
[88] Monk TG, Saini V, Weldon BC, et al. Anesthetic management and one-year mortality after noncardiac surgery. Anesth Analg 2005;100(1):4–10.
[89] Eckenhoff RG, Johansson JS, Wei H, et al. Inhaled anesthetic enhancement of amyloid-beta oligomerization and cytotoxicity. Anesthesiology 2004;101(3):703–9.
[90] Futterer CD, Maurer MH, Schmitt A, et al. Alterations in rat brain proteins after desflurane anesthesia. Anesthesiology 2004;100:302–8.
[91] Culley DJ, Baxter M, Yukhananov R, et al. The memory effects of general anesthesia persist for weeks in young and aged rats. Anesth Analg 2003;96(4):1004–9.
[92] Culley DJ, Baxter MG, Crosby CA, et al. Impaired acquisition of spatial memory 2 weeks after isoflurane and isoflurane-nitrous oxide anesthesia in aged rats. Anesth Analg 2004; 99(5):1393–7.
[93] Culley DJ, Baxter MG, Yukhananov R, et al. Long-term impairment of acquisition of a spatial memory task following isoflurane-nitrous oxide anesthesia in rats. Anesthesiology 2004;100(2):309–14.
[94] Yon JH, Daniel-Johnson J, Carter LB, et al. Anesthesia induces neuronal cell death in the developing rat brain via the intrinsic and extrinsic apoptotic pathways. Neuroscience 2005; 135(3):815–27.
[95] Young C, Jevtovic-Todorovic V, Qin YQ, et al. Potential of ketamine and midazolam, individually or in combination, to induce apoptotic neurodegeneration in the infant mouse brain. Br J Pharmacol 2005;146(2):189–97.
[96] Davidson A, Soriano S. Does anaesthesia harm the developing brain—evidence or speculation? Paediatr Anaesth 2004;14(3):199–200.
[97] Anand KJ, Soriano SG. Anesthetic agents and the immature brain: are these toxic or therapeutic? Anesthesiology 2004;101(2):527–30.
[98] Olney JW, Young C, Wozniak DF, et al. Anesthesia-induced developmental neuroapoptosis. Does it happen in humans? Anesthesiology 2004;101(2):273–5.
[99] Constant I, Seeman R, Murat I. Sevoflurane and epileptiform EEG changes. Paediatr Anaesth 2005;15(4):266–74.
[100] Kerssens C, Sebel PS. To BIS or not to BIS? That is the question. Anesth Analg 2006;102(2): 380–2.
[101] Murat I, Constant I. Bispectral index in pediatrics: fashion or a new tool? Paediatr Anaesth 2005;15(3):177–80.
[102] Bannister CF, Brosius KK, Sigl JC, et al. The effect of bispectral index monitoring on anesthetic use and recovery in children anesthetized with sevoflurane in nitrous oxide. Anesth Analg 2001;92(4):877–81.
[103] Constant I, Leport Y, Richard P, et al. Agitation and changes of bispectral index and electroencephalographic-derived variables during sevoflurane induction in children: clonidine premedication reduces agitation compared with midazolam. Br J Anaesth 2004;92(4): 504–11.
[104] Rodriguez RA, Hall LE, Duggan S, et al. The bispectral index does not correlate with clinical signs of inhalational anesthesia during sevoflurane induction and arousal in children. Can J Anaesth 2004;51(5):472–80.
[105] Chinzei M, Sawamura S, Hayashida M, et al. Change in bispectral index during epileptiform electrical activity under sevoflurane anesthesia in a patient with epilepsy. Anesth Analg 2004;98(6):1734–6.
[106] Drover DR, Lemmens HJ, Pierce ET, et al. Patient state index: titration of delivery and recovery from propofol, alfentanil, and nitrous oxide anesthesia. Anesthesiology 2002;97(1): 82–9.

[107] White PF, Tang J, Ma H, et al. Is the patient state analyzer with the PSArray2 a cost-effective alternative to the bispectral index monitor during the perioperative period? Anesth Analg 2004;99(5):1429–35.
[108] De Cosmo G, Aceto P, Clemente A, et al. Auditory evoked potentials. Minerva Anestesiol 2004;70(5):293–7.
[109] Thornton C, Barrowcliffe MP, Konieczko KM, et al. The auditory evoked response as an indicator of awareness. Br J Anaesth 1989;63(1):113–5.
[110] Newton DE, Thornton C, Konieczko KM, et al. Auditory evoked response and awareness: a study in volunteers at sub-MAC concentrations of isoflurane. Br J Anaesth 1992;69(2): 122–9.
[111] Ekman A, Brudin L, Sandin R. A comparison of bispectral index and rapidly extracted auditory evoked potentials index responses to noxious stimulation during sevoflurane anesthesia. Anesth Analg 2004;99(4):1141–6.
[112] Kreuer S, Bruhn J, Larsen R, et al. Comparison of BIS and AAI as measures of anaesthetic drug effect during desflurane-remifentanil anaesthesia. Acta Anaesthesiol Scand 2004; 48(9):1168–73.
[113] Vereecke HE, Vasquez PM, Jensen EW, et al. New composite index based on midlatency auditory evoked potential and electroencephalographic parameters to optimize correlation with propofol effect site concentration: comparison with bispectral index and solitary used fast extracting auditory evoked potential index. Anesthesiology 2005;103(3):500–7.
[114] Weber F, Zimmermann M, Bein T. The impact of acoustic stimulation on the AEP monitor/2 derived composite auditory evoked potential index under awake and anesthetized conditions. Anesth Analg 2005;101(2):435–9.
[115] Shannon CE. A mathematical theory of communication. Bell System Techn J 1948;27: 623–56.
[116] Viertio-Oja H, Maja V, Sarkela M, et al. Description of the entropy algorithm as applied in the Datex-Ohmeda S/5 Entropy Module. Acta Anaesthesiol Scand 2004;48(2):154–61.
[117] Bruhn J, Bouillon TW, Radulescu L, et al. Correlation of approximate entropy, bispectral index, and spectral edge frequency 95 (SEF95) with clinical signs of "anesthetic depth" during coadministration of propofol and remifentanil. Anesthesiology 2003;98(3): 621–7.
[118] Davidson AJ, Huang GH, Rebmann CS, et al. Performance of entropy and bispectral index as measures of anaesthesia effect in children of different ages. Br J Anaesth 2005;95(5): 674–9.
[119] Davidson AJ, Kim MJ, Sangolt GK. Entropy and bispectral index during anaesthesia in children. Anaesth Intensive Car 2004;32(4):485–93.
[120] Ellerkmann RK, Liermann VM, Alves TM, et al. Spectral entropy and bispectral index as measures of the electroencephalographic effects of sevoflurane. Anesthesiology 2004; 101(6):1275–82.
[121] Iannuzzi M, Iannuzzi E, Rossi F, et al. Relationship between bispectral index, electroencephalographic state entropy and effect-site EC50 for propofol at different clinical endpoints. Br J Anaesth 2005;94(4):492–5.
[122] Vanluchene AL, Struys MM, Heyse BE, et al. Spectral entropy measurement of patient responsiveness during propofol and remifentanil. A comparison with the bispectral index. Br J Anaesth 2004;93(5):645–54.
[123] White PF, Tang J, Romero GF, et al. A comparison of state and response entropy versus bispectral index values during the perioperative period. Anesth Analg 2006;102(1):160–7.
[124] Casati A, Putzu M, Vinciguerra F. A clinical comparison between bispectral index (BIS) and high frequency EEG signal detection (SNAP). Eur J Anaesthesiol 2005;22(1): 75–7.
[125] Anderson RE, Jakobsson JG. Cerebral state monitor, a new small handheld EEG monitor for determining depth of anaesthesia: a clinical comparison with the bispectral index during day-surgery. Eur J Anaesthesiol 2006;23(3):208–12.

[126] Russell IF. The Narcotrend 'depth of anaesthesia' monitor cannot reliably detect consciousness during general anaesthesia: an investigation using the isolated forearm technique. Br J Anaesth 2006;96(3):346–52.

[127] Weber F, Pohl F, Hollnberger H, et al. Impact of the Narcotrend index on propofol consumption and emergence times during total intravenous anaesthesia with propofol and remifentanil in children: a clinical utility study. Eur J Anaesthesiol 2005;22(10): 741–7.

[128] Weber F, Hollnberger H, Gruber M, et al. The correlation of the Narcotrend index with endtidal sevoflurane concentrations and hemodynamic parameters in children. Paediatr Anaesth 2005;15(9):727–32.

[129] Kreuer S, Bruhn J, Stracke C, et al. Narcotrend or bispectral index monitoring during desflurane-remifentanil anesthesia: a comparison with a standard practice protocol. Anesth Analg 2005;101(2):427–34.

[130] Weber F, Gruber M, Taeger K. The correlation of the Narcotrend index and classical electroencephalographic parameters with endtidal desflurane concentrations and hemodynamic parameters in different age groups. Paediatr Anaesth 2005;15(5):378–84.

[131] Grouven U, Beger FA, Schultz B, et al. Correlation of Narcotrend index, entropy measures, and spectral parameters with calculated propofol effect-site concentrations during induction of propofol-remifentanil anaesthesia. J Clin Monit Comput 2004;18(4): 231–40.

[132] Schneider G, Kochs EF, Horn B, et al. Narcotrend does not adequately detect the transition between awareness and unconsciousness in surgical patients. Anesthesiology 2004;101(5): 1105–11.

[133] Weber F, Hollnberger H, Gruber M, et al. Narcotrend depth of anesthesia monitoring in infants and children. Can J Anaesth 2004;51(8):855–6.

[134] Kreuer S, Bruhn J, Larsen R, et al. Application of bispectral index and Narcotrend index to the measurement of the electroencephalographic effects of isoflurane with and without burst suppression. Anesthesiology 2004;101(4):847–54.

[135] Kreuer S, Bruhn J, Larsen R, et al. Comparability of Narcotrend index and bispectral index during propofol anaesthesia. Br J Anaesth 2004;93(2):235–40.

[136] Schultz A, Grouven U, Beger FA, et al. The Narcotrend index: classification algorithm, correlation with propofol effect-site concentrations, and comparison with spectral parameters. Biomed Tech (Berl) 2004;49(3):38–42.

[137] Schmidt GN, Bischoff P, Standl T, et al. Comparative evaluation of Narcotrend, bispectral index, and classical electroencephalographic variables during induction, maintenance, and emergence of a propofol/remifentanil anesthesia. Anesth Analg 2004;98(5):1346–53.

[138] Bauerle K, Greim CA, Schroth M, et al. Prediction of depth of sedation and anaesthesia by the Narcotrend EEG monitor. Br J Anaesth 2004;92(6):841–5.

[139] Kreuer S, Wilhelm W, Grundmann U, et al. Narcotrend index versus bispectral index as electroencephalogram measures of anesthetic drug effect during propofol anesthesia. Anesth Analg 2004;98(3):692–7.

[140] Schmidt GN, Bischoff P, Standl T, et al. Narcotrend and bispectral index monitor are superior to classic electroencephalographic parameters for the assessment of anesthetic states during propofol-remifentanil anaesthesia. Anesthesiology 2003;99(5):1072–7.

[141] Kreuer S, Biedler A, Larsen R, et al. Narcotrend monitoring allows faster emergence and a reduction of drug consumption in propofol-remifentanil anesthesia. Anesthesiology 2003; 99(1):34–41.

[142] Raymondos K, Munte S, Krauss T, et al. Cortical activity assessed by Narcotrend in relation to haemodynamic responses to tracheal intubation at different stages of cortical suppression and reflex control. Eur J Anaesthesiol 2003;20(1):44–51.

[143] Schmidt GN, Bischoff P, Standl T, et al. Narcotrend, bispectral index, and classical electroencephalogram variables during emergence from propofol/remifentanil anaesthesia. Anesth Analg 2002;95(5):1324–30.

[144] Schultz B, Grouven U, Schultz A. Automatic classification algorithms of the EEG monitor Narcotrend for routinely recorded EEG data from general anaesthesia: a validation study. Biomed Tech (Berl) 2002;47(1–2):9–13.

[145] Kreuer S, Biedler A, Larsen R, et al. The Narcotrend—a new EEG monitor designed to measure the depth of anaesthesia. A comparison with bispectral index monitoring during propofol-remifentanil-anaesthesia. Anaesthesist 2001;50(12):921–5.

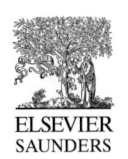

Perioperative Thermoregulation and Temperature Monitoring

Steven R. Insler, DO[a], Daniel I. Sessler, MD[a,b],*

[a]The Cleveland Clinic, 9500 Euclid Avenue, Cleveland, OH 44195, USA
[b]University of Louisville, Louisville, KY, USA

People normally are able to maintain core body temperature (core temperature) within narrow physiological limits. Regulation of core temperature is achieved by means of behavioral and autonomic mechanisms that actively balance heat production and heat loss. These mechanisms are controlled largely from the hypothalamus and depend on the input of afferent neurons from various sites within the body.

Surgery and general anesthesia impair the normal balance between heat production and loss [1–3]. Anesthetic agents, opioids, and sedatives inhibit behavior and autonomic responses, leaving patients essentially poikilothermic. Thus when patients are exposed to cool ambient operating room environments, mild-to-moderate hypothermia is the usual result. Although hypothermia may provide protection against ischemia [4,5], there is ample clinical evidence showing that even mild perioperative hypothermia causes multiple physiologic derangements and leads to adverse outcomes [6–8].

Conversely, hyperthermia also can occur within the perioperative environment, indicating that heat production exceeds heat loss. Although hypothermia is more common than hyperthermia in the perioperative period, hyperthermia (core temperature greater than 38°C) is more dangerous than a comparable degree of cooling. Hyperthermia can result from excessive covering of patients [9], extremely warm operating room temperatures, a febrile response [10,11], or uncontrolled metabolism as occurs during malignant hyperthermia crises.

Supported by NIH Grant GM 061655 (Bethesda, Maryland), the Gheens Foundation (Louisville, Kentucky), the Joseph Drown Foundation (Los Angeles, California), and the Commonwealth of Kentucky Research Challenge Trust Fund (Louisville). Neither author has a personal financial interest related to this review.

* Corresponding author.
 E-mail address: sessler@louisville.edu (D.I. Sessler).

Because temperature disturbances are common, multi-factorial, and serious, it is important that clinicians understand the impact of general anesthesia and surgery on the human thermoregulatory system. Similarly, monitoring temperature accurately is required to make correct diagnoses and provide timely intervention. This article covers normal physiologic temperature regulation, perioperative thermal stress, and techniques of intraoperative temperature monitoring.

Normal thermoregulation

Body core temperature is maintained within a tight range of preset values. Because the speed of chemical reactions varies with temperature, and because normal enzymatic functions occur optimally within a narrow temperature range, normal body functions depend on a relatively constant core body temperature. The core temperature compartment is composed of well-perfused tissues, the temperature of which is higher and more uniform than the rest of the body.

Afferent sensing

The dorsal root ganglia are clusters of sensory neuron cell bodies located in the vertebral column lateral to the spinal column. These neurons are associated with the detection of specific environmental stimuli and can, therefore, be partitioned accordingly. Dorsal root ganglia neurons are considered proprioceptors, low threshold mechanoreceptors, and cells that sense pain, temperature, or both. Thermosensitive neurons detect a temperature range from the noxious (greater than 52°C) to the innocuous (approximately 22 to 40°C). The axons of sensory neurons of the dorsal root ganglia terminate as free nerve endings in the dermal and epidermal layers of the skin. On the basis of their conduction velocities, both the pain and temperature sensing neurons are known to consist of small diameter, slowly conducting, unmyelinated C fibers and larger, rapidly conducting, thinly myelinated A delta fibers [12].

Free nerve endings in the skin are thought to directly sense environmental temperature. A key advance in understanding temperature sensation has come from the cloning and characterization of temperature-activated, transient receptor potential (TRP) ion channels. The activity of many ion channels is thermodynamically modulated by temperature. Thermosensitive TRPs are distinct, in that temperature alone can activate them (Fig. 1). Six of the mammalian TRP vanilloid ion channel subtypes are nonselective cation channels that can be activated by distinct increases or decreases in ambient temperature [13]. These temperature-gated channels are located in sensory neurons that connect the skin to the spinal column and brain by means of the dorsal root ganglia. TRP channels are activated when correct thermal stimuli are received, causing them to open and allow charged ions to cause an electrical potential that signals the brain.

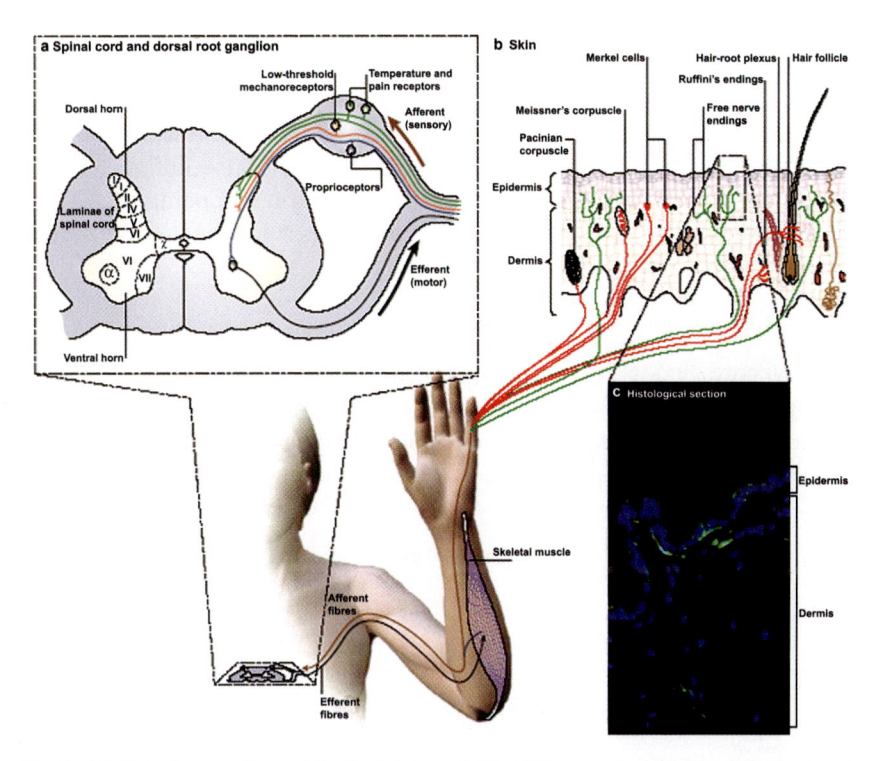

Fig. 1. (A) Spinal nerves formed by the joining of afferent (sensory) and efferent (motor) roots provide peripheral innervation to skin, skeletal muscles, viscera, and glands. Arrows denote the direction of incoming sensory and outgoing motor impulses. The cell bodies of motor neurons are located within the ventral horn (laminae VII – IX) of the spinal cord. Cell bodies of sensory neurons are located in the dorsal root ganglia (DRG). Within the DRG, there are subclasses of sensory neurons known as proprioceptive (*blue*), low threshold mechanosensitive (*red*), and temperature- and pain-sensing neurons (*green*). These neurons project centrally to dorsal horn interneurons (laminae I – VI of the spinal cord) and peripherally to target tissues. Proprioceptive neurons (blue fiber) project to specialized structures within target tissues such as muscle, and sense muscle stretch. (B) Low threshold mechanosensitive neurons (red fibers) project to end organs that transmit mechanical stimuli. Five types of mechanosensitive assemblies have been described and are illustrated. Temperature- and pain-sensing neurons (*green*) do not project to specialized end organs; instead they terminate as free nerve endings in all layers of the skin, and near blood vessels and hair follicles. (C) Section of skin showing free nerve endings (green fiber). (*From* Patapoutian A, Peier AM, Story GM, et al. ThermoTRP channels and beyond: mechanisms of temperature sensation. Nature Reviews Neuroscience 2003;4:530; with permission.)

The TRP vanilloid 3 channel may be unique among the subset, because it is expressed prominently in the skin keratinocytes, activated at temperatures greater than 33°C. Additionally, it exhibits increased responses at higher, noxious temperatures [14]. This finding implies that skin cells might act as a molecular thermometer and be able to sense temperature [14]. Keratinocytes have no direct link to the central nervous system and might communicate to the brain through nonsynaptic contacts with free nerve endings. Free receptors in the skin therefore may be the initial means of detecting environmental temperature changes. In a recent study in mice lacking the TRP vanilloid 3 receptor, Moqrich and colleagues [14] found that these mice had a severe deficit in sensing warm temperatures compared with their normal littermates (Fig. 2). This study suggests that the TRP vanilloid 3 receptor proteins on keratinocytes are detecting warm temperatures. These receptors appear to play an important role in thermoregulation; however, much remains to be discovered about them.

Central regulation

Invertebrate species only can adjust their body temperature using behavioral methods in response to changing environmental conditions. Therefore, they are largely at the mercy of the ambient temperature to which they are exposed. These animals are called poikilothermic, because their core

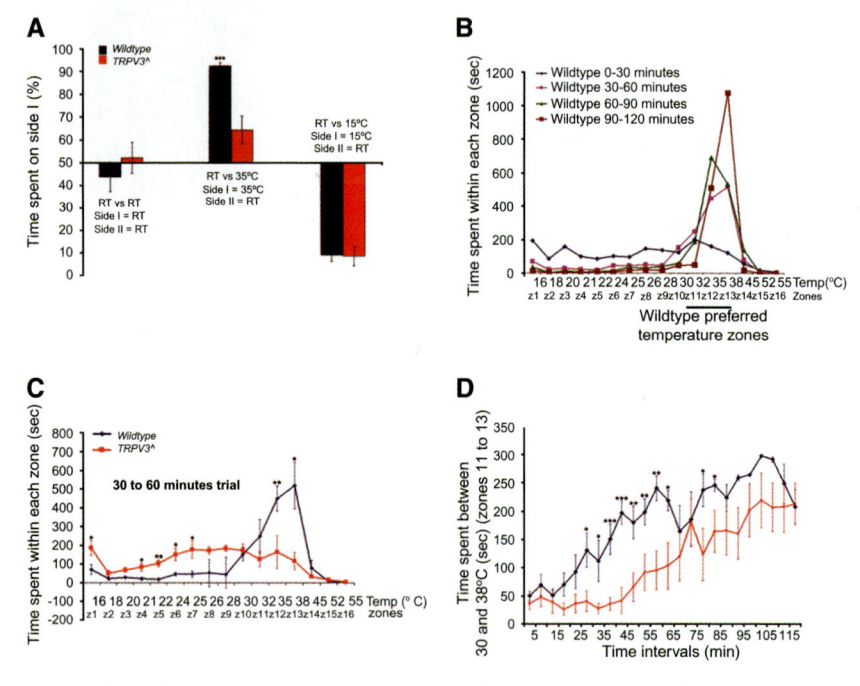

Fig. 2. Mice lacking transient receptor potential vanilloid 3 (TRPV3-/-) channel have a profound deficit in sensing warm temperature in novel thermotaxis assays. (*A*) Behavior of wild-type mice and TRPV3-/- littermates on the temperature choice test. (*B*) Behavior of wild-type mice on the gradient assay over a 2-hour trial shown in 30-minute intervals. (*C*) Behavior of wild-type and TRPV3-/- mice on the gradient from 30 to 60 minutes. (*D*) Time spent within the preferred zones (11 to 13) for wild type and TRPV3-/- mice at each 5-minute interval during the 2-hour trial. (*From* Moqrich A, Hwang SW, Earley TJ, et al. Impaired thermo sensation in mice lacking TRPV3-/-, a heat and camphor sensor in the skin. Science 2005;307(57):1469; with permission.)

temperature fluctuates over a considerable range depending on the environmental temperature. Some vertebrate species have evolved the ability to maintain core temperature by a system of heat production and heat loss that primarily is integrated by the hypothalamus. These homeothermic animals (mammals) strive to maintain core temperature within a narrow range regardless of environmental conditions.

In homeothermic animals, actual body temperatures vary slightly from species to species and to an even lesser extent among individuals. In people, the traditional normal value for oral temperature is 37°C (98.6°F), but the normal human core body temperature (core temperature) undergoes a regular circadian fluctuation of 0.5 to 1.0°C. Core temperature depends more on time of day than activity. It is normally lowest during sleep, slightly higher in the awake, relaxed state, and it rises slightly with activity [15,16] (Fig. 3).

Females have an additional menstrual cycle of temperature variation characterized by a rise in basal temperature related to ovulation. Temperature regulation in young children is less precise, and they may have a more exaggerated diurnal difference than do adults, with higher temperatures in the late afternoon or after physical activity.

Various parts of the body are maintained at different temperatures, with the difference among them influenced by environmental temperature and thermoregulatory vasomotion. The extremities are generally cooler than the rest of the body. Rectal temperature, although generally representative of core temperature, is often somewhat higher than true core temperature, and it varies little with changes in ambient environmental temperature. Oral temperature is generally 0.5°C less than the rectal temperature, but it is influenced by factors including ingestion of hot or cold fluids, gum chewing, smoking, and mouth breathing. Core temperature can be estimated with reasonable accuracy at the axilla and bladder except under extreme thermal stress [17].

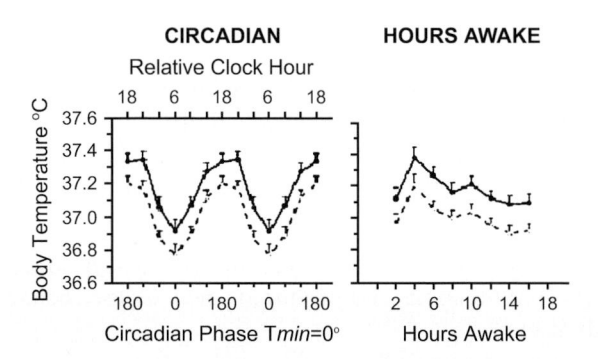

Fig. 3. Average high and low body temperature of 14 subjects across circadian phase (*left*) and hours awake (*right*). (*From* Wright KP, Hull JT, Czeisler CA. Relationship between alertness, performance and body temperature in humans. American Journal of Physiology-Regulatory, Integrative and Comparative Physiology 2002;283:R1372; with permission.)

Precise control of the core temperature is maintained by a thermoregulatory system involving afferent thermal sensing, central control, and efferent defenses [18]. Efferent defenses may be divided broadly into autonomic responses (ie, sweating and shivering) and behavioral responses (ie, seeking warm environment, clothing). Autonomic responses are about 80% dependent on core temperature and largely are regulated by the anterior hypothalamus. Conversely, behavioral modifications are about 50% determined by skin temperature and largely controlled by the posterior hypothalamus [19].

The hypothalamus is the dominant thermoregulatory controller in mammals, but thermoreceptors also are located at other cores sites including the midbrain, medulla, spinal cord, cortex, and deep abdominal and thoracic structures [20]. The skin and core body temperature receptors transmit their input through afferent nerves to the brainstem, especially the preoptic/anterior hypothalamus. Hypothalamic neurons thus play a vital function in co-ordinating most effector mechanisms by efferent connections.

The posterior hypothalamus integrates temperatures from sensory thermoreceptors in the skin and the body core, and regulates afferent thermoregulatory responses [21]. Each of these responses has a core temperature threshold that is dependent on mean skin temperature. When the threshold for a particular response is reached, that response is initiated. Typically, the thresholds for sweating and vasodilation are about 37°C; the threshold for vasoconstriction is about 36.7°C. For nonshivering thermogenesis, it is 36.0°C, and for shivering, it is 35.5°C.

Behavioral modifications as a means of thermoregulation include any behavioral feature that can reduce heat loss or produce heat in a cold environment. Conversely, these modifications include any behavioral feature that inhibits heat gain or causes heat to be released in a warmer environment. These practices might include seeking shade during the hottest part of the day and the use of fire, clothing, and building shelters for warmth.

Heat transfer mechanisms

Mammals constantly produce heat, and, on average, they dissipate as much as they produce to the environment. Body temperature is kept constant so long as heat production equals heat loss. If heat production or loss predominates, hyperthermia or hypothermia will result. The principle components of heat production include:

- Basal metabolic rate, the minimum amount of heat produced to sustain the body's vital functions and produced solely by the chemical reactions of metabolism
- Thermogenesis produced by the digestion of food
- Physical activity (including ventilation and shivering), which produces heat as a by-product of work done
- Hormonal influence on metabolism

For example, the basal metabolic rate will increase when stress hormones of the sympathetic nervous system (eg, epinephrine and norepinephrine) are secreted by the adrenal glands or thyroxine is released from the thyroid gland.

Thermal loss to the environment in people occurs by means of:

- Radiation, the transfer of heat by infrared emanations between the body and surrounding objects
- Conduction, the transfer of heat through direct contact
- Convection, the movement of molecules away from a warm area to a cool area depending on a temperature differential and air flow (wind chill effect)
- Evaporation of sweat from the skin, which reduces body heat by 2.436 kJ/mL sweat produced

It is often useful to consider the human body as an inner core and a peripheral shell. The inner core temperature normally is maintained at approximately 37°C, while the outer shell temperature depends on environmental conditions and vasomotor tone. Regulation of the body core and peripheral shell temperatures is coordinated in the brain by means of several behavioral and autonomic responses. Body core or shell temperature changes are sensed by cutaneous and deep-body thermoreceptors. The nerve supply found just underneath the skin is especially temperature-sensitive. These nerves are considered as either warm or cold receptors. Cold receptors react in the temperature range of approximately -5 to 43°C and are about 10 times as common as warm receptors. Warm receptors operate only at temperatures greater than 30°C (Fig. 4). Peripheral detection of temperature

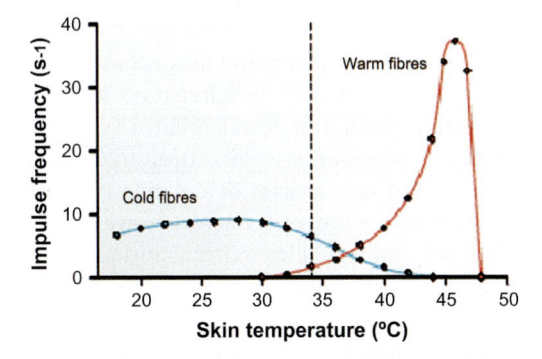

Fig. 4. Average discharge frequency of individual cold and warm sensitive fibers in response to changes in skin temperature. The dotted line indicates the normal skin temperature (33°C). Cold sensitive fibers respond only to cooling, whereas warm sensitive fibers respond to warming. Neither type responds to mechanical stimulation. (*From* Patapoutian A, Peier AM, Story GM, et al. ThermoTRP channels and beyond: mechanisms of temperature sensation. Nature Reviews 2003;4:531; with permission.)

generally is concerned with detecting cold rather than warm temperatures. Skin cooling thus provokes immediate reflexes that initiate shivering, inhibit sweating, and cause skin vasoconstriction to decrease the transfer of body heat to the skin.

Afferent responses

Thermoregulatory responses encompass any physiologic or behavioral mechanism that helps maintain body temperature. In a cold environment, mechanisms act to generate or retain body heat, consequently preventing hypothermia. And in an environment that exceeds body temperature, mechanisms facilitate heat loss to the environment to minimize or prevent hyperthermia.

The principal thermoregulatory responses in people are behavioral defenses [22,23]: sweating [24], precapillary vasodilatation [25], arterio–venous shunt vasoconstriction [26], nonshivering thermogenesis [27], and shivering [28]. Others, such as horripilation (goose bumps) are of little consequence in people. Each response is characterized by its threshold (triggering core temperature), gain (intensity increase with further core temperature deviation), and maximum intensity [29]. Core temperatures between the first autonomic warm response (sweating) and the first autonomic cold defense (vasoconstriction) define the interthreshold range; these temperatures do not initiate autonomic thermoregulatory defenses and hence define the span of normal body temperature at a given time [30].

Most heat exchange of the body with the environment occurs through the skin. Convective and conductive heat loss is controlled by varying cutaneous blood flow. Reducing skin blood flow essentially insulates the body core and limits heat loss. But in a warmer environment, peripheral vasodilatation occurs, which increases blood flow to the periphery and exacerbates heat loss (Fig. 5).

Neural reflex control of cutaneous blood flow is mediated by means of two populations of sympathetic nerves: the adrenergic vasoconstrictor system and a less well-understood sympathetic vasodilator system, which is responsible for 80% to 90% of cutaneous vasodilatation that occurs in response to heat stress [21]. The neural mechanism of cutaneous active vasodilatation apparently is mediated by cholinergic nerves; however, the transmitter is not only acetylcholine, but includes cotransmitters such as vasoactive intestinal peptide and probably other yet-to-be-identified factors [31].

Body fat that is located under the dermis in the subcutaneous layer also may aid in thermoregulation. This fat has several functions. It can act as a source of stored energy, as thermal insulation, and as a source of chemically produced heat. When the fatty acids of this tissue are oxidized to produce energy, a large quantity of heat is produced. The development of a large layer of subcutaneous fat may be an evolutionary adaptation to the loss of body hair and potential cold stress the human ancestor might have experienced.

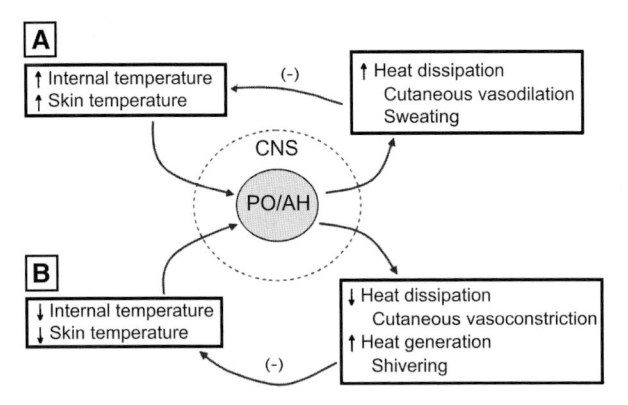

Fig. 5. Negative feedback loops involved in physiologic thermoregulation in humans. Minus signs refer to the correction of the error signal (change in skin or internal temperature) by the appropriate effector response. (*A*) Increases in internal or skin temperatures are sensed by the preoptic/anterior hypothalamus (PO/AH) and result in increased heat dissipation by means of cutaneous vasodilation and sweating, which then correct the original increased temperature. The influence of internal temperature is several times that of skin temperature in the control of these effectors. (*B*) Decreased skin or internal temperature causes reflex decreases in heat dissipation (cutaneous vasoconstriction) and increased heat generation (shivering) to correct the decreases in temperature that initiated those changes. *Abbreviation:* CNS, central nervous system. (*From* Charkoudian N. Skin blood flow in adult human thermoregulation: how it works, when it does not, and why. Mayo Clin Proc 2003;78:604; with permission.)

Perioperative temperature monitoring

Temperature monitoring devices vary according to the type of transducer used and the site to be monitored. The most commonly used transducers are thermistors and thermocouples. Thermistors are composed of electrodes connected to a semiconductive material; the resistance of the material varies nonlinearly according to temperature. Thermocouples consist of a set of bimetal junctions that generate an electromotive force when there is a temperature difference between the two ends of the transducer [32].

A more recent development is monitors that use infrared emission to measure temperature; these are seen commonly in aural canal thermometers (which often are referred to inaccurately as tympanic membrane thermometers). Liquid crystal sensors also can be used to measure skin temperature.

Core temperature is the best single indicator of body temperature. Therefore, all noncore temperature-monitoring sites need to be judged by their ability to accurately assess core temperature. Core temperature monitoring is appropriate for most patients undergoing general anesthesia, to facilitate detection and treatment of fever, malignant hyperthermia, and hypothermia. Although malignant hyperthermia is detected best by a rising $PaCO_2$ out of proportion to minute ventilation, detection of increasing core temperature may help in confirming the diagnosis.

More common than malignant hyperthermia is intraoperative hyperthermia of other etiologies, including excessive warming, infection, blood in the fourth ventricle, and mismatched blood transfusion. Core temperature changes during the first 30 minutes after administering a general anesthetic are sometimes difficult to interpret, because a variable and unpredictable amount of core-to-peripheral redistribution of body heat dominates during this period. Core temperature, however, should be monitored when general anesthesia is expected to last longer than 30 minutes.

Monitoring sites

Pulmonary artery catheters

These allow the measurement of central blood temperature, considered the gold standard for measuring core body temperature [32]. Pulmonary artery catheter measurement thus usually is used as a reference for all other devices. The obvious disadvantage of monitoring pulmonary artery temperature is the high cost and invasiveness of the catheter and the difficulty of insertion. Accordingly, pulmonary artery catheters are reserved for those patients requiring intensive hemodynamic monitoring; a consequence is that pulmonary artery temperatures are rarely available for clinical use.

Esophageal temperature

This usually is monitored with a thermistor or thermocouple that is incorporated into an esophageal stethoscope. Measured properly, esophageal temperature accurately reflects core temperature in almost all conditions. These readings, however, can be artificially affected during general anesthesia by the use of humidified gases [33,34] if the probe is not inserted far enough. The optimal position for the sensor is approximately 45 cm from the nose in adults, which is 12 to 16 cm distal from where the heart and breath sounds are heard best [35]. More proximal positioning can result in falsely decreased temperatures as a result of the proximity to the trachea and the impact of cold, dry gases on the site [34]. Esophageal temperature probes are used frequently for their ease of placement and relatively minimal risk, and because the site is so reliable.

Nasopharyngeal temperature

Nasopharyngeal temperature can be measured with an esophageal probe positioned above the palate, and it is reasonably close to brain and core temperature. Because the eardrum is close to the carotid artery and the hypothalamus, tympanic membrane temperature is a reliable measure of core temperature and often is used as a reference for other sites. This measurement requires that a transducer be placed in contact with the tympanic membrane, which often requires direct visualization with an otoscope for correct positioning and cerumen removal; poor contact or cerumen obstruction can render these readings inaccurate. Older tympanic probes sometimes caused bleeding and perforation of the eardrum [36,37]; fortunately, these problems are not likely to occur with modern probes, which are soft and flexible.

Bladder temperature

This can be measured with a Foley catheter with an attached temperature thermistor or thermocouple. Although bladder temperature is a close approximation of core temperature, the accuracy of this site decreases with low urine output and during surgical procedures of the lower abdomen [38]. Rectal temperature measurement is another site that approximates core temperature, but these readings may be affected by the presence of stool and of bacteria that generate heat [39]; consequently, rectal temperature tends to exceed core temperature. Rectal and bladder temperatures lag behind other central monitoring sites during conditions in which the temperature changes rapidly such as cardiopulmonary bypass surgery. Despite their limitations, bladder and rectal temperature monitors are reasonable choices to use during regional anesthesia, because awake patients can tolerate them.

Skin-temperature measurements

These are potentially confounded by:

- Core-to-peripheral redistribution, which may be seen on anesthetic induction
- Thermoregulatory changes in vasomotor tone triggered when sufficient core hypothermia initiates intraoperative cutaneous vasoconstriction, which can lead to a reduction in skin blood flow and temperature
- Changes in ambient temperature

Ikeda and colleagues, however, evaluated these three conditions in which core-to-skin temperature differences were likely and also considered core-to-skin differences depending on whether thermometers were positioned on the forehead or neck. In fact, there were only slight differences induced by these factors, with the smallest difference of only 0.5 to 1.0°C being on the forehead [40,41].

Axillary temperatures

Axillary temperatures are relatively close to core temperature and may be a reasonable choice in selected patients. But this is the case only if the probe is positioned carefully over the axillary artery and the arms positioned at the patient's side.

Temperature monitoring during cardiopulmonary bypass

Cardiopulmonary bypass constitutes a challenging situation for monitoring temperature because of the rapid and extraordinary degree of heat transferred through the bypass circuit during heating and rewarming. The core compartment goes through the most dramatic temperature changes because of the blood being rapidly reinfused into the mediastinal organs. The thermal changes from the core compartment then are dissipated slowly to the periphery because of the slower nature of heat passing through tissue as opposed to the cardiopulmonary bypass circuit.

During bypass, core-monitoring sites are useful for temperature monitoring (ie, nasopharyngeal, pulmonary artery, tympanic membrane, and distal esophagus). Once full-flow bypass has been established, however, the pulmonary artery catheter may not give an accurate temperature reading because of diminished flow in the central circulation.

Bladder and rectal temperatures often are considered intermediate temperature monitoring sites during bypass, because they lag behind the core sites but change faster than peripheral tissues. During cardiac surgery, bladder temperature equals rectal temperature when urine flow is low, but equals the pulmonary artery temperature when urine flow is high [42]. Because urine flow is such an important determinant of temperature in the cardiac surgery patient, it is best to consider both core and intermediate sites when judging adequacy of rewarming or cooling. Skin temperature, although unrelated to core temperature, may be helpful in evaluating heat distribution between compartments at the end of bypass [43].

Summary

Traditionally, hypothermia has been thought of and used perioperatively as a presumptive strategy to reduce cerebral and myocardial tissue sensitivity to ischemia. Evidence, however, is mounting that maintenance of perioperative normothermia is associated with improved outcomes in patients undergoing all types of surgery, even cardiac surgery.

Ambient environmental temperature is sensed by free nerve endings in the dermal and epidermal layers of the skin, which are the axonal extensions of thermosensitive neurons found in the dorsal root ganglia. Free nerve endings in the skin, by means of transient receptor ion channels that are specifically thermosensitive, also may directly sense environmental temperature. This information is transmitted to the preoptic/anterior hypothalamic region of the brainstem, which coordinates efferent responses to abnormal temperature deviation. People have evolved a highly integrated thermoregulatory system that maintains core body temperature in a relatively narrow temperature range. This system, though, is impaired by the stress of regional and general anesthesia, and the added exposure that occurs during the surgical procedure. When combined, these factors can lead to unwanted thermal disturbances. In a cold operating room environment, hypothermia is the usual perioperative consequence; however, hyperthermia is more dangerous and demands immediate diagnosis.

Intraoperative hypothermia usually develops in three phases. The first is a rapid decrease in core temperature following anesthetic induction, which mostly results from redistribution of heat from the core thermal compartment to the outer shell of the body. This is followed by a slower, linear reduction in the core temperature that may last several hours. Finally, a core temperature plateau is reached, after which core temperature remains virtually unchanged for the remainder of the procedure. The plateau can be passive or result from re-emergence of thermoregulatory control in patients becoming sufficiently hypothermic.

Mild hypothermia in the perioperative period has been associated with adverse outcomes, including impaired drug metabolism, prolonged recovery from anesthesia, cardiac morbidity, coagulopathy, wound infections, and postoperative shivering.

Perioperative temperature monitoring devices vary by transducer type and site monitored. More important than the specific device is the site of temperature monitoring. Sites that are accessible during surgery and give an accurate reflection of core temperature include esophageal, nasopharynx, bladder, and rectal sites. Core temperature also may be estimated reasonably using axillary temperature probes except under extreme thermal conditions.

Rather than taking a passive approach to thermal management, anesthesiologists need to be proactive in monitoring patients in cold operating rooms and use available technology to prevent gross disturbances in the core temperature. Various methods are available to achieve this. Prewarming patients reduces redistribution hypothermia and is an effective strategy for maintaining intraoperative normothermia. Additionally, forced-air warming and circulating water garments also have been shown to be effective. Heating intravenous fluids does not warm patients, but does prevent fluid-induced hypothermia in patients given large volumes of fluid.

This article examined the evolutionary adaptations people possess to combat inadvertent hypothermia and hyperthermia. Because thermal disturbances are associated with severe consequences, the standard of care is to monitor temperature during general anesthesia and to maintain normothermia unless otherwise specifically indicated.

References

[1] Cheney FW. Should normothermia be maintained during major surgery? JAMA 1997; 277(14):1165–6.
[2] Schmied H, Kurz A, Sessler DI, et al. Mild intraoperative hypothermia increases blood loss and allogeneic transfusion requirements during total hip arthroplasty. Lancet 1996;347: 289–92.
[3] Bush HL, Hydo LJ, Fischer E, et al. Hypothermia during elective abdominal aortic aneurysm repair: the high price of avoidable morbidity. J Vasc Surg 1995;21:392–402.
[4] Hypothermia after Cardiac Arrest Study Group. Mild therapeutic hypothermia to improve the neurologic outcome after cardiac arrest. N Engl J Med 2002;346(8):549–56.

[5] Bernard SA, Gray TW, Buist MD, et al. Treatment of comatose survivors of out-of-hospital cardiac arrest with induced hypothermia. N Engl J Med 2002;346(8):557–63.
[6] Kurz A, Sessler DI, Lenhardt R. Perioperative normothermia to reduce the incidence of surgical wound infection and shorten hospitalization. Study of wound infection and temperature group. N Engl J Med 1996;334:1209–15.
[7] Vaughan MS, Vaughan RW, Cork RC. Postoperative hypothermia in adults: relationship of age, anesthesia, and shivering to rewarming. Anesth Analg 1981;60:746–51.
[8] Lenhardt R, Marker E, Goll V, et al. Mild intraoperative hypothermia prolongs postoperative recovery. Anesthesiology 1997;87:1318–23.
[9] Washington DE, Sessler DI, Moayeri A, et al. Thermoregulatory responses to hyperthermia during isoflurane anesthesia in humans. J Appl Physiol 1993;74:82–7.
[10] Simon HB. Hyperthermia. N Engl J Med 1993;329:483–7.
[11] Styrt B, Sugarman B. Antipyresis and fever. Arch Intern Med 1990;150(8):1589–97.
[12] Patapoutian A, Peier AM, Story GM, et al. ThermoTRP channels and beyond: mechanisms of temperature sensation. Nat Rev Neurosci 2003;4(7):529–39.
[13] Xu H, Ramsey IS, Kotecha SA, et al. TRPV3 is a calcium-permeable temperature-sensitive cation channel. Nature 2002;418(6894):181–6.
[14] Moqrich A, Hwang SW, Earley TJ, et al. Impaired thermosensation in mice lacking TRPV3, a heat and camphor sensor in the skin. Science 2005;307(5714):1468–72.
[15] Sessler DI, Lee KA, McGuire J. Isoflurane anesthesia and circadian temperature cycles. Anesthesiology 1991;75:985–9.
[16] Sund-Levander M, Forsberg C, Wahren LK. Normal oral, rectal, tympanic and axillary body temperature in adult men and women: a systematic literature review. Scand J Caring Sci 2002;16(2):122–8.
[17] Cork RC, Vaughan RW, Humphrey LS. Precision and accuracy of intraoperative temperature monitoring. Anesth Analg 1983;62:211–4.
[18] Satinoff E. Neural organization and evolution of thermal regulation in mammals. Science 1978;201:16–22.
[19] Satinoff E, Rutstein J. Behavioral thermoregulation in rats with anterior hypothalamic lesions. J Comp Physiol Psychol 1970;71:77–82.
[20] Passlick-Deetjen J, Bedenbender-Stoll E. Why thermosensing? A primer on thermoregulation. Nephrol Dial Transplant 2005;20(9):1784–9.
[21] Charkoudian N. Skin blood flow in adult human thermoregulation: how it works, when it does not, and why. Mayo Clin Proc 2003;78(5):603–12.
[22] Cabanac M, Dib B. Behavioural responses to hypothalamic cooling and heating in the rat. Brain Res 1983;264:79–87.
[23] Satinoff E, McEwen GN Jr, Williams BA. Behavioral fever in newborn rabbits. Science 976;193:1139–40.
[24] Nadel ER, Pandolf KB, Roberts MF, et al. Mechanisms of thermal acclimation to exercise and heat. J Appl Physiol 1974;37:515–20.
[25] Nadel ER, Cafarelli E, Roberts MF, et al. Circulatory regulation during exercise in different ambient temperatures. J Appl Physiol 1979;46:430–7.
[26] Hales JRS. Skin arteriovenous anastomoses; their control and role in thermoregulation. In: Johansen K, Burggren W, editors. Cardiovascular shunts: phylogenetic, ontogenetic and clinical aspects. Copenhagen (Denmark): Munksgaard; 1985. p. 433–51.
[27] Nedergaard J, Cannon B. The uncoupling protein thermogenin and mitochondrial thermogenesis. New Comprehensive Biochemistry 1992;23:385–420.
[28] Israel DJ, Pozos RS. Synchronized slow-amplitude modulations in the electromyograms of shivering muscles. J Appl Physiol 1989;66:2358–63.
[29] Jessen C, Mayer ET. Spinal cord and hypothalamus as core sensors of temperature in the conscious dog. I. Equivalence of responses. Pflugers Arch 1971;324:189–204.
[30] Sessler DI. Perioperative heat balance. Anesthesiology 2000;92:578–96.

[31] Bennett LA, Johnson JM, Stephens DP, et al. Evidence for a role for vasoactive intestinal peptide in active vasodilatation in the cutaneous vasculature of humans. J Physiol 2003; 552(Pt 1):223–32.
[32] De Witte J, Sessler DI. Perioperative shivering: physiology and pharmacology. Anesthesiology 2002;96(2):467–84.
[33] Siegel MN, Gravenstein N. Passive warming of airway gases (artificial nose) improves accuracy of esophageal temperature monitoring. J Clin Monit 1990;6(2):89–92.
[34] Bissonnette B, Sessler DI, LaFlamme P. Intraoperative temperature monitoring sites in infants and children and the effect of inspired gas warming on esophageal temperature. Anesth Analg 1989;69:192–6.
[35] Erickson RS. The continuing question of how best to measure body temperature. Crit Care Med 1999;27(10):2307–10.
[36] Whitby JD, Dunkin LJ. Cerebral, oesophageal and nasopharyngeal temperatures. Br J Anaesth 1971;43(7):673–6.
[37] Kaufman RD. Relationship between esophageal temperature gradient and heart and lung sounds heard by esophageal stethoscope. Anesth Analg 1987;66:1046–8.
[38] Webb GE. Comparison of esophageal and tympanic temperature monitoring during cardiopulmonary bypass. Analg Anesth 1973;52:729–33.
[39] Wallace CT, Marks WE Jr, Adkins WY, et al. Perforation of the tympanic membrane, a complication of tympanic thermometry during anesthesia. Anesthesiology 1974;41:290–1.
[40] Vaughan MS, Cork RC, Vaughan RW. Inaccuracy of liquid crystal thermometry to identify core temperature trends in postoperative adults. Anesth Analg 1982;61:284–7.
[41] Ikeda T, Sessler DI, Marder D, et al. Influence of thermoregulatory vasomotion and ambient temperature variation on the accuracy of core temperature estimates by cutaneous liquid–crystal thermometers. Anesthesiology 1997;86:603–12.
[42] Rajek A, Lenhardt R, Sessler DI, et al. Tissue heat content and distribution during and after cardiopulmonary bypass at 17 degrees C. Anesth Analg 1999;88:1220–5.
[43] Rajek A, Lenhardt R, Sessler DI, et al. Tissue heat content and distribution during and after cardiopulmonary bypass at 31 degrees C and 27 degrees C. Anesthesiology 1998;88:1511–8.

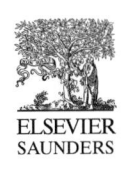

Coagulation Monitoring

Antoine G. Rochon, MD, FRCPC[a],*, Linda Shore-Lesserson, MD[b]

[a]*Department of Anesthesiology, Montreal Heart Institute, 5000 Belanger Street, Montreal, Canada H1T 1C8*
[b]*Department of Anesthesiology Mount Sinai Medical Center New York, NY 10029*

Normal hemostasis protects the organism from hemorrhage and thrombosis. It involves complex and dynamic physiologic processes kept in balance by a system of positive and negative feedback mechanisms. The protagonists at play include: blood vessels, platelets, and coagulation factors; the antagonists include their respective inhibitors and the fibrinolytic system. Traditionally, and for diagnostic purposes, the hemostatic system has been divided into primary and secondary hemostatic events, where, after injury to the vascular endothelium and exposition of collagen, platelets first are involved in the formation of a blood clot, to be solidified subsequently by the fibrin produced from the enzymatic coagulation cascade. In a third phase, and once vascular integrity has been achieved, the fibrinolytic system lyses unnecessary clots, keeping in check coagulation. In recent years, new evidence has given further insights into the in vivo role, mechanism, and sequence of action of the hemostatic actors, and the traditional view of the hemostatic system has been revisited [1,2]. This includes a cell-based model of hemostasis in which tissue factor causes activation of coagulation and the formation of thrombin. Furthermore, the last 10 years have seen the introduction in clinical practice of many new anticoagulants, antiplatelet agents, and procoagulants that render the safe practice of anesthesia and surgery even more challenging. This article discusses current and pertinent perioperative tests and monitors of coagulation, platelet function, and antiplatelet drugs.

Work by Dr. Antoine G. Rochon is supported, in part, by the 2004 Abbott Laboratories Ltd/CAS/CIHR Fellowship in Anesthesia (Grant JAN-73042).
* Corresponding author.
E-mail address: antoine.rochon@icm-mhi.org (A.G. Rochon).

Updated concept of hemostasis

An exhaustive review of the physiology of hemostasis is beyond the scope of this article, but a discussion of the monitors of hemostasis is not possible without the review of certain concepts.

The vascular endothelium provides the first hemostatic barrier. Beyond physically preventing hemorrhage, its surface limits the generation and activity of thrombin and the adhesion of platelets through several interrelated mechanisms, thus preventing inappropriate clotting [3–7].

When there is injury to the endothelium, tissue factor is exposed and interacts with plasma factor VII to activate coagulation and platelets. The sequential activation of coagulation factors model first was proposed by Davie in 1964 [8]. This model envisioned two mutually exclusive activation pathways (an intrinsic and extrinsic) leading to the generation of thrombin. It now is known that the intrinsic and extrinsic pathways are not independent of each other and that coagulation is initiated by the exposition of tissue factor (TF) and the formation of a TF/VIIa complex capable of activating both factor X and factor IX [1]. Thrombin is pivotal to hemostasis. Its major role is to convert fibrinogen to fibrin, but it also activates factors V, VIII, and XI, thus generating more thrombin, and it causes intense activation of platelets.

Tests of coagulation

The best test or monitor of coagulation cannot replace the preoperative medical and hemostatic function history. This preoperative evaluation is by far more cost-effective than systematic test screening. In the presence of a preoperative history of unexplained bleeding diathesis or of a known coagulopathy (acquired or congenital), delaying surgery and consultation with the hematology service for diagnosis and management advice might not only be warranted but also life-saving to the patient.

Most institutions' laboratory coagulation profile includes a platelet count, a fibrinogen concentration, a thrombin time (TT), a prothrombin time (PT), and an activated partial thromboplastin time (aPTT). One should remember that these tests were developed in the era of elucidation and characterization of the coagulation mechanisms. They were not designed to screen and stratify patients for risks of clinical or perioperative bleeding [9–11]. These common laboratory tests will be discussed.

Platelet count

The platelet count is a quantitative measure of single or isolated cells suspended in EDTA solution. This test result gives no information regarding platelet function. A low platelet count may not be synonymous with hemorrhage, and a normal platelet count may not guarantee minimal bleeding.

Most platelet counts are performed by automated cell counters, and results are more reliable than when manually done. Laser technology and automated flow cytology allow the definition of the count of various cell lines by size, morphology, intracellular organelles, and adhesion molecules.

Platelets are the smallest of the human blood cells (3.6 × 0.7 µm). Released by the megakaryocytes of the bone marrow, they are anucleated and discoid-shaped. A platelet count is considered normal if between 150,000 and 450,000 per µL. In addition to their central role in hemostatic and thrombotic processes, they also modulate the inflammatory response and the immune defense and participate in wound healing.

Their role in hemostasis is very complex and becoming increasingly understood. After injury to the vascular endothelium, platelets are recruited to the damaged site to fill in the breach. This occurs in a series of complex and well-orchestrated steps [12]. Platelets first adhere to exposed subendothelial proteins by means of specific glycoproteins (GP). Exposed collagen and exposed von Willebrand factor bind to GPIb and other platelet receptors. Adhesion induces intracellular signaling that results in activation of the platelet, shape change with the formation of pseudopodia, and secretion of the platelets granules content [13,14]. Activated platelets express the fibrinogen receptor (GPIIb/IIIa) in an activated form, allowing aggregation of platelets and formation of the primary hemostatic plug [15]. Furthermore, phospholipids on the platelet surface serve as a substrate for the activation of the coagulation proteases, generation of thrombin, and formation of a stable platelet–fibrin clot [16].

In the presence of normally functioning platelets, a general recommendation of a platelet count of 50,000 per µL is a recommended minimum before elective surgery. A platelet count of 100,000 per µL is recommended for neurosurgery or ophthalmologic procedures involving the posterior segment of the eye. A platelet count of 50,000 per µL is considered sufficient for spinal anesthesia, and a platelet count of 80,000 per µL is considered sufficient for epidurals [17].

Fibrinogen concentration

Fibrinogen concentration is measured using clottable protein methods, end-point detection techniques, or immunochemical tests. The method of Clauss is the most common fibrinogen assay used [18]. This method involves a tenfold dilution of plasma to ensure that fibrinogen is the rate-limiting step in clot formation. An excess of thrombin then is added to the sample and the time to clot formation measured. The clotting time is related inversely to the fibrinogen concentration. Fibrin degradation products, polymerization inhibitors, or other inhibitors of fibrin formation can cause artifactual results, as the Clauss method relies on detection of actual clot. This test is executed with an excess of thrombin, so results will not be affected by small concentrations of heparin.

The whole blood point-of-care (POC) Hemochron (International Technidyne Incorporated, Edison, New Jersey) system offers a fibrinogen assay. A specific test tube contains a lyophilized preparation of human thrombin, snake venom extract, protamine, buffers, and calcium stabilizers. The test tube is incubated with 1.5 mL of distilled water and heated in the Hemochron device for 3 min. Whole blood is diluted by 50% and a volume of 0.5 mL transferred into the specific fibrinogen test tube. The clotting time is measured using standard Hemochron technology. The concentration of fibrinogen is obtained by comparison to a standard curve. Normal fibrinogen concentration of 180 to 220 mg/dL correlates with a clotting time of 54 plus or minus 2.5 seconds. Fibrinogen deficiency of 50 to 75 mg/dL correlates with a clotting time of 150 plus or minus 9.0 seconds.

Compared with the method of Clauss, end-point detection assays rely on the detection of changes in turbidity of plasma after clot formation. Presence of inhibitors will not underestimate the fibrinogen concentration, as this technique does not require the maintenance of a stable cross-linked fibrin product. Immunochemical techniques directly and accurately measure fibrinogen concentrations. They are expensive, time consuming, and require specialized laboratory facilities, however.

Thrombin time

Thrombin time (TT) is the time taken for the conversion of fibrinogen to fibrin when blood or plasma is exposed to thrombin. Detection of fibrin formation using standard laboratory techniques requires incubation of the sampled blood or plasma within a chamber in which an optical or electrical probe sits. Movements of the probe or the generation of an electrical field secondary to the formation of fibrin is sensed by a detector and terminates the test. A POC TT test is manufactured by International Technidyne. 1 mL of whole blood is added to a test tube that contains a lyophilized preparation of thrombin. The detection of fibrin formation uses the standard Hemochron technology. Provided reference normal values for the TT are 39 to 53 seconds for whole blood and 43 to 68 seconds for citrated blood. The TT specifically measures the activity of thrombin and is therefore very sensitive to heparin-induced enhancement of antithrombin III (AT3) activity. Because it excludes the intrinsic and extrinsic coagulation pathway limbs and evaluates the conversion of factor I to Ia, this test is useful in cardiac surgery, after cardiopulmonary bypass (CPB), to differentiate the cause of bleeding when both PT and aPTT are prolonged. The TT is elevated in the presence of heparin, hypofibrinogenemia, dysfibrinogenemia, amyloidosis, or antibodies to thrombin [19]. TT also will be elevated in the presence of fibrin degradation products if the systemic fibrinogen concentration is low.

In the patient given thrombolytics, the TT is an appropriate laboratory test to monitor the degree of fibrinolytic activity. Measurements of the quantity of fibrinogen, plasminogen, or of plasma proteins generated during fibrinolysis are difficult to interpret and yield no prognostic information for dose adjustments. Thrombolytics will invoke the conversion of plasminogen to plasmin, cause clot dissolution, and decrease the concentrations of fibrinogen and fibrin. The TT is useful to monitor these effects. A baseline TT should be measured before institution of thrombolytic therapy, and 3 to 4 hours after therapy is initiated. Prolongation by 1.5 to five times the baseline value should signify effective therapy. Prolongation by greater than seven times the baseline value could put the patient at an increased risk of spontaneous bleeding. Absence of TT prolongation signifies that therapy has failed to activate fibrinolysis.

Activated partial thromboplastin time

The activated partial thromboplastin time (aPTT) tests the integrity of the intrinsic and final coagulation pathways. It is more sensitive to low levels of heparin than the activated clotting time (ACT). Factors IX and X are most sensitive to heparin effects, which explains why the aPTT will be prolonged even at very low heparin concentrations. Thromboplastin is a tissue extract that contains tissue factor and phospholipid. Because the test uses only the phospholipid part as a substitute for the platelet membrane in activating factor XII, it is qualified as partial thromboplastin. Deficiencies of factors XII, XI, IX, VIII, high molecular weight kininogen (HMWK), or kallikrein will prolong the aPTT. To accelerate the PTT reaction, an activator (celite-diatomaceous-earth, kaolin) is added to the test, hence the term activated. Blood is collected in a citrated tube, which arrests coagulation by binding calcium. To initiate the test and activate the intrinsic pathway, thromboplastin, an activator, and calcium are added to plasma, and the time for clot formation is measured. Normal aPTT is 28 to 32 seconds.

Prothrombin time

The prothrombin time (PT) measures the integrity of the extrinsic and common coagulation pathways. Deficiencies in factor VII or vitamin K and therapy with warfarin will cause an elevation in the PT. Inactivation of factor II by large doses of heparin also will prolong the PT. A blood sample is taken in a citrated tube to prevent coagulation. Calcium then is added to the plasma test sample, and thromboplastin is added to initiate clot formation. The time to clot is measured and recorded as the PT. Normal PT values are between 12 and 14 seconds. The international normalized ratio (INR) is a standardized laboratory value that is the ratio of the patient's PT to the result that would have been obtained if the international reference preparation (IRP) had been used instead of the laboratory reagents. Each laboratory uses reagents with a specific sensitivity (international sensitivity index [ISI]) relative to the IRP. The ISI of a particular set of reagents is provided by each manufacturer, so that the INR can be reported and results compared between laboratories.

Bedside tests of coagulation

The aPTT and PT are done on plasma in the laboratory. PT and aPTT tests performed on whole blood are available for use in the operating room or at the bedside. The Hemochron and the Ciba Corning Biotrack 512 (Cardiovascular Diagnostics, Raleigh, North Carolina) are two POC coagulation monitors that allow bedside determination of PT and aPTT.

In patients receiving oral anticoagulant therapy, the Biotrack 512 monitor was found suitable to monitor PT and INR. Reiner and colleagues compared the bedside Biotrack aPTT with the laboratory aPTT and heparin level in patients receiving therapeutic heparinization after interventional cardiac catheterization [20]. They found a strong correlation ($r = 0.89$) between the Biotrack aPTT and the laboratory aPTT. The correlation between the Biotrack aPTT and the heparin level was not strong, probably because of the many other factors that impact on the heparin concentration in vivo, such as heparin neutralization and clearance [21].

Studies comparing the Hemochron and the Ciba Corning Biotrack whole blood PT and aPTT with the laboratory plasma PT and aPTT in the cardiac surgical population have found good accuracy and precision with regard to the PT, but not to the aPTT [19,22].

These POC monitors might be useful to determine the patients at risk of bleeding after cardiac surgery [23], and they have been useful in transfusion algorithms [24,25].

Monitoring fibrinolysis

Fibrinolysis is a normal part of hemostasis that regulates clot formation and dissolution in response to appropriate physiologic stimuli. It also regulates the formation of fibrin, ensuring that coagulation does not proceed unchecked. As hemorrhage is stopped by the fibrin clot, fibrinolysis dissolves the clot when local endothelial healing occurs. Fibrinolysis is mediated by the serine protease plasmin, which is the product of the cleavage of plasminogen by tissue plasminogen activator (tPA). Fibrinolysis is a normal phenomenon in response to clot formation. When it occurs systemically, it represents a pathologic condition.

Fibrinolysis is characterized as primary or secondary. Primary fibrinolysis occurs when fibrinolytic activators are released or produced in excess and do not represent a response to the coagulation process. This occurs during liver transplantation when plasminogen activators are released, during prostate surgery when urokinase is circulating in excess amount, or in the case of exogenous administration of fibrinolytic agents such as streptokinase. With primary fibrinolysis, plasmin cleaves fibrinogen, yielding fibrinogen degradation products. These end products can be measured using immunologic techniques.

Secondary fibrinolysis results from enhanced activation of the coagulation system, as seen during disseminated intravascular coagulation, when both systemic coagulation and fibrinolysis are occurring in excess. During CPB, fibrinolysis is most likely secondary to the microvascular coagulation that is occurring despite attempts at suppression using high doses of heparin [26,27].

Fibrinolysis can be monitored by direct measurement of the clot lysis time (manual or viscoelastic tests) or by measurement of the end products of fibrin degradation.

It should be remembered that these tests of coagulation are done on plasma and not on whole blood, which not only requires time to process but also gives an in vitro evaluation of an in vivo physiologic process. Therefore, their results should be interpreted with caution and not outside the clinical context. Newer POC monitors of coagulation and hemostasis can perform the testing on whole blood. This speeds up results, rendering these tests more useful to the clinician in the acute setting of surgery and bleeding.

Many of the monitors of hemostasis were developed for managing anticoagulation during CPB, and others were developed for monitoring of platelet function and antiplatelet therapy. To date, they rarely have been evaluated outside the realm of cardiac surgery or cardiology, but literature in other fields of study is beginning to emerge.

Hemodilution, hypothermia, and contact activation challenge hemostatic function during CPB in the following ways. Hemodilution results in depletion and dysfunction of coagulation cascade proteases; hypothermia temporarily paralyzes the enzymatic reactions required for coagulation and stimulates fibrinolysis. Contact activation incites microvascular coagulation, thereby upregulating coagulation and fibrinolysis and activating platelets. To mitigate these effects, unfractionated heparin (UH) is used most commonly. Protamine sulfate is given to antagonize heparin anticoagulation at completion of CPB, but protamine, if given in excess, also has antiplatelet and anticoagulant properties. With the use of CPB, monitoring techniques are essential to ensure adequate anticoagulation and adequate heparin neutralization, and to assess platelet function. Coagulation monitoring is associated with decreased hemorrhagic complication and with reduction of transfusion [28].

Heparin concentration and ACT can be used to monitor heparin anticoagulation. The ideal heparin management strategy, however, is not well defined by evidence-based studies, as heparin is not a perfect anticoagulant [29]. Indeed, UH only can inhibit fluid-phase thrombin as opposed to other thrombin inhibitors that can inhibit clot-bound thrombin. UH also causes platelet activation and expression of P-selectin, while the direct thrombin inhibitors do not. The direct thrombin inhibitor bivalirudin increasingly is used as the anticoagulant of choice in interventional cardiology procedures, because ischemic outcomes are comparable to those using heparin, yet bleeding complications are reduced [30]. Another disadvantage to the use of UH is that it requires antithrombin III (AT3) as a cofactor to inhibit factors XIa, Xa, Ixa, and thrombin (IIa). Interpatient differences in AT3 levels and activity therefore can have significant pharmacodynamic impact on the efficacy of heparinization. Recent evidence suggests advantages to the use of direct thrombin inhibitors as an alternative [31], but superiority over heparin as an anticoagulant in cardiac surgery has not been established. A recent randomized controlled trial comparing bivalirudin to heparin in cardiopulmonary bypass demonstrated similar efficacy, transfusion rates, and adverse event rates [32]. Heparin remains the gold standard in cardiopulmonary bypass until more data become available. It is monitored using the ACT. The direct thrombin inhibitors can be monitored using the ACT, but plasma levels of drug are not linearly related to clotting times in the clinical range. A plasma-modified ACT has been shown to be a more direct measure of anticoagulation using direct thrombin inhibitors [33].

Activated clotting time

The ACT is the most frequently used assay to measure heparin's effect during CPB. Different technology measures the ACT in various ways. The Hemochron uses approximately 2 mL of whole blood that is activated by celite, kaolin, glass, or a combination of these activators. A test tube containing a small magnet and a plastic baffle is placed in a rotating tilted well, after manual mixing of the blood sample. A timer is started and as formation of a solid clot occurs, the magnet is engaged and moves away from the dependent portion of the test tube. This interrupts a magnetic field and causes the timer to stop. The ACT is highly susceptible to variations during CPB and does not correlate well with anti-Xa measurement of heparin activity or with heparin concentration during the hypothermia and hemodilution associated with CPB [34–36]. Furthermore, the celite-activated ACT is prolonged by aprotinin and platelet glycoprotein IIb/IIIa antagonists [37,38], and is limited by its tendency to decrease with surgical stress [39]. Nonetheless, safety of CPB was improved significantly by the use of ACT monitoring compared with empiric heparin dosing.

Because heparin concentrations steadily decrease upon institution of CPB while ACT increases [40,41], it is common practice in many institutions to monitor the whole blood heparin concentration in addition to the ACT. Maintenance of the heparin concentration should secure that an appropriate ACT for CPB is not the result of a measurement artifact but of an appropriate plasma concentration of heparin.

Heparin concentration monitoring

The Hepcon (Medtronic, Parker, Colorado) is the most commonly used POC technique that measures whole blood heparin concentration. It uses a protamine titration assay that takes advantage of the anticoagulation property of protamine. Indeed, excess protamine will inhibit clot formation, whereas insufficient protamine will fail to fully antagonize heparin. Therefore, the fastest clot formation will occur in the test channel with the optimal protamine to heparin ratio. Because the protamine concentration in the channels is known, and because 1 mg of protamine will neutralize 100 U of heparin, the heparin concentration can be calculated. It is theorized that higher heparin concentration better suppresses the hemostatic protagonists, and when heparin concentration monitoring is used concomitantly with a strict transfusion algorithm, it has been demonstrated to result in less postoperative bleeding and fewer transfusions of allogenic blood products [42]. Heparin concentration monitoring, however, has been associated with postoperative heparin rebound [43,44] and increased bleeding [45], making the level of evidence supporting heparin concentration monitoring insufficient to be made into a standard of care.

High-dose thrombin time

High-dose thrombin time (HiTT, International Technidyne Incorporated) overcomes some of the limitations of the standard ACT. HiTT is not altered by hemodilution or hypothermia and has been shown to correlate better with heparin concentration than the ACT during CPB [46]. The HiTT exhibits less artifactual modulation, because it measures the effects of heparin at the level of thrombin. With HiTT, a large dose of thrombin is added into the test tube and binds a significant proportion of the heparin-AT3 complexes present during heparinization. The remaining AT3-unbound heparin prolongs the time required for fibrin to form and is measured as HiTT. The Hemochron allows the performance of HiTT. In contrast to the ACT during CPB, HiTT decreases with heparin concentration and is not affected by aprotinin [47]. It also is affected less than ACT by the heparin resistance seen in patients on preoperative heparin infusions [48].

Individualized heparin dosing

More precise control of heparin anticoagulation and of its reversal may reduce blood loss and transfusion in the cardiac surgical patient [49,50]. In vitro assays that measure a patient's heparin sensitivity to a known quantity of heparin and generate a dose–response curve, enabling the calculation of the heparin dose required to attain the target goal, have been introduced.

These assays also make it possible to adjust the protamine dosing to the circulating level of heparin at the end of CPB. The Hepcon (Medtronic) heparin dose response (HDR) is an in vitro heparin dose–response assay that constructs a three-point heparin dose–response curve. From this curve, extrapolation to the desired ACT or heparin concentration will indicate the dose of heparin to be given. With the Hemochron RxDx (International Technidyne), an ACT-based heparin dose–response assay, investigators have been able to significantly lower protamine doses [51] and significantly reduce transfusions and chest tube drainage [52]. Although individualized heparin dosing would appear preferable to weight-based dosing, it is considerably more expensive and not proven to reduce cost of care.

Platelet function

The ability to monitor platelet function has improved greatly, and benefits of platelet function measurements in cardiovascular medicine and in the perioperative period are significant. The heterogeneity of the platelet function defect resulting from CPB has given more insight into its mechanisms [53–61]. Thrombocytopenia rarely causes a bleeding diathesis if platelet function is normal; thus the measurement of platelet count may not be as crucial as the platelet function.

Drug therapy

The use of potent antiplatelet agents is now widespread practice in patients who have cardiac disease. Patients who recently have undergone cardiology interventional procedures or those maintained on anti-thrombotic therapy for months after placement of a drug-eluting stent may present to the anesthesiologist at any time for surgery. For example, antagonists of the glycoprotein IIbIIIa (GPIIb/IIIa) receptor, which mediates platelet–platelet aggregation via fibrinogen bridging, such as Abciximab (Eli Lilly, Indianapolis, Indiana) Eptifibatide (Millenium Pharmaceuticals, Cambridge, Massachusetts) and Tirofiban (Merck & Co, West Point, Pennsylvania), frequently are infused in patients who have undergone a high-risk coronary interventional procedure to prevent thrombus formation in the instrumented coronary artery [62,63].

Furthermore, the thienopyridine ADP receptor antagonists (ticlopidine and clopidogrel) are also effective antiaggregatory agents that have been shown to reduce arterial occlusive events after coronary interventions [64]. Despite the effectiveness of these drugs (GPIIb/IIIa receptor antagonists and ADP receptor antagonists), the antiplatelet effects are not monitored routinely. As the degree of platelet inhibition is, on the one hand, associated with prevention of cardiovascular events [65,66], but on the other hand 'excessive amounts of platelet inhibition are associated with increased bleeding [67,68], monitoring is essential.

Platelet function tests: point of care

Platelet function monitors can be divided into three basic and nonmutually exclusive categories: static tests, dynamic nonactivated tests, and tests of the platelet response to an activating stimulus. Evidence-based supported POC monitors will be discussed.

Static tests of platelet function

Measurement of β-thromboglobulin, ADP release, or determination of the number of receptors present on the platelet surface are punctual and give no information about the dynamic situation encountered in the clinical setting, or about the ability of platelets to respond to an agonist.

Dynamic tests of platelet function

The bleeding time and the thromboelastography (TEG) take into account the time-dependent nature of platelet-mediated hemostasis and better reflect the contribution of platelet function to overall clot formation. Without modification, however, they are nonspecific because of the absence of platelet-specific agonist.

Thromboelastography

The thromboelastography (TEG, Haemoscope Corporation, Niles, Illinois) is a viscoelastic measure of whole blood clotting that can provide, within minutes, information about the integrity of the coagulation cascade, platelet function, platelet–fibrin interactions, and fibrinolysis. The use of TEG can be modified for use in patients receiving heparin, coumadin, fibrinolytic drugs, and antiplatelet agents [27,69–74]. The TEG specifically can identify hemostasis defects. It has been used successfully intraoperatively to better target transfusion therapy [72], and it has been shown to reduce chest tube drainage and transfusion requirements in cardiac and liver transplant surgical patients when concomitantly used with a transfusion algorithm [75–81].

A small volume of whole blood (360 µL) is placed into an oscillating cuvette at physiological temperature, and a piston connected to a transducer and oscillograph is immersed into the blood sample. The movement of the piston becomes coupled to the oscillating cuvette. As the blood clots, a signature tracing is generated, giving the following parameters: reaction time (R value), coagulation time (K value), α angle, maximum amplitude (MA), and amplitude 60 min after the maximal amplitude (A60). These parameters measure fibrin formation, fibrinogen turnover, speed of clot formation, platelet–fibrin interactions, and fibrinolysis, respectively.

The TEG recently has been modified to allow improved monitoring capabilities. The time required for development of MA is shortened by the use of recombinant human tissue factor as an activator to accelerate the rate of thrombin formation. Information about clot strength and platelet function is obtained in 5 to 10 minutes. Furthermore, in vitro addition of a large dose of abciximab to the test cuvette enhances the diagnostic ability of TEG to discriminate between hypofibrinogenemia and platelet dysfunction as a cause of decreased MA [80,81]. A new assay called the Platelet Mapping Assay (Haemoscope Corporation, Niles, Illinois) allows for the thromboelastographic measurement of platelet function in patients on specific platelet antagonistic drugs. The Platelet Mapping Assay incorporates arachidonic acid into the assay to measure patient responsiveness to aspirin, and another assay incorporates ADP to measure the patient response to clopidogrel (an ADP antagonist) [82].

Tests of platelet response to an agonist stimulus

The newest group of platelet function tests includes POC monitors specifically designed to measure agonist-induced platelet-mediated hemostasis.

The Hemostatus (Medtronic Incorporated), platelet-activated clotting time, was a measure of the ACT without platelet activator, and compared this value to the ACT obtained when increasing concentrations of a platelet-activating factor (PAF) were added. The percentage of reduction of the ACT caused by the addition of PAF was related to the ability of platelets to be activated and shortened clotting time [83]. This assay was performed using a specific Hemochron cartridge approved by the US Food and Drug Administration for monitoring platelet function during cardiac surgery. This test is no longer supported commercially.

The Ultegra (Accumetrics, San Diego, California), was designed to measure the platelet response to a thrombin receptor agonist peptide (TRAP). It measures TRAP activation-induced platelet agglutination of fibrinogen-coated beads with an optical detection system. Because the GPIIb/IIIa receptor mediates fibrinogen-platelet binding, this monitor is particularly useful to measure the receptor inhibition in patients given GPIIb/IIIa inhibitors [84–88]. The recent introduction of Ultegra cartridge systems to measure the effects of aspirin and clopidogrel make this system attractive for use in the preoperative patient.

The Clot Signature Analyzer (CSA, Xylum, Scarsdale, New York) measures the distal pressure in a synthetic vessel as whole blood maintained under the constant driving pressure of 60 mm Hg is forced out into it. The time to restoration of this distal pressure is a function of the development of a platelet plug; hence the time for initial closure is a measure of platelet function. This POC monitor is not yet commercially available, but it has been used experimentally to measure platelet reactivity [89–92] and to characterize the CPB-induced platelet dysfunction [93].

The Platelet Function Analyzer, PFA-100 (Dade Behring, Miami, Florida) monitor conducts a modified in vitro bleeding time. Whole blood is drawn through a chamber by vacuum, and is perfused across an aperture in a collagen membrane coated with an agonist (epinephrine or ADP). Platelet adhesion and formation of aggregates will seal the aperture, thus indicating the closure time measured by the PFA-100 [94,95]. Although the preoperative PFA-100 closure time significantly correlates with postoperative blood loss (r = 0.41, P = .022) [96] in the cardiac surgical population, the assay has a high intraoperative negative predictive value, yet a low positive predictive value [97]. The PFA-100, therefore, may be more useful in detecting pharmacologic platelet dysfunction before cardiac surgery or to detect hypercoagulability after CPB [98].

The Plateletworks (Helena Laboratories, Beaumont, Texas) uses a platelet count ratio to assess platelet reactivity. A Coulter counter measures the platelet count in a tube containing standard EDTA and in tubes containing platelet agonists (eg, ADP, collagen, or arachidonic acid). The ratio of the activated platelet count to the nonactivated platelet count is a function of the reactivity of the platelets. This assay was proven useful to provide platelet count, and to measure the platelet dysfunction that accompanies CPB [99]. Plateletworks also has been used to study the pharmacokinetics and pharmacodynamics of clopidogrel in conjunction with other drug therapy [100], and in the perioperative period [101].

Platelet aggregometry

A photo-optical instrument is used to measure light transmittance through a sample of platelet-rich plasma. After platelet aggregation has been induced with an agonist, the light transmittance will be increased, as aggregated platelet will decrease the turbidity of the sample. Correlation between postoperative platelet aggregation and 3-hour postoperative bleeding was found in one ex vivo study using platelet-rich plasma [102]. Platelet aggregation also can be measured in whole blood by using an impedance measurement technique. This assay does not have the same precision or reproducibility as light transmittance aggregometry. It is useful in the perioperative period, however, because it uses whole blood.

Summary

Monitoring hemostasis is now possible by different modalities, of which the point of care devices seem most helpful to the clinician in the operating room. Most of these monitors are being used in the cardiac population, and their significance in other fields remains to be assessed.

References

[1] Glesen PL, Nemerson Y. Tissue factor on the loose. Semin Thromb Hemost 2000;26:379–84.
[2] Roberts HR, Monroe DM, Escobar MA. Current concepts of hemostasis. Anesthesiology 2004;100:722–30.

[3] Thompson EA, Salem HH. Inhibition by human thrombomodulin of factor Xa-mediated cleavage of prothrombin. J Clin Invest 1986;78(1):13–7.
[4] Cines DB, Polack ES, Buck CA, et al. Endothelial cells in physiology and in the pathophysiology of vascular disorders. Blood 1998;91:3627–61.
[5] Esmon CT, Fukudome K. Cellular regulation of the protein C pathway. Semin Cell Biol 1995;6(5):259–68.
[6] Broze GJ Jr. Tissue factor pathway inhibitor. Thromb Haemost 1990;74(1):90–3.
[7] Marcum JA, Rosenberg RD. Anticoagulantly active heparin-like molecules from vascular tissue. Biochemistry 1984;23(8):1730–7.
[8] Davie EW, Ratnoff OD. Waterfall sequence for intrinsic blood clotting. Science 1964;164: 1310–2.
[9] Eika C, Havig O, Godal HC. The value of preoperative haemostatic screening. Scand J Haematol 1978;21:349–54.
[10] Kaplan EB, Sheiner LB, Boeckmann AJ. The usefulness of preoperative laboratory screening. JAMA 1985;253:3576–81.
[11] Rodgers RP, Levin J. A critical reappraisal of the bleeding time. Semin Thromb Hemost 1995;21:21–6.
[12] Jurk K, Kehrel BE. Platelets: physiology and biochemistry. Semin Thromb Hemost 2005; 31(4):381–92.
[13] Shattil SJ, Ginsberg MH, Brugge JS. Adhesive signaling in platelets. Curr Opin Cell Biol 1994;6:695–704.
[14] Fox JE. The platelet cytoskeleton. Thromb Haemost 1993;70:884–93.
[15] Phillips DR, Law D, Scarborough RM. Glycoprotein IIb-IIIa in platelet aggregation: an emerging target for the prevention of acute coronary thrombotic occlusions. Arch Pathol Lab Med 1998;122:811–2.
[16] Monroe DM, Hoffman M, Roberts HR. Platelets and thrombin generation. Arterioscler Thromb Vasc Biol 2002;22:1381–9.
[17] Samama CM, Djoudi R, Lecompte T, et al. Perioperative platelet transfusion: recommendations of the Agence française de sécurité sanitaire des produits de santé (AFSSaPS) 2003. Can J Anesth 2005;52:30–7.
[18] Clauss A. [Rapid physiological coagulation method in determination of fibrinogen]. Acta Haematol 1957;17:237–46 [in English].
[19] Reich DL, Yanakakis MJ, Vela-Cantos FP, et al. Comparison of bedside coagulation monitoring tests with standard laboratory tests in patients after cardiac surgery. Anesth Analg 1993;77:673–9.
[20] Reiner JS, Coyne KS, Lundergan CF, et al. Bedside monitoring of heparin therapy: comparison of activated clotting time to activated partial thromboplastin time. Cathet Cardiovasc Diagn 1994;32(1):49–52.
[21] Bain B, Forster T, Sleigh B. Heparin and the activated partial thromboplastin time - a difference between the in vitro and in vivo effects and implications for the therapeutic range. Am J Clin Pathol 1980;74:668–73.
[22] Samama CM, Quezada R, Riou B, et al. Intraoperative measurement of activated partial thromboplastin time and prothrombin time with a new compact monitor. Acta Anaesthesiol Scand 1994;38:232–7.
[23] Nuttall GA, Oliver WC, Beynen FM, et al. Determination of normal versus abnormal activated partial thromboplastin time and prothrombin time after cardiopulmonary bypass [see comments]. J Cardiothorac Vasc Anesth 1995;9:355–61.
[24] Despotis GJ, Santoro SA, Spitznagel E, et al. Prospective evaluation and clinical utility of on-site monitoring of coagulation in patients undergoing cardiac operation. J Thorac Cardiovasc Surg 1994;107:271–9.
[25] Despotis GJ, Grishaber JE, Goodnough LT. The effect of an intraoperative treatment algorithm on physicians' transfusion practice in cardiac surgery [see comments]. Transfusion 1994;34:290–6.

[26] Muller N, Popov-Cenic S, Buttner W, et al. Studies of fibrinolytic and coagulation factors during open heart surgery. II. Postoperative bleeding tendency and changes in the coagulation system. Thromb Res 1975;7:589–98.
[27] Umlas J. Fibrinolysis and disseminated intravascular coagulation in open heart surgery. Transfusion 1976;16:460–3.
[28] Jaberi M, Bell WR, Benson DW. Control of heparin therapy in open-heart surgery. J Thorac Cardiovasc Surg 1974;67:133–41.
[29] Aggarwal A, Sobel BE, Schneider DJ. Decreased platelet reactivity in blood anticoagulated with bivalirudin or enoxaparin compared with unfractionated heparin: implications for coronary intervention. J Thromb Thrombolysis 2002;13:161–5.
[30] Doggrell S. Can bivalirudin and provisional GP IIb/IIIa blockade REPLACE heparin and planned glycoprotein IIb/IIIa blockade during percutaneous coronary intervention? Expert Opin Pharmacother 2003;4(8):1431–3.
[31] Weitz JI, Crowther MA. New anticoagulants: current status and future potential. Am J Cardiovasc Drugs 2003;3(3):201–9.
[32] Dyke CM, Smedira NG, et al. A comparison of bivalirudin to heparin with protamine reversal inpatients undergoing cardiac surgery with cardiopulmonary bypass: the EVOLUTION-ON study. J Thorac Cardiovasc Surg 2006;131(3):533–9.
[33] Zucker ML, Koster A, et al. Sensitivity of a modified ACT test to levels of bivalirudin used during cardiac surgery. J Extra Corpor Technol 2005;37(4):364–8.
[34] Metz S, Keats AS. Low activated coagulation time during cardiopulmonary bypass does not increase postoperative bleeding. Ann Thorac Surg 1990;49:440–4.
[35] Culliford AT, Gitel SN, Starr N, et al. Lack of correlation between activated clotting time and plasma heparin during cardiopulmonary bypass. Ann Surg 1981;193:105–11.
[36] Wang JS, Lin CY, Karp RB. Comparison of high-dose thrombin time with activated clotting time for monitoring of anticoagulant effects of heparin in cardiac surgical patients. Anesth Analg 1994;79:9–13.
[37] Wang JS, Lin CY, Hung WT, et al. Monitoring of heparin-induced anticoagulation with kaolin-activated clotting time in cardiac surgical patients treated with aprotinin. Anesthesiology 1992;77:1080–4.
[38] Ammar T, Scudder LE, Coller BS. In vitro effects of the platelet glycoprotein IIb/IIIa receptor antagonist c7E3 Fab on the activated clotting time [see comments]. Circulation 1997;95:614–7.
[39] Gravlee GP, Whitaker CL, Mark LJ, et al. Baseline activated coagulation time should be measured after surgical incision. Anesth Analg 1990;71:549–53.
[40] Despotis GJ, Summerfield AL, Joist JH, et al. Comparison of activated coagulation time and whole blood heparin measurements with laboratory plasma anti-Xa heparin concentration in patients having cardiac operations. J Thorac Cardiovasc Surg 1994;108:1076–82.
[41] Martindale SJ, Shayevitz JR, D'Errico C. The activated coagulation time: suitability for monitoring heparin effect and neutralization during pediatric cardiac surgery. J Cardiothorac Vasc Anesth 1996;10:458–63.
[42] Despotis GJ, Joist JH, Hogue CW Jr, et al. More effective suppression of hemostatic system activation in patients undergoing cardiac surgery by heparin dosing based on heparin blood concentrations rather than ACT. Thromb Haemost 1996;76:902–8.
[43] Gravlee GP, Haddon WS, Rothberger HK, et al. Heparin dosing and monitoring for cardiopulmonary bypass. A comparison of techniques with measurement of subclinical plasma coagulation. J Thorac Cardiovasc Surg 1990;99:518–27.
[44] Gravlee GP, Rogers AT, Dudas LM, et al. Heparin management protocol for cardiopulmonary bypass influences postoperative heparin rebound but not bleeding. Anesthesiology 1992;76:393–401.
[45] Rochon AG, Stone ME, et al. A comparison of two heparin management devices for cardiopulmonary bypass. Anesthesiology 2005;101:A-393.

[46] Wang JS, Lin CY, Karp RB. Comparison of high-dose thrombin time with activated clotting time for monitoring of anticoagulant effects of heparin in cardiac surgical patients. Anesth Analg 1994;79:9–13.
[47] Tabuchi N, Njo TL, Tigchelaar I, et al. Monitoring of anticoagulation in aprotinin-treated patients during heart operation. Ann Thorac Surg 1994;58:774–7.
[48] Shore-Lesserson L, Manspeizer HE, Bolastig M, et al. Anticoagulation for cardiac surgery in patients receiving preoperative heparin: use of the high-dose thrombin time. Anesth Analg 2000;90:813–8.
[49] Jobes DR, Aitken GL, Shaffer GW. Increased accuracy and precision of heparin and protamine dosing reduces blood loss and transfusion in patients undergoing primary cardiac operations. J Thorac Cardiovasc Surg 1995;110:36–45.
[50] Despotis GJ, Joist JH, Hogue CW Jr, et al. The impact of heparin concentration and activated clotting time monitoring on blood conservation. A prospective, randomized evaluation in patients undergoing cardiac operation [see comments]. J Thorac Cardiovasc Surg 1995;110:46–54.
[51] Shore-Lesserson L, Reich DL, DePerio M. Heparin and protamine titration do not improve haemostasis in cardiac surgical patients [see comments]. Can J Anaesth 1998;45:10–8.
[52] Jobes DR, Aitken GL, Shaffer GW. Increased accuracy and precision of heparin and protamine dosing reduces blood loss and transfusion in patients undergoing primary cardiac operations. J Thorac Cardiovasc Surg 1995;110:36–45.
[53] Adelman B, Michelson AD, Loscalzo J, et al. Plasmin effect on platelet glycoprotein Ib-von Willebrand factor interactions. Blood 1985;65:32–40.
[54] Michelson AD, Barnard MR. Thrombin-induced changes in platelet membrane glycoproteins Ib, IX, and IIb-IIIa complex. Blood 1987;70:1673–8.
[55] Michelson AD, Barnard MR. Plasmin-induced redistribution of platelet glycoprotein Ib. Blood 1990;76:2005–10.
[56] Rohrer MJ, Kestin AS, Ellis PA, et al. High-dose heparin suppresses platelet alpha granule secretion. J Vasc Surg 1992;15:1000–8 [discussion 1008–9].
[57] Kestin AS, Valeri CR, Khuri SF, et al. The platelet function defect of cardiopulmonary bypass [see comments]. Blood 1993;82:107–17.
[58] John LC, Rees GM, Kovacs IB. Reduction of heparin binding to and inhibition of platelets by aprotinin. Ann Thorac Surg 1993;55:1175–9.
[59] John LC, Rees GM, Kovacs IB. Inhibition of platelet function by heparin. An etiologic factor in postbypass hemorrhage. J Thorac Cardiovasc Surg 1993;105:816–22.
[60] Michelson AD, MacGregor H, Barnard MR, et al. Reversible inhibition of human platelet activation by hypothermia in vivo and in vitro. Thromb Haemost 1994;71:633–40.
[61] Khuri SF, Valeri CR, Loscalzo J, et al. Heparin causes platelet dysfunction and induces fibrinolysis before cardiopulmonary bypass [see comments]. Ann Thorac Surg 1995;60: 1008–14.
[62] Steinhubl SR, Kottke-Marchant K, Moliterno DJ, et al. Attainment and maintenance of platelet inhibition through standard dosing of abciximab in diabetic and nondiabetic patients undergoing percutaneous coronary intervention. Circulation 1999;100: 1977–82.
[63] Steinhubl SR, Ellis SG, Wolski K, et al. Ticlopidine pretreatment before coronary stenting is associated with sustained decrease in adverse cardiac events: data from the Evaluation of Platelet IIb/IIIa Inhibitor for Stenting (EPISTENT) Trial. Circulation 2001; 103:1403–9.
[64] Bertrand ME, Rupprecht HJ, Urban P, et al. Double-blind study of the safety of clopidogrel with and without a loading dose in combination with aspirin compared with ticlopidine in combination with aspirin after coronary stenting: the Clopidogrel Aspirin Stent International Cooperative Study (CLASSICS). Circulation 2000;102:624–9.
[65] Steinhubl SR, Talley JD, Braden GA, et al. Point of care measured platelet inhibition correlates with a reduced risk of an adverse cardiac event after percutaneous coronary

intervention: results of the GOLD (AU-Assessing Ultegra) multi-center study. Circulation 2001;103:2572–8.
[66] Barragan P, Bouvier J, Roquebert P, et al. Resistance to thienopyridines: clinical detection of coronary stent thrombosis by monitoring of vasodilator-stimulated phosphoprotein phosphorylation. Catheter Cardiovasc Interv 2003;59:295–303.
[67] Lefkovits J, Ivanhoe RJ, Califf RM, et al. Effects of platelet glycoprotein IIb/IIIa receptor blockade by a chimeric monoclonal antibody (abciximab) on acute and six-month outcomes after percutaneous transluminal coronary angioplasty for acute myocardial infarction. EPIC investigators. Am J Cardiol 1996;77:1045–51.
[68] Brown DL, Fann CS, Chang CJ. Meta-analysis of effectiveness and safety of abciximab versus eptifibatide or tirofiban in percutaneous coronary intervention. Am J Cardiol 2001;87:537–41.
[69] Tuman KJ, Spiess BD, McCarthy RJ, et al. Comparison of viscoelastic measures of coagulation after cardiopulmonary bypass. Anesth Analg 1989;69:69–75.
[70] Tuman KJ, McCarthy RJ, Djuric M, et al. Evaluation of coagulation during cardiopulmonary bypass with a heparinase-modified thromboelastographic assay. J Cardiothorac Vasc Anesth 1994;8:144–9.
[71] Nuttall GA, Oliver WC, Ereth MH, et al. Coagulation tests predict bleeding after cardiopulmonary bypass [see comments]. J Cardiothorac Vasc Anesth 1997;11:815–23.
[72] Greilich PE, Alving BM, O'Neill KL, et al. A modified thromboelastographic method for monitoring c7E3 Fab in heparinized patients. Anesth Analg 1997;84:31–8.
[73] Cherng YG, Chao A, Shih RL, et al. Preoperative evaluation and postoperative prediction of hemostatic function with thromboelastography in patients undergoing redo cardiac surgery. Acta Anaesthesiol Sin 1998;36:179–86.
[74] Mousa SA, Bozarth JM, Seiffert D, et al. Using thromboelastography to determine the efficacy of the platelet glycoprotein IIb/IIIa antagonist, roxifiban, on platelet/fibrin-mediated clot dynamics in humans. Blood Coagul Fibrinolysis 2005;16:165–71.
[75] Spiess BD, Gillies BS, Chandler W, et al. Changes in transfusion therapy and re-exploration rate after institution of a blood management program in cardiac surgical patients. J Cardiothorac Vasc Anesth 1995;9:168–73.
[76] Kang Y. Transfusion based on clinical coagulation monitoring does reduce hemorrhage during liver transplantation [see comments]. Liver Transpl Surg 1997;3:655–9.
[77] Kang Y. Coagulation and liver transplantation: current concepts. Liver Transpl Surg 1997;3:465–7.
[78] Lesserson L, Manspeizer HE, DePerio M, et al. Thromboelastography-guided transfusion algorithm reduces transfusions in complex cardiac surgery. Anesth Analg 1999;88:312–9.
[79] Nuttall GA, Oliver WC, Santrach PJ, et al. Efficacy of a simple intraoperative transfusion algorithm for nonerythrocyte component utilization after cardiopulmonary bypass. Anesthesiology 2001;94:773–81 [discussion 5A–6A].
[80] Mousa SA, Khurana S, Forsythe MS. Comparative in vitro efficacy of different platelet glycoprotein IIb/IIIa antagonists on platelet-mediated clot strength induced by tissue factor with use of thromboelastography: differentiation among glycoprotein IIb/IIIa antagonists. Arterioscler Thromb Vasc Biol 2000;20:1162–7.
[81] Kettner SC, Panzer OP, Kozek SA, et al. Use of abciximab-modified thromboelastography in patients undergoing cardiac surgery. Anesth Analg 1999;89:580–4.
[82] Craft RM, Chavez JJ, Bresse SJ, et al. A novel modification of the Thromboelastograph assay, isolating platelet function, correlates with optical platelet aggregation. J Lab Clin Med 2004;143(5):301–9.
[83] Bode AP, Lust RM. Masking of heparin activity in the activated coagulation time (ACT) by platelet procoagulant activity. Thromb Res 1994;73:285–300.
[84] Coller BS, Folts JD, Scudder LE, et al. Antithrombotic effect of a monoclonal antibody to the platelet glycoprotein IIb/IIIa receptor in an experimental animal model. Blood 1986;68:783–6.

[85] Coller BS, Lang D, Scudder LE. Rapid and simple platelet function assay to assess glycoprotein IIb/IIIa receptor blockade. Circulation 1997;95:860–7.
[86] Smith JW, Steinhubl SR, Lincoff AM, et al. Rapid platelet-function assay: an automated and quantitative cartridge-based method. Circulation 1999;99:620–5.
[87] Steinhubl SR, Talley JD, Braden GA, et al. Point of care measured platelet inhibition correlates with a reduced risk of an adverse cardiac event after percutaneous coronary intervention: results of the GOLD (AU-Assessing Ultegra) multi-center study. Circulation 2001;103:2572–8.
[88] Serebruany VL, Malinin AI, Ziai W, et al. Effects of clopidogrel and aspirin in combination versus aspirin alone on platelet activation and major receptor expression in patients after recent ischemic stroke. Stroke 2005;36:2289–92.
[89] Kovacs IB, Mayou SC, Kirby JD. Infusion of a stable prostacyclin analogue, iloprost, to patients with peripheral vascular disease: lack of antiplatelet effect but risk of thromboembolism [see comments]. Am J Med 1991;90:41–6.
[90] John LC, Rees GM, Kovacs IB. Reduction of heparin binding to and inhibition of platelets by aprotinin. Ann Thorac Surg 1993;55:1175–9.
[91] Ikarugi H, Taka T, Nakajima S, et al. Norepinephrine, but not epinephrine, enhances platelet reactivity and coagulation after exercise in humans. J Appl Physiol 1999;86:133–8.
[92] Fricke W, Kouides P, Kessler C, et al. A multi-center clinical evaluation of the Clot Signature Analyzer. J Thromb Haemost 2004;2:763–8.
[93] Griffin MJ, Rinder HM, Smith BR, et al. The effects of heparin, protamine, and heparin/protamine reversal on platelet function under conditions of arterial shear stress. Anesth Analg 2001;93:20–7.
[94] Kundu SK, Heilmann EJ, Sio R, et al. Description of an in vitro platelet function analyzer–PFA-100. Semin Thromb Hemost 1995;21:106–12.
[95] Mammen EF, Comp PC, Gosselin R, et al. PFA-100 system: a new method for assessment of platelet dysfunction. Semin Thromb Hemost 1998;24:195–202.
[96] Wahba A, Sander S, Birnbaum DE. Are in vitro platelet function tests useful in predicting blood loss following open-heart surgery? Thorac Cardiovasc Surg 1998;46:228–31.
[97] Slaughter TF, Sreeram G, Sharma AD, et al. Reversible shear-mediated platelet dysfunction during cardiac surgery as assessed by the PFA-100 platelet function analyzer. Blood Coagul Fibrinolysis 2001;12:85–93.
[98] Lasne D, Fiemeyer A, Chatellier G, et al. A study of platelet functions with a new analyzer using high shear stress (PFA 100) in patients undergoing coronary artery bypass graft. Thromb Haemost 2000;84:794–9.
[99] Carville DG, Schleckser PA, Guyer KE, et al. Whole blood platelet function assay on the ICHOR point-of-care hematology analyzer. J Extra Corpor Technol 1998;30:171–7.
[100] Lau WC, Waskell LA, Watkins PB, et al. Atorvastatin reduces the ability of clopidogrel to inhibit platelet aggregation: a new drug–drug interaction. Circulation 2003;107:32–7.
[101] Craft RM, Chavez JJ, Snider CC, et al. Comparison of modified Thromboelastograph and Plateletworks whole blood assays to optical platelet aggregation for monitoring reversal of clopidogrel inhibition in elective surgery patients. J Lab Clin Med 2005;145:309–15.
[102] Ray MJ, Hawson GA, Just SJ, et al. Relationship of platelet aggregation to bleeding after cardiopulmonary bypass. Ann Thorac Surg 1994;57:981–6.

Monitoring Hepatic and Renal Function

Vivek Moitra, MD, Geraldine Diaz, DO,
Robert N. Sladen, MB,ChB, MRCP(UK),
FRCP(C), FCCM*

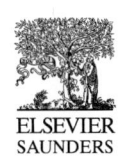

Department of Anesthesiology, College of Physicians & Surgeons of Columbia University, PH 527-B, 630 West 168th Street, New York, NY 10032, USA

MONITORING HEPATIC FUNCTION

Liver disease represents a serious risk factor for patients requiring anesthesia and surgery. The degree of risk depends on the etiology of liver disease (acute or chronic), severity of hepatic dysfunction, type of surgery, and urgency of the procedure [1,2]. Overt physiologic manifestations may not be apparent until liver disease is quite advanced, but even subclinical liver disease increases perioperative morbidity and mortality. Thus, detection of early hepatic dysfunction requires astute clinical skill. Substantial medical progress in the diagnosis and treatment of portal hypertension has extended the lives and functional activity of patients with cirrhosis, so that the prevalence of liver disease within the population is increasing, and its manifestations are muted [3]. At the same time, an increasing number of patients with liver disease will require preoperative assessment for elective and emergent surgical procedures. Indeed, Jackson and colleagues estimated as many as 10% of patients with end-stage liver disease (ESLD) require surgery during their last 2 years of life [4].

The estimation of hepatic dysfunction and assessment of perioperative risk are made complex, because even a diseased liver may have substantial functional reserve, and there is no clinical assay (such as renal glomerular filtration rate) to quantify specific hepatic metabolic capacity. Acute hepatic decompensation after surgery remains poorly understood and frequently is not predicted preoperatively by the deviation of hepatic function tests from normal. Available data principally include retrospective studies of cirrhotic patients undergoing emergent or semiemergent abdominal procedures and

---

* Corresponding author.
E-mail address: rs543@columbia.edu (R.N. Sladen).

case series. Few if any prospective studies are performed with the intent of evaluating perioperative risk [2,5,6]. Thus, evaluation of hepatic risk remains an inexact science dependent upon attentive physical examination, precise history, interpretation of indirect laboratory testing, and a fundamental understanding of the extrahepatic manifestations of liver disease.

Clinical evaluation: the first monitor

Liver dysfunction may result from an acute insult, a chronic process of hepatocyte injury, or an acute exacerbation of a chronic condition. Early acute and chronic liver disease may share similar presentations; namely, transaminitis, mild hyperbilirubinemia, or impaired coagulation. It is therefore important to recognize these early manifestations and identify the underlying etiology of liver dysfunction to stratify perioperative risk [6,7].

A detailed history and astute physical examination often will provide invaluable information on the etiology of liver failure. Patients should be questioned about prior blood transfusion, travel, jaundice, infectious diarrhea, recent surgery, intravenous drug abuse, tattoos, high-risk sexual behavior, potential contact with individuals who are jaundiced or suffering from viral symptoms, medications, and alcohol use (quantity, frequency, and length). Patients with known liver disease may manifest worsening function by symptoms of profound fatigue, malaise, bloody or coffee ground emesis, pruritus, abdominal distension, sexual dysfunction, altered sleep patterns (day/night reversal), or behavioral changes (encephalopathy). The family history may suggest hemochromatosis (heart disease, liver failure, diabetes, or liver cancer), Wilson's disease, or alpha-1-antitrypsin deficiency (chronic obstructive pulmonary disease).

On physical examination, jaundice, scleral icterus, encephalopathy (asterixis), and coagulopathy are common to both acute and chronic liver failure. Chronic liver disease is suggested by the finding of palmar erythema, testicular atrophy, gynecomastia, spider nevi, ascites, caput medusae, and a small, firm liver on palpation. Associated poor skin turgor, skeletal muscle atrophy, and loss of adipose tissue are typical of the malnutrition associated with chronic liver disease. Findings that imply acute liver failure include hepatosplenomegaly, hepatic tenderness, and central nervous symptoms consistent with cerebral edema (eg, agitation, nuchal rigidity, or papilledema) [7].

Acute liver disease

Fulminant hepatic failure and intracranial pressure monitoring

Fulminant hepatic failure (FHF) is the clinical manifestation of acute, overwhelming liver injury. The most common causes include acute viral hepatitis, massive acetaminophen ingestion in a suicide attempt, inadvertent ingestion of hepatotoxins such as the mushroom *Amanita phylloides*, or acute exacerbations of autoimmune hepatitis. It is characterized by hyperbilirubinemia, severe coagulopathy, encephalopathy, and impaired immunoregulation. Management of these critically ill patients is largely supportive. Surgical and anesthetic considerations are limited to liver transplantation and the rare performance of a total hepatectomy with porto-caval shunt in anticipation of transplantation [6–8].

Considerations for monitoring are dictated by the fundamental goals of clinical management: metabolic support, prevention of sepsis, and management of cerebral edema. Sepsis and cerebral herniation are the principal causes of mortality in FHF. The pathophysiology of cerebral edema in acute liver failure has not been elicited completely. It is multi-factorial, and includes impairment of cerebral blood flow autoregulation and an osmotic effect from accumulation of glutamine in the brain [9]. Placement of an intracranial pressure (ICP) monitor has been advocated for managing these patients. Safe insertion requires correction of coagulopathy with fresh frozen plasma, cryoprecipitate, or recombinant factor VII, and platelet transfusion. The sheer volume of blood product required may exacerbate cerebral edema. Conclusive data do not exist for ICP monitoring to be considered standard-of-care. Although ICP monitoring does assist in intraoperative management during the transplant procedure, the reported incidence of complications is high, ranging from 10% to 20%, and ICP monitoring has not demonstrated significantly improved outcomes [10].

Acute hepatitis

Acute hepatitis is transient, typically reversible, hepatic dysfunction resulting from viral, toxin (drug, alcohol), autoimmune, or ischemic injury. Historic data report high perioperative mortality (greater than 10%) from surgical procedures that typically were performed to distinguish medical from surgical hyperbilirubinemia [11]. Current diagnostic imaging, augmented by the capacity to perform transjugular liver biopsy to assess parenchyma injury and evidence of recovery, have virtually eliminated the need for surgical exploration [12]. As a result, management of acute hepatitis centers upon supportive care and the prevention of further insults. Surgery should be reserved for life-threatening conditions with a specific diagnosis. Elective and urgent surgery should be postponed until active inflammation (transaminitis) and cellular dysfunction (direct hyperbilirubinemia, coagulopathy) resolve. Once hepatic function has improved, perioperative risk is diminished, and routine procedural monitoring with a heightened awareness of the patient's history becomes sufficient [6].

An important caveat is the onset of acute hepatitis in the setting of pre-existing liver disease. This typically occurs with alcoholic hepatitis but also may be observed in patients who have a history of autoimmune liver disease or obesity. Underlying chronic liver disease impairs hepatic metabolic and regenerative capacity and contributes to the historically poor outcome observed with alcoholic hepatitis. Thus, in the patient who has acute hepatitis, preoperative assessment for evidence of chronic liver disease is obligatory and should be supported by diagnostic imaging or transjugular liver biopsy as necessary. Monitoring of these patients mirrors that of chronic liver disease.

Chronic and end-stage liver disease

Chronic liver disease or ESLD with portal hypertension and cirrhosis secondary to chronic hepatitis account for most liver disease in North America [5]. Surgery frequently is indicated in this population. The indications for elective surgery must be evaluated carefully, because high postoperative morbidity and mortality can result from primary hepatic failure or complications of the extrahepatic manifestations of chronic liver disease. The risk of postoperative hepatic failure in cirrhosis is directly proportional to the degree of hepatic dysfunction and the magnitude and urgency of the surgical procedure [6]. Compared with laparotomy, minimally invasive and interventional radiologic procedures decrease blood loss and reduce perioperative complications. Emergent or urgent surgery, particularly abdominal surgery, is tolerated poorly.

Extrahepatic manifestations of end-stage liver disease

Extrahepatic manifestations of ESLD involve the neurologic, cardiac, pulmonary, endocrine, renal, hematologic, and immunologic systems, and their dysfunction greatly contributes to morbidity and mortality after surgery.

Hepatic encephalopathy and arterial ammonia

The severity of hepatic encephalopathy (grade 1: confabulation; 2: confusion, asterixis; 3: stupor; 4: coma) is an important prognostic determinant of outcome after surgery. Its primary mechanism is postulated to be accumulation of neurologic toxins, particularly ammonia, whose hepatic clearance is impaired. There are multiple other disturbances, however. Catecholamine synthesis is impaired, and phenylalanine (a precursor of dopamine) is converted to octopamine, a false neurotransmitter. Branched-chain amino acids are oxidized selectively by muscle, and aromatic amino acids accumulate. One such, tryptophan, is the precursor of 5-hydroxy tryptamine (serotonin), which is a neurodepressor and may contribute to stupor. Impaired function of endogenous neurotransmitters including gamma-aminobutyric acid (GABA), glutamate, and nitric oxide, may contribute further to encephalopathy [13]. Heme degradation products are cleared inadequately and may act as endogenous activators of central GABA receptors [14]. In this regard, benzodiazepines should be used with extreme caution to avoid central GABA-benzodiazepine receptor activation.

The arterial ammonia level traditionally has been measured as a guide to the degree of encephalopathy. An elevated ammonia level, however, correlates little between patients or within the same patient under different physiologic stresses, and an increasing or decreasing trend may be more meaningful than absolute levels. A history of hepatic encephalopathy or prior requirement for medications such as lactulose, neomycin, or rifaximin suggests that the patient has severe underlying liver disease. This should prompt the anesthesiologist to question the necessity for an elective procedure, because encephalopathy predisposes to a postoperative course complicated by immobility, combativeness, lack of cooperation, difficulty achieving extubation, and risk of aspiration [15]. Postponement of all but absolutely emergent surgical procedures is warranted. When surgery cannot be avoided, it is prudent to initiate aggressive medical management of encephalopathy with lactulose (if gut function is normal), neomycin (in the absence of renal dysfunction), rifaximin, and a low-protein diet [16]. Surgical blood loss intensifies postoperative encephalopathy, so it is preferable whenever feasible to use minimally invasive techniques, laparoscopy, or interventional radiology. It is important to correct hypokalemic alkalosis, because it promotes conversion of ionized ammonium to nonionized ammonia, which crosses the blood–brain barrier and exacerbates central nervous system dysfunction [8].

Hyperdynamic circulation and cardiac assessment

The cardiac manifestations of chronic liver disease are substantial and must be appreciated to avert serious potential morbidity. Approximately 70% of patients who have ESLD demonstrate hyperdynamic cardiac physiology characterized by elevated cardiac index, decreased systemic vascular resistance, low blood pressure, normal-to-increased stroke volume, and a mildly elevated heart rate [17]. This is postulated to result from chronic splanchnic vasodilation secondary to impaired hepatic clearance of circulating vasoactive mediators, including nitric oxide. In addition to the generalized vasodilatation that occurs within the large vessels of the body, there is derangement of the microcirculation, resulting in arteriovenous shunting at the capillary level.

Cardiac evaluation should include assessment of function and screening for coronary artery disease. Electrocardiograms typically demonstrate evidence of ventricular hypertrophy, right heart strain, sinus tachycardia, and electrolyte-associated arrhythmias [18]. Ascites, fatigue, and pulmonary manifestations of chronic liver disease prevent most patients from performing an exercise stress test. Today, dobutamine stress echocardiography is the preferred modality for assessing coronary artery disease, pulmonary hypertension, and cardiomyopathy [1].

Patients with ESLD who do not manifest a hyperdynamic circulation have a distinctly worse perioperative outcome, and they should prompt a thorough cardiac work-up [19]. The etiology may be primary cardiac disease or liver-associated cardiomyopathy from hemochromatosis or alcoholic liver disease. Cardiac catheterization in this patient population frequently reveals coronary artery disease that requires correction before major abdominal surgery.

Pulmonary dysfunction and lung function tests

Pulmonary manifestations of ESLD are common and may involve elements of restrictive disease, obstructive disease, or ventilation–perfusion mismatch [20]. Restrictive disease is induced by anasarca, pleural effusions, hepatic hydrothorax, and ascites, and is the most common etiology of hypoxemia in these patients. Hepatic hydrothorax occurs in approximately 5% of patients who have ESLD, typically on the right side [21]. Preoperative drainage is not recommended in the absence of hypoxemia, because the effusion rapidly reaccumulates. Medical management initially includes diuretics and fluid restriction. Symptomatic pleural effusion is treated optimally with the performance of a transjugular intrahepatic portosystemic shunt (TIPS). Repeated thoracentesis predisposes to hemorrhage, septal formation, and parenchymal entrapment. Conversely, drainage by means of an indwelling catheter may be complicated by infection, electrolyte imbalance, substantial protein loss, and fistula formation [20]. Asymptomatic pleural effusions require careful assessment with positional changes during induction and maintenance of anesthesia; symptomatic pleural effusions should prompt evaluation of the necessity for immediate surgery. If immediate surgery is mandated, ultrasound-guided thoracentesis offers the most expeditious results, but reaccumulation should be anticipated.

Ascites is a marker of irreversible liver failure and is a relative contraindication to elective surgery. Its clinical implications are more serious than hepatic hydrothorax alone. Ascites and hepatic hydrothorax decrease functional residual capacity and predispose to rapid desaturation during anesthetic induction in the supine patient. Perioperative aspiration potential is high because of ascites-induced increases in intragastric pressure and altered gastric motility. There is a constant risk of spontaneous bacterial peritonitis and bacteremia. Large fluid shifts during the performance of abdominal procedures increase the need for volume transfusion and the risk of acute pulmonary edema or respiratory distress syndrome. Management of ascites and hepatic hydrothorax is always difficult. Aggressive diuresis may impair hepatic (and renal) perfusion further, so careful sodium and water restriction, together with aldosterone antagonists, provides the mainstay of therapy. TIPS is reserved for failed medical therapy and helps to avoid the morbidity associated with repeated paracentesis [22].

Patients who have ESLD may have incidental obstructive lung disease as a consequence of smoking or alpha-1-antitrypsin deficiency.

Hepatopulmonary syndrome (HPS) is diagnosed in approximately 5% of patients who have ESLD. It is caused by intrapulmonary arteriovenous fistulae in a similar fashion to spider nevi, with microscopic and macroscopic right-to-left shunting and hypoxemia, with little response to high-inspired oxygen fraction (FiO$_2$) [21]. HPS may present as platypnea (dyspnea in the upright position), but orthodeoxia (worsening oxygen saturation when changing from the supine to the upright position) is pathognomonic. Clubbing of fingers and spider nevi also may be present. The diagnosis of HPS is confirmed by contrast echocardiography or Technetium-99-labeled macroaggregated albumin scan, and subclassified as microscopic or macroscopic. Type I HPS is characterized by diffuse microscopic pulmonary vascular dilatations not evident on pulmonary angiogram; hypoxemia is responsive to high FiO$_2$. Type II HPS manifests as macroscopic pulmonary vascular dilatations visible by pulmonary angiography, but it does not respond to high FiO$_2$ and is unlikely to reverse after liver transplantation. These patients should be referred to specialized centers, as their perioperative management is extraordinarily difficult [23].

Portopulmonary hypertension (PPH) develops in 2% to 4% of patients who have ESLD. Diagnostic criteria include portal hypertension, mean pulmonary artery pressure (MPAP) greater than 25 mmHg, normal pulmonary capillary wedge pressure, and pulmonary vascular resistance greater than 120 dyne/s/cm [24]. PPH is postulated to result from the action of vasoconstrictive or prothrombotic substances normally cleared by the liver. Severe PPH (MPAP greater than 50 mmHg) is a life-threatening condition that leads to right ventricular failure and hypoxemia [21]. It is an absolute contraindication to surgery. Symptomatic PPH patients with MPAP less than 50 mmHg may tolerate surgery if pulmonary pressures are responsive to pulmonary vasodilators such as prostaglandins (epoprostenol), phosphodiesterase inhibitors (sildenafil), or endothelin antagonists (bosentan). Unresponsive or symptomatic PPH is an absolute contraindication to elective surgery regardless of MPAP.

Pulmonary evaluation of the patient who has ESLD includes a chest radiogram, spirometry, pulmonary function tests, and arterial blood gas analysis. Pneumonia, diaphragmatic elevation secondary to ascites, and pleural effusion are identified easily by chest radiograph. A bubble contrast echocardiogram can differentiate patients who have hypoxemia caused by HPS from those with V/Q mismatch, although it cannot estimate the degree of shunting. In HPS, bubbles injected in the right ventricle appear in the left ventricle within approximately three heartbeats, whereas in V/Q mismatch, the bubbles are absorbed by the lungs and do not reach the left circulation [21]. Administration of 100% oxygen with arterial blood gas analysis can distinguish type I (responsive) from type II (unresponsive) HPS.

Because the chest radiograph is so frequently abnormal, V/Q scans are often extraordinarily difficult to interpret. Pulmonary angiography and CT are tolerated poorly in this patient population. These are uncomfortable tests for patients who cannot remain recumbent for long periods of time, and the risk of contrast nephropathy is high [25]. In most cases, an astute history and physical examination in combination with chest radiograph, spirometry, arterial blood gas, and echocardiography typically provide adequate information to proceed with major surgery.

Endocrine and nutritional dysfunction

The endocrine disturbance in chronic liver disease is characterized by altered glucose metabolism and nutrient use. In cirrhosis, 60% to 80% of patients demonstrate impaired glucose tolerance, insulin resistance, hyperinsulinemia, and increased catabolism. Hyperinsulinemia probably occurs as a result of both increased pancreatic beta cell secretion and decreased hepatic clearance. About 10% to 15% of cirrhotic patients develop type II diabetes from decreased insulin secretion, possibly related to pancreatic burn out or infiltrations such as hemochromatosis [26].

The liver is essential for normal nutrient absorption and protein use. Biochemical evidence of impaired protein synthesis and depleted lean body mass, with decreased prealbumin, retinol binding protein and transferring, occurs early in liver failure. Hypoalbuminemic, protein calorie malnutrition (kwashiorkor) is exacerbated by malabsorption secondary to impaired biliary function and additional protein losses through tissue edema and ascites. Low oncotic pressure predisposes to ascites, anasarca, electrolyte imbalance, and impaired gastrointestinal (GI) function. Recurrent sepsis caused by spontaneous bacterial peritonitis or impaired hepatic immune responses increases circulating inflammatory mediators, catabolism, and impaired protein calorie use. The altered enterohepatic circulation leads to fat malabsorption, steatorrhea and absorptive diarrhea, electrolyte imbalance, and fat-soluble vitamin deficiencies [27].

Hematologic abnormalities and coagulopathy

Hematologic manifestations of ESLD include anemia, thrombocytopenia, and impaired coagulation.

Anemia is caused by malnutrition, anemia of chronic disease, bleeding, or renal failure. Patients respond well to erythropoietin analogs when they are given in conjunction with appropriate nutritional support and medical prophylaxis against GI bleeding from portal hypertension (endoscopic banding, beta-blocker prophylaxis, or proton pump inhibitors).

The coagulopathy of liver disease is multi-factorial and includes alterations in vitamin K metabolism, impaired synthesis of coagulation factors, low-grade disseminated intravascular coagulation secondary to subclinical hemorrhage, enhanced fibrinolytic activity, and quantitative and qualitative platelet dysfunction.

Coagulation studies are integral to the assessment of hepatic function and reserve. With the exception of factor VIII and von Willebrand factor, all clotting factors are synthesized in the liver. The severity of coagulopathy is related directly to the degree of liver disease. Vitamin K-dependent factors (II, VII, IX, X) are affected initially, followed by a broader, more complex coagulopathy. Factor VII has the shortest half-life of the vitamin K dependent factors, approximately 8 hours. Thus, the earliest manifestation of coagulopathy is a prolonged prothrombin time (or international normalized ratio, INR), and there is a demonstrable association between increased prothrombin time and mortality in patients undergoing major surgery [3]. Correction of an elevated prothrombin time by the administration of vitamin K is an important prognostic indicator that a patient may tolerate major surgery. Conversely, failure to normalize the prothrombin time after administration of vitamin K is an absolute contraindication to all but emergent surgery, because it indicates a high risk of acute postoperative liver failure. Thromboelastography may be useful in evaluating complex coagulopathy and guiding administration of blood products in situations such as emergency surgery in a cirrhotic patient progressing to hepatic failure [28].

Thrombocytopenia is typically the result of splenic sequestration, peripheral destruction, and bone marrow depression. Increased platelet counts are observed with the successful treatment of portal hypertension (TIPS, surgical shunt, liver transplantation) and appropriate nutritional support. When thrombocytopenia is secondary to portal hypertension, platelet transfusion is not indicated as prophylaxis but may be required in the setting of active hemorrhage. Platelet function is altered with the onset of renal insufficiency and the hepatorenal syndrome. For these conditions, prophylactic platelet transfusion and administration of desmopressin are indicated for major surgical procedures and interventions [29].

Hepatorenal syndrome and renal evaluation

Renal function inevitably is compromised in patients who have liver disease. The hyperdynamic vasodilatory state shifts the renal autoregulatory curve rightwards and places the kidneys at risk for hypoperfusion during hypotension or sepsis. Intravascular hypovolemia induced by ascites triggers the release of aldosterone, which promotes salt and water retention and exacerbates edema. Renal hypoperfusion activates the renin-angiotensin-aldosterone axis, afferent arteriolar vasoconstriction, and further reduction in glomerular filtration rate (GFR) [1]. Antidiuretic hormone (arginine vasopressin) also is activated by renal hypoperfusion and promotes water retention and oliguria.

Hepatorenal syndrome (HRS) is a frequent complication of advanced ESLD; in type I, clinical deterioration is slow, and in type II, it is rapid [30]. There are numerous different mechanisms. Endotoxin in the gut normally is inactivated by conjugated bilirubin, and when absorbed into the portal circulation, it is engulfed by hepatic Kupffer cells. In ESRD, conjugated bilirubin is deficient, Kupffer cells are dysfunctional and portosystemic shunting results in the delivery of endotoxin to the renal circulation, where it induces vasoconstriction and direct tubular damage. Splanchnic vasodilatation decreases effective intravascular volume and further alters renal blood flow [31,32]. The result is an intensely prerenal syndrome, characterized by azotemia, oliguria, and low urinary sodium (less than 10 mEq/L). Urinary sediment is normal, and the fractional excretion of sodium is low.

Before the widespread implementation of liver transplantation, HRS heralded irreversible liver failure. HRS, however, is a functional prerenal failure. The kidneys are histologically normal and will start to function normally when transplanted into a patient with normal hepatic function, or when the liver itself is transplanted successfully.

HRS is an absolute contraindication to elective, nontransplant surgery. The intravascular fluid shifts of anesthesia and major surgery exacerbate the intravascular volume depletion, and there is a high risk of acute postoperative liver failure.

Laboratory evaluation of liver disease

Liver function tests

Alanine aminotransferase (ALT) and aspartate aminotransferase (AST) are enzymes present in the cytosol of hepatocytes. They are released during hepatocellular injury, and therefore they serve as markers of hepatocellular damage rather than hepatic function. They are abnormal in up to 36% of patients with no clinically apparent liver dysfunction. In advanced liver disease, these enzymes may be normal or mildly elevated, because of a paucity hepatocytes to release the enzymes.

Alkaline phosphatase elevation is a marker for cholestasis and biliary obstruction. This abnormality, however, is not specific for liver disease, as the enzyme is also present in many other tissues.

Albumin is produced in the liver and is a marker of hepatic synthetic function. It also may be decreased in chronic disease states or malnutrition. Albumin levels, however, may be normal in acute liver dysfunction because of albumin's long half-life (2 to 3 weeks).

Child-Turcotte-Pugh classification

The Child-Turcotte-Pugh classification is a widely used tool for assessing the degree of liver dysfunction [33]. There are five variables, including encephalopathy, ascites, prothrombin time, albumin, and bilirubin, each with a score of 1 to 3 depending on the degree of abnormality. Thus, the available scores are 5 to 15, with a class grouping of A (mild dysfunction, score 5 to 6), B (moderate dysfunction, score 7 to 9), or C (severe dysfunction, score 10 to 15). There is a direct relationship between the Child-Turcotte-Pugh score and 3-month mortality: 4%, 14%, and 51% respectively [34]. Although this method has been used to assess the degree of hepatic dysfunction and in stratifying risk for surgery, it has been criticized for having two subjective variables (encephalopathy and ascites). Its usefulness as a means of allocating donor organs is limited by the lack of distinction between mildly and severely abnormal values and the existence of only three classes of disease severity.

Model of end-stage liver disease score

The model of end-stage liver disease (MELD) score initially was developed to provide prognostic information before the TIPS procedure [35]. In Feb 2002, the United Network for Organ Sharing (UNOS) determined that the MELD score would provide recipient priority for allocating donor organs. The MELD score has been validated in numerous patient cohorts, and it is being tested to specifically examine outcomes in patients undergoing surgery [34]. It uses three laboratory values (bilirubin, creatinine, and the INR) to assign a value from 6 to 40, which corresponds to the 90-day mortality risk from liver failure. It thus can determine the severity of liver disease and urgency of need for donor organs [36]. The superiority of the MELD score over the Child-Turcotte-Pugh score as a predictor of evaluation for transplant candidacy is suggested by an 11% decrease in the number of deaths while waiting for transplant in the first year of its implementation [37].

Summary

Patients who are asymptomatic with minimal liver abnormalities (eg, Child's class A, or MELD less than 11) often do well with elective surgery and should not be overinvestigated at the risk of delaying a necessary procedure. Patients with moderate or symptomatic cirrhosis (eg, Child's class B, or MELD 12 to 15) are at risk for perioperative morbidity and mortality, and the risks and benefits of elective surgery must be considered carefully. Elective surgery is contraindicated in the presence of acute viral hepatitis, acute alcohol hepatitis, fulminant hepatic failure, severe chronic hepatitis, severe coagulopathy, and severe extrahepatic complications (eg, hypoxemia, cardiomyopathy, heart failure, acute renal failure) [5]. Surgery in patients who have Child's class C cirrhosis (or MELD greater than 15) should be restricted to life-threatening emergency or liver transplantation; if other procedures are required, these patients should be referred to a center performing liver transplantation for evaluation and medical management.

MONITORING RENAL FUNCTION

Introduction

For the anesthesiologist, the mainstay of perioperative renal monitoring remains the measurement of urine output. Urine output, however, may bear little if any relationship to what is really going on in the kidney. The blood urea nitrogen (BUN) and serum creatinine (S_{Cr}) are simple, useful measures of renal excretory function, but their interpretation is subject to many limitations, especially when renal function is changing rapidly.

Because 25% of the cardiac output goes to the kidneys, one can use global hemodynamics (ie, cardiac output) to make educated guesses about renal perfusion. It is not clinically practicable, however, to measure renal blood flow (RBF). Moreover, in acute tubular necrosis (ATN), which may be induced by an abrupt and transient decrease in RBF, the lesion persists despite normalization of renal hemodynamics.

GFR is the most important index of intrinsic renal function, and still the most reliable means of detecting early renal injury. It often is deduced by S_{Cr}-based nomograms that are simple to do but are quite inaccurate when GFR is rapidly changing. Accurate estimation of fluctuations in GFR requires clearance techniques that involve some effort.

Tubular function is the easiest to measure. It can provide considerable information about the renal response to hypovolemia and hypervolemia and helps distinguish prerenal oliguria from ATN. It does not quantitate renal reserve, however. There are numerous established and investigational tests that reveal subclinical tubular injury, but they may or may not relate to renal outcome.

Urine output

Perioperative oliguria usually is defined as a urine flow rate less than 0.5 mL/kg/h, and often taken to imply renal dysfunction. In most situations, perioperative oliguria is an appropriate prerenal response to intravascular hypovolemia and a component of the physiologic response to surgical stress [38]. Hypovolemia may be absolute, as a consequence of acute hemorrhage, severe diarrhea, vomiting or fluid restriction; or relative, as occurs in congestive heart failure, sepsis and liver failure. In response (and exacerbated by surgical stress), the sympathoadrenal and renin-angiotensin-aldosterone systems and antidiuretic hormone activate the renal tubules to avidly reabsorb water and sodium. Although RBF and GFR are autoregulated, urine flow is not, and it declines when blood pressure falls. For all these reasons, prerenal oliguria is almost inevitable during anesthesia and surgery. With postoperative restoration of intravascular volume and blood pressure and cessation of stress, the stimulus to the tubules abates, and normal urinary flow resumes.

Postrenal oliguria implies urinary tract obstruction at the level of the renal pelvis, ureters, bladder, urethra, or urinary catheter. Although it typically manifests as anuria, acute renal failure may occur with subtotal obstruction and persistent, albeit decreased, urine flow.

Perioperative ATN (so-called intrarenal oliguria) may indeed be anuric (zero flow) or oliguric (urinary flow rate less than 15 mL/hr), but more often, it is nonoliguric (15 to 80 mL/h) or even polyuric (greater than 80 mL/h). More recently, an attempt was made to unify the definition of acute renal failure by the RIFLE (Risk, Injury, Failure, Loss, End-stage renal disease) criteria, based on changes in S_{Cr} and urine flow. The first three categories are defined in part by oliguria (< 0.5 mL/kg/h) for 6, 12, and 24 hrs respectively. This, however, does not consider that nonoliguric renal failure (NORF) is the most common manifestation of ATN today.

In sum, perioperative oliguria is common, almost always prerenal in nature, and rarely implies acute renal failure. On the other hand, the absence of oliguria does not exclude it. Urine output is far less reliable an indicator of renal function than GFR.

Blood urea nitrogen

When amino acids are deaminated, their NH_2 groups form ammonia (NH_3), which is converted to urea in the liver. Urea nitrogen is a small, uncharged molecule that is not protein-bound and is cleared rapidly by glomerular filtration. It also is reabsorbed by the tubules so BUN does not correlate directly with GFR, but is a marker of symptomatic azotemia.

The relationship between BUN and S_{Cr} is usually around 10:1. An increase >20:1 implies the existence of a prerenal syndrome. There are numerous factors, however, that influence BUN independently of renal function and GFR.

Elevation of BUN out of proportion to decreases in GFR occurs whenever there is increased protein breakdown and formation of urea nitrogen. This includes absorption of blood from the GI tract, steroid-induced catabolic activity, major trauma, and sepsis. Conversely, a misleadingly low BUN occurs with cachexia, malnutrition, and severe liver disease, the last because of inability to convert ammonia to urea.

Serum creatinine

S_{Cr} reflects the balance between creatinine production by muscle and creatinine excretion by the kidney, which is dependent on the GFR. When these processes are in equilibrium, and renal function is stable, S_{Cr} is a useful marker of GFR.

The relationship between S_{Cr} and GFR is inverse and exponential; that is, a doubling of the S_{Cr} implies a halving of the GFR. At the lower range of normal, an increase in S_{Cr} from 0.8 to 1.6 mg/dL may not generate much attention, but it indicates a 50% decrease in GFR. An understanding of this relationship is essential to the early diagnosis of acute renal injury and possible therapeutic intervention. A much larger S_{Cr} increase (eg, from 4 to 8 mg/dL) also represents a 50% decrease in GFR, but by this time, it is too late for anything other than dialysis.

There are many caveats to the interpretation of S_{Cr} as a reflection of GFR, even in steady-state situations. The most commonly used method to measure creatinine is the Jaffé reaction, a chromogenic assay affected by glucose, protein, ketones, and ascorbic acid. Ketoacidosis, barbiturates, and cephalosporin antibiotics may artifactually increase measured S_{Cr} up to

100%, and cimetidine and trimethaprim block its secretion by the tubule. N-Acetylcysteine, an antioxidant advocated as a renoprotective agent in contrast nephropathy [39], has been found to decrease S_{Cr} levels, which may in part account for its apparently beneficial effect on renal function [40].

Large changes in GFR may occur within the normal range without any concomitant change in S_{Cr}. GFR predictably declines with age, from about 125 mL/min in a healthy 20-year-old person, to about 60 mL/min in an 80-year-old person (or a 60-year-old person with atherosclerosis [41]). Because S_{Cr} does not begin to increase above normal levels until the GFR declines below 50 mL/min, changes in GFR induced by aging are not reflected in the S_{Cr}. Put simply, a 20-year-old person and an 80-year-old person may both have S_{Cr} within normal limits, but the older patient will have half the GFR, or renal reserve, of the younger.

Although the creatinine generation rate is relatively consistent in a given individual, it varies with muscle mass, rate of catabolism, physical activity, and protein intake [42]. In a cachectic patient with depleted muscle mass, creatinine generation may be so feeble that S_{Cr} remains subnormal (less than 0.9 mg/dL) even in the face of a markedly decreased GFR (less than 25 mL/min) [43].

Because creatinine is soluble and freely distributes through the total body water, S_{Cr} is diluted by the 10% to 15% increases in total body water that occur with fluid administration and retention during major surgery. It is not uncommon to encounter the phenomenon whereby S_{Cr} increases from for example 1.2 to 1.5 mg/dL from the first to second postoperative day. This may be thought to represent acute renal injury, but closer examination might reveal a preoperative S_{Cr} of 1.5 mg/dL. The improved S_{Cr} on postoperative day 1 is a result of hemodilution, and the worsening S_{Cr} on day 2 is simply the result of re-equilibration to baseline with fluid mobilization, diuresis, and decreased total body water.

S_{Cr} is a very unreliable marker of GFR when renal function is changing rapidly. If a transient renal insult (eg, suprarenal aortic cross-clamping) causes creatinine excretion to cease, S_{Cr} will remain at baseline, and it may take days before a new equilibrium is established at which S_{Cr} represents zero GFR. Then, when renal function recovers, it may take days before creatinine excretion again exceeds creatinine production and S_{Cr} starts to decline. In fact, it may still increase for a few days while GFR is recovering [41]. In established oliguric acute renal failure, S_{Cr} is directly proportional to the creatinine generation rate, so that even though GFR is consistently low, there is wide variability of S_{Cr}.

Renal plasma flow and renal blood flow

It is impractical to place renal flow probes in patients, so renal plasma flow (RPF) and RBF most often are measured indirectly by clearance techniques. These are based on the Fick principle [44], which states that the amount of a substance x excreted by the kidney equals the amount delivered in the arterial supply minus the amount in the venous return. The urinary excretion rate (mg/min) of substance x is the product of its urinary concentration (mg/dL) and the urine flow rate (mL/min). The amount of substance x delivered to the kidney is the product of its arterial concentration and RBF, and the amount returning the product of its venous concentration and RBF. In practice, however, RBF and venous return are not measured. Instead, the removal of substance x from the plasma by the kidney is expressed by the concept of clearance (C), defined as the virtual volume of plasma cleared of substance x in mL/min. If it is assumed that the concentration of substance x is similar in the renal artery and vein, clearance of substance x (C_x) in mL/min may be calculated as its urinary excretion rate (mg/min) divided by its venous concentration (mg/mL). That is, $C_x = U_x \times V/P_x$, where U_x is the urinary concentration of x (mg/mL), V is the urinary flow rate (mL/min), and P_x is the venous concentration of x (mg/mL).

Para-amino hippurate (PAH) is an organic anion filtered by the glomerulus and secreted by the tubule that is cleared almost completely from the plasma in a single pass through the kidney. Thus, clearance of PAH (C_{PAH}) represents RPF. The test, however, is laborious and requires intravenous and urinary catheters. A PAH infusion is set up to maintain a steady-state PAH concentration of about 2 mg/dL, together with a carefully timed catheter urine collection. Because 10% of the RPF bypasses the peritubular capillaries, C_{PAH} underestimates the true RPF, so it is known as the effective RPF. In young healthy adults, effective RPF is about 660 mL/min/1.73 m^2.

Effective RBF may be calculated using the hematocrit (Hct) (ie, RPF/1 − Hct). For example, if effective RPF is 600 mL/min, and Hct is 30% (0.3), effective RBF is 600/0.7 (ie, 860 mL/min).

Unfortunately, C_{PAH} is an unreliable indicator of RPF during surgical stress, because hypovolemia and oliguria induce sequestration of PAH in the kidney. Ironically, the most important limitation of C_{PAH} is renal injury, because about 80% of PAH is cleared by tubular secretion. In the presence of proximal tubular injury, PAH secretion declines, and C_{PAH} underestimates RPF [45].

Access to the renal vein (eg, during major abdominal vascular surgery) allows measurement of arterial and renal vein PAH and calculation of the renal extraction of PAH (E_{PAH}), an index of proximal tubular function. For example, if renal function is normal, E_{PAH} approaches 100%, and renal vein PAH is close to zero. With worsening proximal tubular function, E_{PAH} progressively declines, and renal vein PAH concentration progressively increases.

Glomerular filtration rate

It has become recognized that the development of ischemic or nephrotoxic ATN involves several distinct phases [46]. In the initiation phase, epithelial and vascular cell injury results in a rapid decline in GFR. The extension phase involves exacerbation of epithelial and endothelial cell injury, apoptosis, and necrosis. During the maintenance phase, the injury becomes stabilized, with the beginning of cellular reorganization that culminates in the recovery phase. Because the initiation phase is so often transient, the extension phase is the most important window of opportunity for therapeutic intervention that might reverse renal injury, lending importance to the accurate detection of rapid declines in GFR [47].

Serum creatinine-based nomograms

It has become quite popular in clinical investigations to estimate GFR using nomograms based on population studies that use SCr, age, weight, and gender. One example is that formulated by Cockroft and Gault [48]: GFR = (140 − age) × weight in kg/SCr × 72. For females, the derived GFR is multiplied by 0.85. A more complex nomogram is based on a study called Modification of Diet in Renal Disease (MDRD) [49], where GFR = 170 × $SCr^{-0.999}$ × $age^{-0.176}$ × $BUN^{-0.170}$ × $albumin^{0.318}$. For females, the derived GFR is multiplied by 0.762, and for black patients, GFR is multiplied by 1.18.

In the Cockroft-Gault formula, estimated GFR is dependent on the body weight used. In obese or edematous patients, total body weight is much greater than the lean body mass from which creatinine is derived, so the formula overestimates GFR. In cachectic patients with depleted lean body mass, creatinine production is so low that S_{Cr} is often less than 1.0 mg/dL, and again the formula overestimates true GFR. Accuracy is restored by incorporating ideal body weight from a nomogram and S_{Cr} corrected to 1.0 mg/dL if less than 1.0 mg/dL [50]. The MDRD nomogram is independent of body weight but liable to the fluctuations induced by changing relationships between BUN and S_{Cr}, and all S_{Cr}-based nomograms are subject to the same limitations as S_{Cr} itself in reflecting rapid changes in GFR.

Inulin clearance

Clearance is also the most commonly used technique to estimate GFR, using compounds that are filtered predominantly by the glomerulus and neither secreted nor reabsorbed by the renal tubules. Inulin, an inert polyfructose sugar, is just such a compound, and inulin clearance (C_{IN}) is considered the gold standard estimate of GFR. C_{IN} is measured identically to C_{PAH} and requires a continuous inulin infusion to establish a steady-state plasma concentration of 15 to 20 mg/dL. Like C_{PAH}, however, the test is laborious; the inulin assay is time-consuming, and it is not used in clinical care. Normal values for C_{IN} (expressed as mL/min/1.73m^2) are 110 to 140 in males and 95 to 125 in females. Sodium iothalamate, a radiocontrast dye, has been substituted for inulin and facilitates accurate assessment of rapid changes in GFR in acute renal injury [47].

The fractional relationship between C_{IN} and C_{PAH} is called the filtration fraction, and it expresses that fraction of the RPF filtered by the glomerulus (GFR/RPF). With a normal GFR of 125 mL/min and RPF of 660 mL/min, the filtration fraction is 0.2. An increase in filtration fraction indicates that GFR is increased relative to RPF. This could be achieved by efferent arteriolar constriction or afferent arteriolar dilation and maintains glomerular filtration pressure in the face of decreased RPF. Conversely, a decrease in filtration fraction implies that GFR is decreased relative to RPF by afferent arteriolar constriction or efferent arteriolar dilation.

Creatinine clearance

Creatinine is the endogenous end product of creatine phosphate metabolism. It is generated from muscle at a very uniform rate and is handled by the kidney similarly to inulin. Thus, creatinine clearance (C_{Cr}) provides a simple, inexpensive bedside estimate of GFR. A single blood sample is drawn for S_{Cr} at the midpoint of a carefully timed urine collection, and C_{Cr} in mL/min is calculated from $U_{CR} \times V/P_{CR}$ where U_{CR} is the urine creatinine (mg/dL), V the urinary flow rate (mL/min), and P_{CR} equals S_{Cr} (mg/dL).

The C_{Cr} is far more accurate in tracking rapid alterations in GFR than S_{Cr} itself, or S_{Cr}-based nomograms. This is because changes in GFR immediately alter the creatinine excretion rate, which is incorporated into the C_{Cr} as $U_{CR} \times V$. Bedside use of C_{Cr} was restricted formerly by the erroneous belief that a prolonged (12 to 24-hour) urine collection is necessary to eliminate error induced by residual urine in the bladder. Not only is this collection tedious and cumbersome, but if renal function rapidly declines over 24 hours, S_{Cr} could increase from, say, 1 to 2 mg/dL from the beginning to the end of the urine collection. A C_{Cr} based on an S_{Cr} drawn during the midpoint of the collection would average out the changes in GFR and not truly represent dynamic renal function.

In fact, precise timing, not the duration, of the urine collection is the critical issue. In catheterized patients with urine flow rates greater than 15 mL/hr, a C_{Cr} obtained with a 2-hour urine collection gives values equivalent to those obtained with a 22-hour collection [51]. Moreover, a short urine collection enables rapid, repeated estimates of GFR to be obtained, so that in the example, a 2-hour C_{Cr} obtained at the beginning and end of the 24-hour period would truly reflect the halving of GFR represented by a doubling of the S_{Cr} from 1 to 2 mg/dL.

Even short, timed C_{Cr} requires meticulous measurement and reporting of urine volume, the most common source of laboratory error. There is considerable variation in the normal range of C_{Cr} within and between individuals, and diurnally. However, its variability diminishes as GFR declines; in fact, loss of variability of C_{Cr} is a clue to deteriorating renal function. Unlike inulin, 20% of creatinine is secreted by the proximal tubule, so C_{Cr} overestimates GFR. As the GFR declines, tubular secretion of creatinine increases, and the error is compounded. Administration of cimetidine, which blocks tubular secretion of creatinine, actually improves the accuracy of C_{Cr} at low GFR. When SCr is very high, it is excreted into the gut and undergoes extrarenal metabolism by intestinal organisms.

For these reasons, an isolated C_{Cr} is not as useful as serial estimations in revealing alterations in renal function and prognosis. It is most valuable in guiding the dosing of renally excreted, potentially nephrotoxic aminoglycoside antibiotics (gentamicin, tobramycin, amikacin) or calcineurin antagonists (cyclosporine A, tacrolimus). The GFR may decline to less than 50% of normal before S_{Cr} increases above the normal range, so an observed decrease in C_{Cr} may allow down-adjustment of drug dosing before nephrotoxicity becomes established and the drug accumulates even further.

Plasma clearance

Plasma clearance is an alternate method for measuring GFR that avoids the necessity for a simultaneous urine collection. It involves an intravenous bolus dose or infusion of a marker, followed by multiple plasma levels to calculate the disappearance rate of the marker. A limitation of the methodology, however, is that it depends on achievement of a steady-state plasma concentration of the marker, which is difficult to achieve with rapid changes in GFR [47].

Numerous markers are used, including nonradioactive inulin and iothalamate, and radioisotopes such as Cr^{51}-ethylenediamine tetra-acetic acid (EDTA), Tc^{99m}-diethylenetriamine penta-acetic acid (DTPA), and ^{125}I-iothalamate. The latter, which uses measurement of decay in radiation, has shown promise in the rapid assessment of GFR.

Tubular function tests

Tubular function tests measure urinary concentrating ability and sodium and urea handling. They help to distinguish prerenal versus intrarenal oliguria; in other words, they distinguish hypovolemia from ATN.

In prerenal oliguria, tubular function is activated to retain salt and water, resulting in concentrated urine, low in sodium. Normalization of hemodynamic status reverses oliguria and tubular activation (with the notable exceptions of sepsis and liver failure). The administration of potent diuretics may override tubular conservation, resulting in dilute urine, high in sodium (natriuresis), rendering the test uninterpretable. In this situation, analysis of urea handling is more reliable. Moreover, if intravascular hypovolemia is severe enough, tubular sodium retention persists despite the administration of diuretics such as low-dose dopamine [52], emphasizing that diuretics are not a substitute for rehydration!

In ATN, concentrating ability and sodium conservation are lost, resulting in dilute urine with high sodium that is not reversed by restoration of renal blood flow. In nonoliguric renal failure (NORF), however, which accounts as for up to 75% of cases of ATN [53], the intrarenal pattern of tubular function (dilute urine with high sodium) is less distinct from that of the prerenal syndrome.

Urinary concentrating ability

Concentrating ability is activated early in dehydration, and lost early in tubular injury (ie, it is a sensitive barometer of tubular function). In prerenal states, urinary osmolar concentration is increased markedly; in ATN, the ability to concentrate urine may be lost 24 to 48 hours before S_{Cr} or BUN start to increase.

Urine-to-plasma osmolar ratio

The normal tubular response to dehydration is to concentrate the urine and increase urine osmolality from greater than or equal to 450 mOsm/kg. Therefore a prerenal syndrome is indicated by a urine-to-plasma osmolar ratio (U:P_{OSM}) of greater than or equal to 1.5 (ie, $\geq$450: 300 mOsm/kg). Loss of concentrating ability (isosthenuria) is revealed by a U:P_{OSM} = 1.0 (ie, 300: 300 mOsm/kg), and dilute urine in the presence of oliguria implies loss of tubular function. Isosthenuria, however, can be induced in a prerenal state when diuretics are administered.

Free water clearance

Free water clearance (C_{H_2O}) is a measure of renal water regulation by tubular dilution or concentration of urine. In essence, free water is cleared by the tubules in response to hypervolemia (positive free water clearance), or retained in response to hypovolemia (negative free water clearance). The kidney's capacity for water regulation is enormous, and C_{H_2O} can vary from + 18L to −8L/day [54].

It is calculated by subtracting the solute or osmolar clearance (C_{Osm}) from the urinary flow rate (V), ie, C_{H_2O} = V − C_{Osm} mL/min. This implies that when urine is dilute, and flow is greater than osmolar clearance, C_{H_2O} is positive. When urine flow is concentrated and less than osmolar clearance, C_{H_2O} is negative. Negative C_{H_2O}, ie, free water retention, also known as tubular conservation of water (TC_{H_2O}) [45]. This represents the volume of fluid that would have to be added to the urine to make U_{Osm} = P_{Osm}. In ATN, when urine flow equals osmolar clearance, C_{H_2O} is zero (isosthenuria).

Water conservation

Urine-to-plasma creatinine ratio

Normally, about 98% of water filtered by the glomerulus is abstracted by the tubules, so that urine creatinine (U_{Cr}) is much greater than S_{Cr}. The urine-to-plasma (U:P) creatinine ratio is an index of the proportion of water filtered by the glomerulus that is abstracted by the distal tubule, and it is increased considerably in severe prerenal states. In contrast, with severe tubular dysfunction, the ratio declines to <20:1.

The application of the U:P creatinine is illustrated by the example of two patients with oliguria and S_{Cr} elevated to 2.0 mg/dL. In patient A, U_{Cr} is 100 mg/dL, and in patient B, it is 20 mg/dL. Patient A likely has a prerenal state, because tubular water abstraction is high (U:P creatinine = 50:1). Patient B likely has ATN, because tubular water abstraction is impaired (U:P creatinine = 10:1).

Sodium conservation

Urine sodium

Dehydration or hypovolemia markedly stimulates tubular sodium reabsorption, and in the prerenal syndrome, oliguria is characterized by a very low urinary sodium (U_{Na}), less than 20 mEq/L. Typically, this response is reversed by restoration of intravascular volume. In two situations, however, sepsis and the hepatorenal syndrome of liver failure, refractory oliguria with low U_{Na} persists despite aggressive fluid resuscitation. The pathogenesis is multi-factorial, but common to both is endotoxemia, which induces renal vasoconstriction and avid tubular sodium reabsorption.

In ATN, oliguria is associated with elevated U_{Na} (greater than 60 mEq/L), a reflection of the loss of tubular sodium reabsorption. High U_{Na}, however, may occur when diuretics that overcome tubular sodium conservation are administered in a prerenal state, so in this situation U_{Na} is not helpful in diagnosing ATN. Persistence of low U_{Na} in the face of diuretic therapy implies the existence of an intense prerenal state [52].

Fractional excretion of sodium

Fractional excretion of sodium (FENa) is an additional means of evaluating tubular responses to hypo- and hypervolemia. FENa expresses sodium clearance (C_{Na}) as a percentage of C_{Cr}. The implication is that in hypovolemia, C_{Na} and FENa decline to reflect tubular sodium conservation; in hypervolemia, the opposite occurs.

FENa is calculated using the standard clearance equations: ($U_{Na} \bullet V/P_{Na}$)/($U_{Cr} \bullet V/P_{Cr}$) × 100%. Because urine flow rate (V) is identical in the numerator and denominator, the equation is simplified to (U_{Na}/P_{Na})/(U_{Cr}/P_{Cr}) × 100%, so FENa is calculated from a spot sample of blood and urine without requiring a timed urine collection.

During dehydration or hypovolemia, sodium clearance and FENa are decreased to less than 1% of C_{Cr}. When tubular conservation of sodium is lost in ATN, FENa increases to greater than 3% of C_{Cr}. Just as with U_{Na}, however, FENa may be misleadingly increased after diuretic therapy.

Urea handling

Fractional excretion of urea

Unlike sodium, tubular handling of urea is subject to passive forces and is influenced little by diuretic therapy [55]. Indeed, compared with FENa, the fractional excretion of urea nitrogen (FEUN) has proven more robust in the diagnosis of prerenal syndrome despite diuretic therapy. It is calculated identically to FENa; FEUN = $(U_{UN}/BUN)/(U_{Cr}/P_{Cr}) \times 100\%$, where UUN is the urinary urea nitrogen. In a prerenal syndrome with or without diuretic therapy, FEUN is less than 35%; in ATN it is 50% or greater.

Indices of tubular injury

Beta$_2$-microglobulin

Beta$_2$-microglobulin is a small protein component of the major histocompatibility complex, found on the surface of almost all cells. It normally is filtered by the glomerulus, and then it undergoes partial tubular reabsorption. As such, it is helpful in distinguishing glomerular from tubular injury. In glomerular injury, serum beta$_2$-microglobulin levels increase, and urine levels decrease (an early sign of rejection in renal transplantation) [56].

In primary tubular injury, reabsorption is lost, so urinary levels of beta$_2$-microglobulin increase, and blood levels decline. In a study where cardiopulmonary bypass (CPB) with pulsatile flow was used, there was a significant decrease in plasma renin activity, but urinary beta$_2$-microglobulin increased on CPB with pulsatile or non-pulsatile flow [57]. The implication is that although pulsatile flow maintains better renal perfusion, it does not prevent a subclinical renal tubular injury. The relationship between increased urinary beta$_2$-microglobulin and subsequent ATN, however, has not been characterized.

Urinary N-acetyl beta D-glucosaminidase

The assay of increased urinary concentrations of the tubular enzyme, N-acetyl beta D-glucosaminidase (NAG), is a well-established method of identifying subclinical tubular injury. Urinary NAG levels, or the ratio of its isoenzymes, have been used in the early detection of rejection in transplant patients, or to follow the course of chronic renal disease (eg, lupus nephritis) [58]. However, there are few data on the relationship between tubular enzymuria and acute renal outcome, such as the need for postoperative renal replacement therapy.

Neutrophil gelatinase-associated lipocalin

Neutrophil gelatinase-associated lipocalin (NGAL) is a small polypeptide expressed in proximal tubular cells, whose mRNA undergoes dramatic upregulation after ischemic tubular injury [59]. NGAL is protease resistant and readily detected in tiny amounts of urine. Additionally, it appears almost immediately after renal injury, preceding the appearance of NAG and beta$_2$-microglobulin. Urinary NGAL has been demonstrated to increase significantly within 2 hours of CPB in pediatric or adult patients who subsequently went on to develop a 50% increase in postoperative S$_{Cr}$, which reached its peak only 1 to 3 days after surgery [60,61]. These data suggest that urinary NGAL may represent an early, sensitive, noninvasive urinary biomarker for ischemic and nephrotoxic renal injury.

References

[1] Garg RK. Anesthetic considerations in patients with hepatic failure. Int Anesthesiol Clin 2005;43:45–63.
[2] Rizvon MK, Chou CL. Surgery in the patient with liver disease. Med Clin North Am 2003; 87:211–27.
[3] Ziser A, Plevak DJ, Wiesner RH, et al. Morbidity and mortality in cirrhotic patients undergoing anesthesia and surgery. Anesthesiology 1999;90:42–53.
[4] Jackson FC, Christophersen EB, Peternel WW, et al. Preoperative management of patients with liver disease. Surg Clin North Am 1968;48:907–30.
[5] Friedman LS. The risk of surgery in patients with liver disease. Hepatology 1999;29:1617–23.
[6] Suman A, Carey WD. Assessing the risk of surgery in patients with liver disease. Cleve Clin J Med 2006;73:398–404.
[7] Gaglio P, Aron J, Brown R. Fulminant hepatic failure. In: Al Knawy B, Wiesner RH, Shiffman ML, editors. Hepatology: a practical approach. Philadelphia: Elsevier; 2004. p. 315–30.
[8] Riordan S, Williams R. Transplantation for fulminant hepatic failure. In: Busuttil RW, Klintmalm GB, editors. Transplantation of the liver. 2nd edition. Philadelphia: Elsevier Saunders; 2005. p. 161–75.
[9] Blei A, Larsen FS. Pathophysiology of cerebral edema in fulminant hepatic failure. J Hepatol 1999;31:771–6.
[10] Raghavan M, Marik P. Therapy of intracranial hypertension in patients with fulminant hepatic failure. Neurocrit Care 2006;4:179–89.
[11] Patel T. Surgery in the patient with liver disease. Mayo Clin Proc 1999;74:593–9.
[12] Sass DA, Shakil AO. Fulminant hepatic failure. Liver Transpl 2005;11:594–605.
[13] Cordoba J. Glutamine, myo-inositol, and brain edema in acute liver failure. Hepatology 1996;23:1291–2.
[14] Ruscito BJ, Harrison NL. Hemoglobin metabolites mimic benzodiazepines and are possible mediators of hepatic encephalopathy. Blood 2003;102:1525–8.
[15] Keegan MJ, Plevak DS. Preoperative assessment of the patient with liver disease. Am J Gastroenterol 2005;100:2116–27.
[16] Morgan M. The treatment of chronic hepatic encephalopathy. Hepatogastroenterology 1991;38:377–87.
[17] Glauser F. Systemic hemodynamic and cardiac function changes in patients undergoing orthotopic liver transplantation. Chest 1990;98:1210–5.
[18] Moller S, Henriksen JH. Cirrhotic cardiomyopathy: a pathophysiological review of circulatory dysfunction in liver disease. Heart 2002;87:9–15.
[19] Nasraway SA, Klein RD, Spanier TB, et al. Hemodynamic correlates of outcome in patients undergoing orthotopic liver transplantation: evidence for early postoperative myocardial depression. Chest 1995;107:218–24.
[20] Mohamed R, Freeman JW, Guest PJ, et al. Pulmonary gas exchange abnormalities in liver transplant candidates. Liver Transpl 2002;8:802–8.
[21] Krowka M. Hepatopulmonary syndromes. In: Maddrey WC, Schiff ER, Sorrell MF, editors. Transplantation of the liver. Philadelphia: Lippincott Williams & Wilkins; 2001. p. 405–16.
[22] Sharma P, Vargas H, Rakela J. Monitoring and care of the patient before liver transplantation. In: Busuttil RW, Klintmalm G, editors. Transplantation of the liver. 2nd edition. Philadelphia: Elsevier; 2005. p. 473–90.

[23] Schenk P, Schoniger-Hekele M, Fuhrmann V, et al. Prognostic significance of the hepatopulmonary syndrome in patients with cirrhosis. Gastroenterology 2003;125:1042–52.
[24] Kuo PC, Plotkin JS, Gaine S, et al. Portopulmonary hypertension and the liver transplant candidate. Transplantation 1999;67:1087–93.
[25] Mai ML, Gonwa TA. Pretransplantation evaluation: pulmonary, cardiac, and renal. Transplant Liver 1996;307–14.
[26] Shmueli E, Record CO, Alberti KG. Liver disease, carbohydrate metabolism and diabetes. Baillieres Clin Endocrinol Metab 1992;6:719–43.
[27] Hasse J. Nutritional aspects of adult liver transplantation. In: Busuttil RW, Klintmalm GB, editors. Transplantation of the liver. Philadelphia: Elsevier; 2005. p. 491–506.
[28] Clayton DG, Miro AM, Kramer DJ, et al. Quantification of thromboelastographic changes after blood component transfusion in patients with liver disease in the intensive care unit. Anesth Analg 1995;81:272–8.
[29] Wiklund RA. Preoperative preparation of patients with advanced liver disease. Crit Care Med 2004;32:S106–15.
[30] Kramer L, Horl W. Hepatorenal syndrome. Semin Nephrol 2002;22:290–301.
[31] Cardenas A, Arroyo V. Hepatorenal syndrome. Ann Hepatol 2003;2:23–9.
[32] Gines P, Cardenas A, Arroyo V, Rodes J. Management of cirrhosis and ascites. N Engl J Med 2004;350:1646–54.
[33] Child C, Turcotte J. Surgery and portal hypertension. Philadelphia: Saunders; 1964.
[34] Farnsworth N, Fagan SP, Berger DH, et al. Child-Turcotte-Pugh versus MELD score as a predictor of outcome after elective and emergent surgery in cirrhotic patients. Am J Surg 2004;188:580–3.
[35] Malinchoc M, Kamath PS, Gordon FD, et al. A model to predict poor survival in patients undergoing transjugular intrahepatic portosystemic shunts. Hepatology 2000;31:864–71.
[36] Forman L, Lucey M. Predicting the prognosis of chronic liver disease: an evolution from CHILD to MELD. Hepatology 2001;33:473–5.
[37] United Network for Organ Sharing. Available at: www.UNOS.org/SharedContent Documents/MELD-PELD.pdf.
[38] Sladen RN. Oliguria in the ICU. Systematic approach to diagnosis and treatment. Anesthesiol Clin North America 2000;18:739–52 [viii.].
[39] Tepel M, Zidek W. N-Acetylcysteine in nephrology; contrast nephropathy and beyond. Curr Opin Nephrol Hypertens 2004;13:649–54.
[40] Hoffmann U, Fischereder M, Kruger B, et al. The value of N-acetylcysteine in the prevention of radiocontrast agent-induced nephropathy seems questionable. J Am Soc Nephrol 2004; 15:407–10.
[41] Myers BD, Miller DC, Mehigan JT, et al. Nature of the renal injury following total renal ischemia in man. J Clin Invest 1984;73:329–41.
[42] Moran SM, Myers BD. Course of acute renal failure studied by a model of creatinine kinetics. Kidney Int 1985;27:928–37.
[43] Doolan PD, Alpen EL, Theil GB. A clinical appraisal of the plasma concentration and ndogenous clearance of creatinine. Am J Med 1962;32:65–81.
[44] Kasiske BL, Keane WF. Laboratory assessment of renal disease: clearance, urinalysis and renal biopsy. In: Brenner BM, editor. Brenner & Rector's the kidney. 6th edition. Philadelphia: WB Saunders; 2000. p. 1129–70.
[45] Stanton BA, Koeppen BM. Elements of renal function, physiology. 4th edition. In: Berne RM, Levy MN, editors. . St Louis (MO): Mosby; 1998. p. 677–98.
[46] Molitoris BA. Transitioning to therapy in ischemic acute renal failure. J Am Soc Nephrol 2003;14:265–7.
[47] Dagher PC, Herget-Rosenthal S, Ruehm SG, et al. Newly developed techniques to study and diagnose acute renal failure. J Am Soc Nephrol 2003;14:2188–98.
[48] Cockroft DW, Gault MH. Prediction of creatinine clearance from serum creatinine. Nephron 1976;16:31–41.

[49] Levey AS, Bosch JP, Lewis JB, et al. A more accurate method to estimate glomerular filtration rate from serum creatinine: a new prediction equation. Modification of Diet in Renal Disease Study Group. Ann Intern Med 1999;130:461–70.
[50] Robert S, Zarowitz BJ, Peterson EL, et al. Predictability of creatinine clearance estimates in critically ill patients. Crit Care Med 1993;21:1487–95.
[51] Sladen RN, Endo E, Harrison T. Two-hour versus 22-hour creatinine clearance in critically ill patients. Anesthesiology 1987;67:1013–6.
[52] Bryan AG, Bolsin SN, Vianna PT, et al. Modification of the diuretic and natriuretic effects of a dopamine infusion by fluid loading in preoperative cardiac surgical patients. J Cardiothorac Vasc Anesth 1995;9:158–63.
[53] Allgren RL, Marbury TC, Rahman SN, et al. Anaritide in acute tubular necrosis. N Engl J Med 1997;336:828–34.
[54] Stanton BA, Koeppen BM. Control of body fluid osmolality and volume. In: Berne RM, Levin HR, editors. Physiology. 4th edition. St Louis (MO): Mosby; 1998. p. 715–43.
[55] Carvounis CP, Nisar S, Guro-Razuman S. Significance of the fractional excretion of urea in the differential diagnosis of acute renal failure. Kidney Int 2002;62:2223–9.
[56] Garcia-Garcia M, Garcia-Valero J, Mourad G, et al. Urinary and serum beta 2-microglobulin in living related kidney donors and in renal failure. Contrib Nephrol 1995;112:77–82.
[57] Canivet JL, Larbuisson R, Damas P, et al. Plasma renin activity and urine beta 2-microglobulin during and after cardiopulmonary bypass: pulsatile vs nonpulsatile perfusion. Eur Heart J 1990;11:1079–82.
[58] Price RG. Urinary N-acetyl-beta-D-glucosaminidase (NAG) as an indicator of renal disease. Curr Probl Clin Biochem 1979;9:150–63.
[59] Mishra J, Ma Q, Prada A, et al. Identification of neutrophil gelatinase-associated lipocalin as a novel early urinary biomarker for ischemic renal injury. J Am Soc Nephrol 2003;14: 2534–43.
[60] Mishra J, Dent C, Tarabishi R, et al. Neutrophil gelatinase-associated lipocalin (NGAL) as a biomarker for acute renal injury after cardiac surgery. Lancet 2005;65:1231–8.
[61] Wagener G, Jan M, Kim M, et al. Association between increases in urinary neutrophil gelatinase-associated lipocalin and acute renal dysfunction after adult cardiac surgery. Anesthesiology 2006;105:485–91.

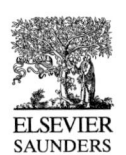

Index

Note: Page numbers of article titles are in **boldface** type.

A

A-Line AEP Monitor/2, for monitoring depth of anesthesia, 811–812

Activated clotting time, 846

Activated partial thromboplastin time, 843

Acute liver disease, perioperative monitoring in patients with, 858–860

Aggregometry, platelet, 851

American Society of Anesthesiologists (ASA), guidelines for intraoperative monitoring with transesophageal echocardiography, 737–740

Ammonia, arterial, perioperative monitoring of, in patients with hepatic encephalopathy, 860–861

Anesthesia, depth of, consequences of too much or too little, 801–809
   monitoring for, **793–822**
      BIS algorithm, 794
         alternatives to, 810–814
         clinical validation of, 794–795
         drugs and, 796–797
         in pediatric patients, 809–810
         movement, 795–796
         muscle action potentials and other high-frequency artifacts, 797–800
         paradoxical delta activity, 801

Anesthesiologists, role in cost-effectiveness analysis of medical technology, 685–687

Arterial ammonia, perioperative monitoring of, in patients with hepatic encephalopathy, 860–861

Arterial pressure monitoring, direct, **717–735**
   abnormal pressure waveform morphology, 724–725
   central *vs.* peripheral, 723
   complications of, 721
   effects of respiratory cycle on, 724–725
   indications for, 721
   normal arterial waveform morphology, 722–723

Assessment, of medical technology, **677–696**
   and the anesthesiologist, 685–687
   applicability to anesthesiology, 692–693
   application of Blue Cross criteria, 687–688
   cost effectiveness, 678–680
   fiscal analysis, 690–692
   left ventricular assist devices, 683–685
   regulatory approval of, 688
   scientific evidence on health outcomes, 689
   tissue plasminogen activator as template for, 680–683

Axillary temperature, perioperative monitoring of, 833

B

Beta-2 microgulobulin, perioperative monitoring of, as indicator of tubular injury, 877

Bioimpedance, 771–773

Bladder temperature, perioperative monitoring of, 833

Blood velocity, measurement of, with cardiac ultrasound and esophageal Doppler devices, 767–769

Blue Cross Blue Shield Association, criteria for technology assessment, 687–688

Brain, intraoperative monitoring of spinal cord and, **777–791**
   brainstem auditory evoked potentials, 788
   electromyography, 785–788
   impact on the anesthesiologist, 788–789
   motor evoked potentials, 782–785

882 INDEX

Brain (*continued*)
    somatosensory evoked potential, 778–782

Brainstem auditory evoked potentials, intraoperative monitoring of, 788

Bundle branch blocks, electrocardiographic monitoring of, 706–709

C

Cardiac assessment, perioperative monitoring of, in patients with chronic liver disease, 861–862

Cardiac output, measurement of, with Fick principle, 764–766

Cardiac ultrasound, measurement of blood velocity of, 767–769

Cardiopulmonary bypass, temperature monitoring during, 834

Cardiopulmonary resuscitation, transesophageal echocardiography-based diagnosis in patients undergoing, 743

Cardiovascular surgery, intraoperative transesophageal echocardiography during, **737–753**

Central venous pressure monitoring, **717–735**
    abnormal waveform morphology, 730–732
    complications, 726–728
    indications, 725–726
    interpretation of, 728–729
    normal waveform morphology, 729–730

Child-Turcotte-Pugh classification, for liver dysfunction, 866–867

Chronic liver disease, perioperative monitoring in patients with, 860–866

Clearance techniques, perioperative monitoring of, 872–874

Coagulation monitoring, **839–856**
    activated clotting time, 846
    drug therapy and, 848
    heparin concentration monitoring, 847
    high-dose thrombin time, 847
    individualized heparin dosing, 847–848
    monitoring fibrinolysis, 844–846
    platelet function, 848
    platelet function tests, 849–851
        dynamic tests, 849
        platelet aggregometry, 851
        static tests, 849
        tests of platelet response to agonist stimulus, 850–851
        thromboelastography, 849–850
    test of coagulation, 840–844
        activated partial thromboplastin time, 843
        bedside, 844
        fibrinogen concentration, 841–842
        platelet count, 840–841
        prothrombin time, 843–844
        thrombin time, 842–843
    update concept of hemostasis, 840

Coagulopathy, perioperative monitoring of, in patients with chronic liver disease, 864–865

Conduction defects, electrocardiographic monitoring of, 704–706

Congenital heart defects, intraoperative transesophageal echocardiography during surgical repair of, 746–747

Cost effectiveness, analysis of, for left ventricular assist devices, 683–685
    of medical technology, 678–680

Creatinine clearance, perioperative monitoring of, 873–874

Creatinine, serum, perioperative monitoring of, 869–870

CSM Monitor, for monitoring depth of anesthesia, 813

D

Datex-Ohmeda S/5 Entropy Model, for monitoring depth of anesthesia, 812–813

Depth, of anesthesia, consequences of too much or too little, 801–809
    monitoring for, **793–822**
        BIS algorithm, 794
            alternatives to, 810–814
            clinical validation of, 794–795
        drugs and, 796–797
        in pediatric patients, 809–810
        movement, 795–796
        muscle action potentials and other high-frequency artifacts, 797–800
        paradoxical delta activity, 801

Direct pressure measurement, technical aspects of, 717–721
    catheter transducer system, 717–720

Direct (*continued*)
pressure transducer setup, 720–721

Doppler device, esophageal, for measurement of blood velocity, 767–769

E

Echocardiography, transesophageal (TEE), assessment of left ventricular systolic function with, **755–762**
global function, 757–759
left ventricle-focused examination, 755–757
segmental function, 759–761
intraoperative monitoring with, **737–753**
indications, 738
indications and class I recommendations, 738–748
risks of, 748–749
training in, 749–751

Electrocardiography (ECG), 697–715
components of ECG analysis, 697–704
conduction defects and blocks, 704–706
electrolyte, thyroid, and temperature effects, 709–711
fascicular and bundle branch blocks, 706–709
implications of, 713–714
ischemia, 711–713

Electroencephalography (EEG), monitoring depth of anesthesia with, **793–822**

Electrolytes, effects on electrocardiographic monitoring, 709–711

Electromyography, intraoperative monitoring of, 785–788

Encephalopathy, hepatic, perioperative monitoring of arterial ammonia in patients with, 860–861

End-stage liver disease, perioperative monitoring in patients with, 860–866

Endocarditis, intraoperative transesophageal echocardiography during surgical intervention for, 747

Endocrine dysfunction, perioperative monitoring of, in patients with chronic liver disease, 864

Entropy, in monitoring depth of anesthesia, 812

Esophageal Doppler device, for measurement of blood velocity, 767–769

Esophageal temperature, perioperative monitoring of, 832

Evidence, scientific, for medical technology effect on health outcomes, 689–690

F

Fascicular blocks, electrocardiographic monitoring of, 706–709

Fibrinogen concentration, 841–842

Fibrinolysis, monitoring of, 844–846

Fick principle, measurement of cardiac output using, 764–766

Fiscal analysis, in assessment of medical technology, 690–692

Free water clearance, perioperative monitoring of, 875

Fulminant hepatic failure, perioperative monitoring in patients with, 858–859

G

Global left ventricular function, transesophageal echocardiography in assessment of, **755–762**

Glomerular filtration rate, perioperative monitoring of, 871–872

H

Hematologic abnormalities, perioperative monitoring of, in patients with chronic liver disease, 864–865

Hemodynamics, renal, perioperative monitoring of, 870–871

Hemostasis, updated concept of, 840

Heparin concentration monitoring, 847

Heparin dosing, individualized, 847–848

Hepatic encephalopathy, perioperative monitoring of arterial ammonia in patients with, 860–861

Hepatic function, perioperative monitoring of, **857–880**
acute liver disease, 858–860
chronic and end-stage liver disease, 860–866
clinical evaluation, 858
laboratory evaluation of liver disease, 866–867

Hepatitis, acute, perioperative monitoring in patients with, 859–860

Hepatorenal syndrome, perioperative monitoring of, in patients with chronic liver disease, 865–866

High-dose thrombin time, 847

Hyperdynamic circulation, perioperative monitoring of, in patients with chronic liver disease, 861–862

Hypotension, intraoperative transesophageal echocardiography in diagnosis of, 741–743

I

Intracranial pressure monitoring, perioperative, in patients with fulminant hepatic failure, 858–859

Intraoperative monitoring. *See also* Monitoring., of the brain and spinal cord, **777–791**
    brainstem auditory evoked potentials, 788
    electromyography, 785–788
    impact on the anesthesiologist, 788–789
    motor evoked potentials, 782–785
    somatosensory evoked potential, 778–782
    with transesophageal echocardiography, **737–753**

Inulin clearance, perioperative monitoring of, 872–873

Ischemia, electrocardiographic diagnosis of, 711–713

K

Kidneys. *See* Renal function.

L

Left ventricular assist devices, cost-effectiveness analysis of, 683–685

Left ventricular systolic function, assessment of, with transesophageal echocardiography, **755–762**
    global function, 757–759
    left ventricle-focused examination, 755–757
    segmental function, 759–761

Lipocalin, neutrophil gelatinase-associated, perioperative monitoring of, 877–878

Liver function tests, 866

Liver. *See* Hepatic function.

Lung function tests, perioperative, in patients with chronic liver disease, 862–864

M

Medical technology. *See* Technology.

Mitral valve repair, intraoperative transesophageal echocardiography in, 743–744

Monitoring, during anesthesia and surgery, arterial and central venous pressure, 717–735
    assessment of technology for, **677–696**
    brain and spinal cord, **777–791**
    coagulation, **839–856**
    electrocardiography, **697–715**
    for depth of anesthesia, **793–822**
    hepatic and renal function, **857–880**
    thermoregulation and temperature, **823–837**
    tissue perfusion, noninvasive technologies for, **763–775**
    transesophageal echocardiography, intraoperative monitoring with, **737–753**
    of left ventricular global and segmental systolic function, **755–762**

Motor potential, intraoperative monitoring of, 782–785

N

Narcotrend Monitor, for monitoring depth of anesthesia, 813

Nasopharyngeal temperature, perioperative monitoring of, 832–833

Neurophysiologic monitoring, intraoperative, **777–791**
    brainstem auditory evoked potentials, 788
    electromyography, 785–788
    impact on the anesthesiologist, 788–789
    motor evoked potentials, 782–785
    somatosensory evoked potential, 778–782

Neutrophil gelatinase-associated lipocalin, perioperative monitoring of, 877–878

Nutritional dysfunction, perioperative monitoring of, in patients with chronic liver disease, 864

P

Plasma clearance, perioperative monitoring of, 874

Platelet count, 840–841

Platelet function tests, 849–851
    dynamic tests, 849
    platelet aggregometry, 851
    static tests, 849
    tests of platelet response to agonist stimulus, 850–851
    thromboelastography, 849–850

Pressure monitoring systems, during anesthesia, **717–735**
    arterial blood pressure measurement, 721–725
    central venous pressure measurement, 725–732
    direct pressure measurement, technical aspects, 717–721

Prothrombin time, 843–844

Pulmonary artery catheters, site for perioperative temperature monitoring, 832

Pulmonary dysfunction, perioperative monitoring of, in patients with chronic liver disease, 862–864

Pulse contour analysis technique, 769–771

R

Regulatory approval, of medical technology, 688

Renal blood flow, perioperative monitoring of, 870–871

Renal function, perioperative monitoring of, **857–880**
    clearance techniques, 872–874
    glomerular nutrition rate, 871–872
    indices of tubular injury, 877–878
    renal hemodynamics, 870–871
    serum urea nitrogen and serum creatinine, 869–870
    sodium conservation, 876
    tubular function tests, 874–875
    urea handling, 876–877
    urine output, 868–869
    water conservation, 875–876

Renal plasma flow, perioperative monitoring of, 870–871

Ross procedure, for valve replacement, intraoperative transesophageal echocardiography in, 745–746

S

SEDLine Monitor, for monitoring depth of anesthesia, 810–811

Segmental left ventricular function, transesophageal echocardiography in assessment of, **755–762**

Serum creatinine, perioperative monitoring of, 869–870
    nomograms, 872

Serum urea nitrogen, perioperative monitoring of, 869

Skin temperature, perioperative monitoring of, 833

Snap Monitor, for monitoring depth of anesthesia, 813

Society of Cardiovascular Anesthesiologists (SCA), guidelines for intraoperative monitoring with transesophageal echocardiography, 737–740

Sodium conservation, perioperative monitoring of, 876

Somatosensory evoked potential, intraoperative monitoring of, 778–782

Spinal cord, intraoperative monitoring of brain and, **777–791**
    brainstem auditory evoked potentials, 788
    electromyography, 785–788
    impact on the anesthesiologist, 788–789
    motor evoked potentials, 782–785
    somatosensory evoked potential, 778–782

T

Technology, medical, assessment of, **677–696**
    and the anesthesiologist, 685–687
    applicability to anesthesiology, 692–693
    application of Blue Cross criteria, 687–688
    cost effectiveness, 678–680
    fiscal analysis, 690–692
    left ventricular assist devices, 683–685
    regulatory approval of, 688
    scientific evidence on health outcomes, 689
    tissue plasminogen activator as template for, 680–683

Temperature, effects on
electrocardiographic monitoring,
709–711
perioperative monitoring, **823–837**
during cardiopulmonary bypass,
834
monitoring sites, 832–833
normal thermoregulation and,
824–831
afferent responses, 830–831
afferent sensing, 824–826
central regulation, 826–828
heat transfer mechanisms,
828–830

Thermoregulation, normal, 824–831
afferent responses, 830–831
afferent sensing, 824–826
central regulation, 826–828
heat transfer mechanisms,
828–830
perioperative, and temperature
monitoring, **823–837**
during cardiopulmonary bypass,
834
monitoring sites, 832–833

Thrombin time, 842–843

Thromboelastography, 849–850

Thyroid, effects on electrocardiographic
monitoring, 709–711

Tissue perfusion, noninvasive technologies
for monitoring, **763–775**
bioimpedance, 771–773
cardiac output using Fick
principle, 764–766
measurement of blood velocity,
766–769
pulse contour analysis, 769–771

Tissue plasminogen activator, as template
for technology assessment, 680–683

Training, in transesophageal
echocardiography, 749–751

Transesophageal echocardiography,
assessment of left ventricular systolic
function with, **755–762**
global function, 757–759
left ventricle-focused
examination, 755–757
segmental function, 759–761
intraoperative monitoring with,
737–753
indications, 738
indications and class I
recommendations,
738–748
risks of, 748–749
training in, 749–751

Tubular function tests, perioperative
monitoring of, 874

U

Ultrasound, cardiac, measurement of blood
velocity of, 767–769

Urea, perioperative monitoring of serum
urea nitrogen, 869

Urea handling, perioperative monitoring of,
876–877

Urine concentrating ability, perioperative
monitoring of, 875

Urine output, perioperative monitoring of,
868–869

Urine-to-plasma osmolar ratio,
perioperative monitoring of, 875

V

Valve replacement surgery, intraoperative
transesophageal echocardiography in,
745–746

Venous pressure. *See* Central venous
pressure.

W

Water conservation, perioperative
monitoring of, 875–876

United States Postal Service
Statement of Ownership, Management, and Circulation

1. Publication Title	2. Publication Number	3. Filing Date
Anesthesiology Clinics of North America	0 8 8 9 - 8 5 3 7	9/15/06

4. Issue Frequency	5. Number of Issues Published Annually	6. Annual Subscription Price
Mar, Jun, Sep, Dec	4	$180.00

7. Complete Mailing Address of Known Office of Publication (Not printer) (Street, city, county, state, and ZIP+4)	Contact Person
Elsevier Inc. 360 Park Avenue South New York, NY 10010-1710	Sarah Carmichael
	Telephone (215) 239-3681

8. Complete Mailing Address of Headquarters or General Business Office of Publisher (Not printer)
Elsevier Inc., 360 Park Avenue South, New York, NY 10010-1710

9. Full Names and Complete Mailing Addresses of Publisher, Editor, and Managing Editor (Do not leave blank)
Publisher (Name and complete mailing address)
John Schrefer, Elsevier Inc., 1600 John F. Kennedy Blvd. Suite 1800, Philadelphia, PA 19103-2899
Editor (Name and complete mailing address)
Rachel Glover, Elsevier Inc., 1600 John F. Kennedy Blvd. Suite 1800, Philadelphia, PA 19103-2899
Managing Editor (Name and complete mailing address)
Catherine Bewick, Elsevier Inc., 1600 John F. Kennedy Blvd. Suite 1800, Philadelphia, PA 19103-2899

10. Owner (Do not leave blank. If the publication is owned by a corporation, give the name and address of the corporation immediately followed by the names and addresses of all stockholders owning or holding 1 percent or more of the total amount of stock. If not owned by a corporation, give the names and addresses of the individual owners. If owned by a partnership or other unincorporated firm, give its name and address as well as those of each individual owner. If the publication is published by a nonprofit organization, give its name and address.)

Full Name	Complete Mailing Address
Wholly owned subsidiary of	4520 East-West Highway
Reed/Elsevier Inc., US holdings	Bethesda, MD 20814

11. Known Bondholders, Mortgagees, and Other Security Holders Owning or Holding 1 Percent or More of Total Amount of Bonds, Mortgages, or Other Securities. If none, check box ➤ None

Full Name	Complete Mailing Address
N/A	

12. Tax Status (For completion by nonprofit organizations authorized to mail at nonprofit rates) (Check one)
The purpose, function, and nonprofit status of this organization and the exempt status for federal income tax purposes:
☒ Has Not Changed During Preceding 12 Months
☐ Has Changed During Preceding 12 Months (Publisher must submit explanation of change with this statement)

(See Instructions on Reverse)

PS Form 3526, October 1999

---

13. Publication Title	14. Issue Date for Circulation Data Below
Anesthesiology Clinics of North America	June, 2006

15. Extent and Nature of Circulation		Average No. Copies Each Issue During Preceding 12 Months	No. Copies of Single Issue Published Nearest to Filing Date
a. Total Number of Copies (Net press run)		2,350	2,100
b. Paid and/or Requested Circulation	(1) Paid/Requested Outside-County Mail Subscriptions Stated on Form 3541. (Include advertiser's proof and exchange copies)	998	881
	(2) Paid In-County Subscriptions Stated on Form 3541 (Include advertiser's proof and exchange copies)		
	(3) Sales Through Dealers and Carriers, Street Vendors, Counter Sales, and Other Non-USPS Paid Distribution	567	510
	(4) Other Classes Mailed Through the USPS		
c. Total Paid and/or Requested Circulation [Sum of 15b. (1), (2), (3), and (4)]	➤	1,565	1,391
d. Free Distribution by Mail (Samples, complimentary, and other free)	(1) Outside-County as Stated on Form 3541	102	111
	(2) In-County as Stated on Form 3541		
	(3) Other Classes Mailed Through the USPS		
e. Free Distribution Outside the Mail (Carriers or other means)			
f. Total Free Distribution (Sum of 15d. and 15e.)	➤	102	111
g. Total Distribution (Sum of 15c. and 15f)	➤	1,667	1,502
h. Copies not Distributed		683	598
i. Total (Sum of 15g. and h.)	➤	2,350	2,100
j. Percent Paid and/or Requested Circulation (15c. divided by 15g. times 100)		93.88%	92.61%

16. Publication of Statement of Ownership
☒ Publication required. Will be printed in the December 2006 issue of this publication.
☐ Publication not required

17. Signature and Title of Editor, Publisher, Business Manager, or Owner
Jodi Palucci – Executive Director of Subscription Services
Date 9/15/06

I certify that all information furnished on this form is true and complete. I understand that anyone who furnishes false or misleading information on this form or who omits material or information requested on the form may be subject to criminal sanctions (including fines and imprisonment) and/or civil sanctions (including civil penalties).

Instructions to Publishers

1. Complete and file one copy of this form with your postmaster annually on or before October 1. Keep a copy of the completed form for your records.
2. In cases where the stockholder or security holder is a trustee, include in items 10 and 11 the name of the person or corporation for whom the trustee is acting. Also include the names and addresses of individuals who are stockholders who own or hold 1 percent or more of the total amount of bonds, mortgages, or other securities of the publishing corporation. In item 11, if none, check the box. Use blank sheets if more space is required.
3. Be sure to furnish all circulation information called for in item 15. Free circulation must be shown in items 15d, e, and f.
4. Item 15h, Copies not Distributed, must include (1) newsstand copies originally stated on Form 3541, and returned to the publisher, (2) estimated returns from news agents, and (3), copies for office use, leftovers, spoiled, and all other copies not distributed.
5. If the publication has Periodicals authorization as a general or requester publication, this Statement of Ownership, Management, and Circulation must be published; it must be printed in any issue in October or, if the publication is not published during October, the first issue printed after October.
6. In item 16, indicate the date of the issue in which this Statement of Ownership will be published.
7. Item 17 must be signed.

Failure to file or publish a statement of ownership may lead to suspension of Periodicals authorization.

PS Form 3526, October 1999 (Reverse)

Moving?

Make sure your subscription moves with you!

To notify us of your new address, find your **Clinics Account Number** (located on your mailing label above your name), and contact customer service at:

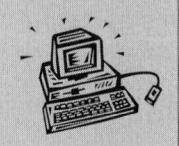

E-mail: elspcs@elsevier.com

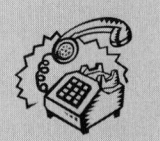

800-654-2452 (subscribers in the U.S. & Canada)
407-345-4000 (subscribers outside of the U.S. & Canada)

Fax number: 407-363-9661

Elsevier Periodicals Customer Service
6277 Sea Harbor Drive
Orlando, FL 32887-4800

*To ensure uninterrupted delivery of your subscription, please notify us at least 4 weeks in advance of move.

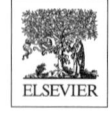

ELSEVIER